The Gift of Participation

A Guide to Making Informed Decisions About Volunteering for a Clinical Trial

The Gift of Participation

A Guide to Making Informed Decisions About Volunteering for a Clinical Trial

Second Edition

Kenneth Getz

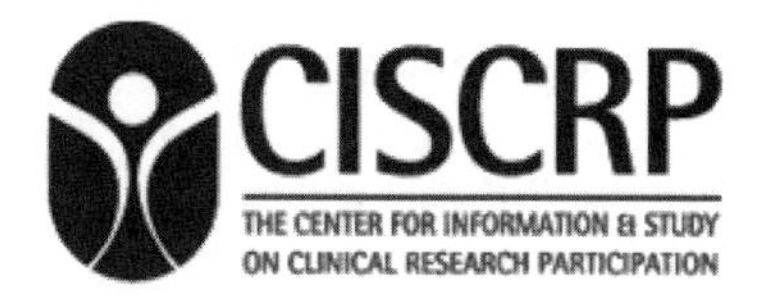

The Gift of Participation: A Guide to Making Informed Decisions About Volunteering for a Clinical Trial
By Kenneth Getz

Printed in the United States.
1 2 3 4 5 10 09 08 07 06

For more information contact: The Center for Information and Study on Clinical Research Participation, 56 Commercial Wharf East, Boston, MA 02110; 617-725-2750.

Cover and copy design by Paul Gualdoni, Jr.

ISBN 978-0-615-15664-4

To the millions of people who give the gift of
participation in clinical trials each year;
and to the rest of us who admire them for doing so.

TABLE OF CONTENTS

FOREWORD

In 2007, I introduced a resolution in the House of Representatives—House Resolution 248—honoring and recognizing the sacrifice, commitment, and contributions of clinical trial participants. Volunteers participating in clinical research play an invaluable role in advancing scientific knowledge and conquering disease, and these participants deserve recognition by the general public.

My personal experience of having someone close to me affected by cancer spurred my introduction of this resolution. Cancer imposes a tremendous toll on its victims and their family members. Clinical trials on new medicines to treat cancer offer the hope of new approaches to prevent and to treat this debilitating disease.

The contributions of clinical trial participants have led to the promising prospect of developing treatments and potential cures for not only cancer, but for a wide range of illnesses including Alzheimer's disease, diabetes, and heart disease. Unfortunately, the general public is not aware of the benefits of clinical trials, and too many patients are not even aware that they are eligible to participate in these trials. Too many people have little or no knowledge about clinical trial research and the participation process.

As a member of Congress, I recognized the importance of a significant investment of federal funding for medical research to derive new treatments and cures. Throughout my service in Congress, I strongly supported efforts by the federal government to improve medical research. These advances, however, would not have been possible without the participation of clinical trial volunteers. I introduced my resolution in the House of Representatives in order to honor these individuals. Without their participation, without their brave contributions, the United States would not be on the cutting edge of medical research.

If you were diagnosed in 1999 with chronic myeloid leukemia (CML), you probably would not be alive today. Only thirty percent of patients survived five years after diagnosis. You would have had two treatment options: a risky bone-marrow transplant; or daily injections of interferon, a drug whose side effects are often compared to a bad case of the flu. Given the same diagnosis today, you would take a daily pill that targets the cancerous cells directly, causing few side effects and likely driving your cancer into remission. This breakthrough, targeted approach is highly effective and precise.

This same success story has been repeated in many disease areas: deaths from HIV/AIDS have fallen by seventy percent in the United States since 1996. Blood-pressure medicines have prevented millions of hospitalizations. This decade, the rates of heart attack and heart failure have been cut nearly in half through better diagnosis and treatment.

We all know the potential benefits medicines can bring—from preventing strokes to improving mobility to easing pain. But where do these life-enhancing and life-saving medicines come from? Researchers are currently working on more than two and a half thousand new medical therapies in clinical trials. These therapies offer great hope to patients and their families and friends. Patients today can help make those new medicines a reality through participation in clinical trials. These volunteers are truly heroic; their actions have the potential to save the lives of many future patients and to improve overall public health.

In closing, I would like to give a heartfelt thanks to the millions of clinical trial volunteers who give the gift of participation each year. These courageous individuals deserve our honor and respect. I also want to recognize and applaud the efforts of the Center for Information and Study on Clinical Research Participation in educating patients and the public about the importance of clinical trials and the vital role they play in improving public health. It is my hope that this organization's efforts, and the information included in this educational book—*The Gift of Participation*—will help further the public's understanding and appreciation. I am pleased to offer my continued support and encouragement for the vital contributions of clinical trial participants.

Former Congressman Rick Boucher (D-VA; 1983 to 2011)

THE GIFT OF PARTICIPATION

It is said that the most profound gifts are given anonymously, without assurance of any direct personal benefit.

This is the gift of participation in clinical research.

It is true that many people initially sign up for clinical trials in order to gain access to a new or potentially better treatment option. But over the course of a clinical trial, the two-million-plus people who participate each year realize that their participation matters far more to other individuals, from their family members to future patients.

It is a brave and selfless act. The profound decision to participate may bring hope to the individual participating, but often it does not. Still, something new is always learned from each clinical research study. The act of participation benefits public health and advances medical knowledge, regardless of whether or not an investigational treatment is safe and effective.

In 2004 I founded the Center for Information and Study on Clinical Research Participation (CISCRP) to provide outreach and education to those individuals considering participation in clinical trials. Based in the Boston area, this nonprofit organization is also dedicated to encouraging the public, government employees, and health and research professionals to recognize and appreciate the profound gift that participation brings to all of us.

Your purchase of this book is another way of showing appreciation for the gift of participation. Proceeds from all book sales will be donated to CISCRP and will support educational initiatives to assist those contemplating or carrying out the heroic act of volunteering in clinical trials.

Ken Getz

ACKNOWLEDGMENTS

Thank you to the many clinical trial participants who shared their experiences for this book. I wish all of them many years of good health. Their unflagging patience after so many questions helped to illuminate the profound gift of participation in medical research. Their stories also simplified the task of creating wisdom from words, insights, and impressions.

Thank you to the clinical research professionals, medical professionals, and other stakeholders who shared their ideas and expertise. Special gratitude is owed to Angela Bates in the National Institute of Health's Office of Research on Women's Health for directing me toward helpful resources. I thank Gary Chadwick, Pharm.D., M.P.H., at the University of Rochester, for helping me better understand the legislative monstrosity known as HIPAA. Thanks to Deborah Zarin, M.D., director of ClinicalTrials.gov at the National Library of Medicine, for her assistance in describing the evolution of the ever-expanding, publicly accessible clinical trials database. A very special thank you to Myrl Weinberg, president of the National Health Council in Washington, D.C., for her thoughtful insights and encouragement.

I'm grateful to David Korn, M.D., senior vice president of biomedical and health sciences research with the Association of American Medical Colleges, for his help with the sections on accreditation of human research programs and medical information privacy. Thank you to Alan Milstein, a Pennsauken, N.Y., lawyer, for his perspective on the problems inherent in modern research.

As for the chapter on vulnerable populations, I wish to acknowledge the helpfulness of Steve Hirschfeld, M.D., Ph.D., medical officer with the Food and Drug Administration (FDA); Philip Walson, M.D., director of the clinical pharmacology division and clinical trials office at Cincinnati Children's Hospital; and Anne Zajicek, M.D., Pharm.D., pediatric medical officer with the National Institute of Child Health and Human Development. I appreciate the many hours contributed to this project by Kathleen Quinn and Susan Cruzan in the FDA's Office of Public Affairs; Carolyn Hommel with the FDA's Good Clinical Practice Program; Patricia El-Hinnawy in the Department of Health and Human Services's (DHHS's) Office for Human Research Protections; and DHHS's Office of Minority

Health Resource Center. Thanks to Robert Temple, M.D., associate director for medical policy in the Center for Drug Evaluation and Research (CDER); Diane Murphy, M.D., CDER's associate director for pediatrics; and David Lepay, M.D., senior advisor for clinical science in the Office of the Commissioner. Thanks also go out to Dr. Margaret Miller, manager of science programs, and Susan Wood, M.D., director, in the FDA's Office of Women's Health. I am similarly grateful to Michael Carome, M.D., director of the OHRP's division of oversight compliance, and Bill Hall, in the HHS Office of the Assistant Secretary for Public Affairs, for their prompt response to information requests.

Thank you to the many experts who assisted me in understanding clinical trial risk. Among them: Adil Shamoo, Ph.D., co-founder of Citizens for Responsible Care and Research; Arthur Caplan, director of the Center for Bioethics at the University of Pennsylvania; Dan Schuster, M.D., associate dean for clinical research at Washington University in St. Louis; Leonard Glantz, professor of health law at Boston University School of Public Health; Joseph Lau, M.D., professor of medicine at New England Medical Center; and Patrick McNeilly, compliance oversight coordinator in the Office for Human Research Protections (OHRP). Much thanks to John Paling, Ph.D., a Gainesville, Fla.-based risk communication consultant for his unique perspective on understanding risk.

Thank you to those who helped demonstrate through case examples the enormous value clinical-trial volunteers bring to the science of drug development, the everyday practice of medicine, and the health and well-being of people around the globe. For this I am indebted to David Canter, M.D., the researcher who headed up the Lipitor Development Team for Pfizer; John Tsai, M.D., the Lipitor medical team leader; and Laurie Letvak, M.D., who heads up medical affairs globally for Gleevec on behalf of Novartis.

Thank you to my family for their patience and support during the many hours I spent sequestered in my study conducting research and writing chapters. Thank you to Laura Faden and Jennifer Kim at the Tufts Center for the Study of Drug Development for their assistance in pulling together data and metrics presented throughout this book. I wish to thank Roni Thaler, Rachel Stanley, Diane Simmons, Natale Vayaran, and the many professionals at CISCRP whose collective dedication to educating and informing the public and patient communities about clinical research participation and the important role that it plays in advancing public health were an inspiration. Thank you to Jeffrey Zuckerman for copyediting and proofreading this second edition. Thank you to Paul Gualdoni for the cover and copy design.

Lastly, my deepest thanks and appreciation to Deborah Borfitz, for all of her invaluable assistance in research, interviews, and preparations for this book.

CHAPTER ONE

Recognizing the Gift of Participation

Behind every medicine and treatment are people who gave the gift of participation in clinical trials. Without people to volunteer for clinical trials, the world would be a far different place. New diseases would flourish. Well-known diseases—many of which are managed today with medication and lifestyle changes—would instead cripple, disfigure, or kill. Flu epidemics would rage unchecked. Many adults and children stricken with cancer would be buried or facing the end of life as opposed to fighting the disease, and living long, productive lives.

Doctors would have no scientific basis for advising patients to lower their blood pressure or cholesterol, for example. Doctors would have no knowledge helping them determine what medication, diet, or exercise plan to prescribe.

Without the gift of participation in clinical trials, medicine and public health would be reduced to folklore.

Around the world, people are living longer, healthier, and happier lives because people they never met volunteered for clinical trials. Volunteers help researchers explore promising leads for targeting the cause of illness, for relieving the symptoms of disease, and for improving the human condition. Even when researchers find that they are pursuing false leads, study participants play an important role because their experiences guide researchers to better paths. The gift of participation helps researchers and doctors learn about what works and what doesn't work in treating illnesses and conditions. The impact of clinical trial participation is both immediate and ongoing as it continues long after participation has ended and researchers and medical professionals build on the knowledge gained from that clinical trial. There are innumerable examples of the profound impact that the gift of participation contributes to public health.

Several well-known examples illustrate the enormous value of information and knowledge that comes from volunteers in clinical trials.

The Framingham Heart Study: Prevention Is Possible

A remarkable number of discoveries about the development and progression of heart disease has come out of the long-running Framingham Heart Study, one of the most important in the history of medicine. It changed the once-common view that people who develop a disease are simply unlucky and can do nothing to influence their health status. In fact, the study coined the phrase "risk factor," radically and forever changing the way doctors care for their patients. Suddenly, people were given personal responsibility for reducing their risk for a heart attack or stroke. And doctors started talking in terms of "ideal" rather than "normal" cholesterol and blood pressure levels, which meant that people had even lower levels to target.

The study began in 1948, shortly after cardiovascular disease was recognized as an American epidemic. So far, it has involved three generations of study participants, as well as researchers from the National Heart, Lung, and Blood Institute (NHLBI) and the Boston University School of Medicine. The chief goal is learning how and why people who develop heart disease differ from those who escape it. As it turns out, the answer is only partly determined by lifestyle and traditional risk factors. It is also rooted in our DNA. The first round of participants were 5,209 healthy men and women, ages 30–62, from the town of Framingham, MA. In 1971, a second-generation group (the Offspring Cohort) comprising 5,124 of the original participants' adult children and their spouses were enrolled. In 1995, 500 members of Framingham's minority population were recruited to participate and the number continues to grow. The intent is to help health officials understand how, and if, risk factors for heart and other diseases are the same or different among minorities than among the first two, mostly white cohorts. More recently, the Framingham Heart study began enrolling children of the Offspring Cohort to better understand how genetic factors relate to cardiovascular disease. The goal is to recruit and examine 3,500 grandchildren of the original group.

Participation in the study involves a number of procedures. Every two years, study participants are given a thorough, four-hour medical evaluation that includes a medical history, physical examination, lifestyle questionnaire, blood and urine tests, electrocardiogram

(EKG), pulmonary function test, and use of new diagnostic technologies such as bone densitometry (for monitoring osteoporosis) and echocardiography (an ultrasound examination of the heart).

Since its inception, more than 1,200 scientific papers have been published that cite the Framingham Heart Study. Among the study's noteworthy contributions:

It identified risk factors associated with heart disease and stroke

Before the Framingham Heart Study, most doctors thought atherosclerosis (hardening of the arteries) and high blood pressure were normal outcomes of the aging process. It was also commonly thought that women and the elderly tolerated hypertension (high blood pressure) well.

Early on in the study, cholesterol level, blood pressure, and electrocardiogram abnormalities were found to increase the risk of heart disease. A strong positive association was made between low-density lipoprotein (LDL or "bad") cholesterol and heart disease. Conversely, high-density lipoprotein (HDL) levels had a powerful inverse and protective effect. It did not matter whether a person was male or female.

During most of the study's first 50 years, important milestones were being routinely produced. Back in 1959, for example, some heart attacks were discovered to be "silent," causing no pain. In 1970, hypertension was found to increase the risk of stroke and, in 1978, atrial fibrillation (a condition in which the heart beats irregularly) was named a culprit. In 1976, menopause was shown to increase the risk of heart disease. In 1978, psychosocial factors were found to affect heart disease. In 1981, filter cigarettes were found to give no protection against coronary artery disease, as was commonly believed. A major report was also issued on the relationship of diet and heart disease. In 1994, an enlarged left ventricle (one of two lower chambers of the heart) was shown to increase risk of stroke. In 1996, the progression from hypertension to heart failure was described.

Thanks to Framingham Heart Study participants, risk prediction formulas were developed to calculate a patient's risk for developing coronary heart disease over the course of ten years. The risk is determined by assessing multiple risk factors, such as hypertension, high cholesterol, smoking, and diabetes, which tend to work together to cause disease. The test provides physicians and their patients with a single number that shows how the patient's risk compares to the average or optimal risk scores for their age and gender brackets. Strategies can then be implemented to modify risk factors contributing to an elevated risk for disease.

A risk-prediction formula has also been developed to estimate the risk of stroke following the first occurrence of atrial fibrillation. Estimates are based on data from the Framingham Heart Study and look at baseline risk factors such as age, systolic blood pressure, and prior stroke.

Although the study participants are primarily white, the importance of the major identified risk factors for cardiovascular disease have been shown in other studies to apply almost universally among racial and ethnic groups, according to the NHLBI.

It demonstrated the effect of lifestyle on the development of heart disease

Before the Framingham Heart Study, many aspects of the American lifestyle had been contributing to high rates of disease and disability. Doctors did not realize that changing certain behaviors—including cigarette smoking and sedentary living—would help patients avoid or reverse the underlying causes of serious heart and vascular conditions.

The study convincingly showed that smokers were at increased risk of having a heart attack or experiencing a sudden death, and that the risk was related to the number of cigarettes smoked each day. According to the study, quitting promptly cut that risk in half.

The Framingham Heart Study also demonstrated that exercise had a protective effect on the heart and that weight gain, coupled with a lack of exercise, increased cardiovascular risk factors like hypertension and diabetes. An association of type "A" (driven and high-strung) behavior with heart disease was also reported.

The findings generated a revolution in preventive medicine, including national awareness campaigns and greater medical emphasis on early detection and treatment of cardiovascular risk factors.

It contributed to understanding about how diseases begin

Researchers gained numerous insights into the epidemiology of heart failure, peripheral arterial disease, stroke, and arrhythmia (irregular heartbeat). As the original study participants aged, researchers also learned a great deal about dementia, cancer, arthritis, osteoporosis, hearing, and eye disorders. In 1987, for example, estrogen replacement therapy was found to reduce the risk of hip fractures in post-menopausal women.

Over time, the focus of investigation shifted to better understanding the biological differences between LDL and HDL cholesterol. Today, researchers are working to identify the genes that regulate how cholesterol is handled within the human body. The chief question confronting them is how genes contribute to common metabolic disorders such as obesity, hypertension, diabetes, and Alzheimer's. The answers will come, in part, from a DNA library of blood samples amassed from over 5,000 individuals in the Framingham Heart Study. Researchers are also scanning samples from 1,800 members of the largest families in the study, looking for genes that control the major risk factors for heart disease and other conditions.

Framingham researchers now suspect hypertension may develop differently in men and women. In men but not women, for example, a link has been found between a particular gene and high blood pressure. Some researchers are currently trying to better understand a gene that appears to protect individuals of both sexes from getting heart disease in hopes of developing new therapies to help those lacking this protective genetic trait. Others are looking for the location of a gene that appears to increase the risk for heart disease so that those harboring it can be advised to modify their diets or other lifestyle habits to reduce that risk.

Other potential risk factors are also actively under investigation. A high level of the amino acid homocysteine, for example, is thought to contribute to heart disease, stroke, and a reduced flow of blood to the hands and feet. Genetics play a role, but so does diet. Eating meals high in folic acid and B-vitamins favorably affects the levels of homocysteine. Framingham researchers are also investigating whether viruses and other infectious agents, including chlamydia and a bacterium that causes stomach ulcers, play a role in damaging healthy blood vessels.

It documented information about the incidence of heart disease in women and identified female-specific risk factors

Based on data gathered during the Framingham Heart Study, it was determined that coronary heart disease was the most prevalent cardiovascular event in both sexes. While men experienced coronary events twice as often as women, the gap narrowed with advancing age. In women, chest pain (angina) was the most common initial symptom. In men, it was a heart attack. When heart attack was the first coronary event, it was more likely to go unrecognized in women than men. Coronary attacks were also more often fatal in women.

Data analysis showed that, in addition to menopause, risk factors unique to women included the potency of having diabetes. One of the many lessons of the Framingham study is that Type II diabetes is more prevalent in women than in men, and is for women more closely associated with cardiovascular disease.

Very active women were found to have the most protection against heart disease—a factor previously known to be true only for men. And women who smoked heavily were found to be less likely to quit than men.

Clinical Trials with Lipitor: Advance Understanding of Cholesterol

The Framingham Heart Study led to the development of a whole new class of drugs known as statins, which interfere with the manufacture of cholesterol—including the bad (LDL) cholesterol. One of the latest statins to hit pharmacy shelves is Lipitor (Atorvastatin). On its way to market, a new definition of a "normal" cholesterol reading emerged. "What's normal for many people is too high for those with heart disease," said David Canter, MD, the researcher who headed up the Lipitor Development Team for Pfizer. "That's a huge piece of knowledge that clinical trial participants gave to all of us."

Moreover, the benefit of lowering cholesterol with drugs like Lipitor doesn't "bottom out," as was once believed, Canter added. "It keeps going lower. For anyone who has heart disease, their cholesterol should be under 100. We couldn't make that statement ten years ago." With Lipitor, doctors are comfortable increasing doses, if necessary, to achieve better cholesterol-lowering results because in trials and actual clinical practice it has proven safe to do so.

A total of 3,520 patients participated in 21 clinical trials of Lipitor prior to its approval by the Food and Drug Administration (FDA) in December 1996. About 1,000 of these volunteers were put either on a placebo or a comparator drug. Relative to other statins already on the market, Lipitor's superior cholesterol-lowering ability was obvious to the FDA after the first few hundred volunteers were actively participating in the trials, said Canter. It took another three years, and many more study volunteers, to demonstrate that the extra benefit did not come at a cost to patient safety. In fact, Lipitor was shown to lower cholesterol better than other drugs taken at significantly higher doses. Within three months of Lipitor's approval, roughly half a million people in the U.S. were taking the drug. It has been known since the early 1990s that, if LDL cholesterol can be lowered by about 35%, heart disease risk can be meaningfully reduced, said Canter. Clinical studies found that Lipitor could lower bad cholesterol between 39% and 60%. It also could reduce total cholesterol 29%–45% and, for patients with multiple risk factors for heart disease, reduce the risk of heart attack by more than one third.

"We learn efficacy/benefits of a drug as a group, but safety as an individual," said Canter. Some of the 140-odd adverse events listed on Lipitor's label occurred in a single study volunteer. "With clinical trials, we collect data on every small symptom. Nothing is filtered out." In placebo-controlled studies, for instance, 270 patients given a sugar pill reported getting a headache. At a 10mg dose of the actual drug, slightly more than 5% of 863 patients had the same complaint. Among those getting 20mg of Lipitor, more than 16% of participants reported a headache, but there were only 36 volunteers at that dose level. Will the average person taking Lipitor get headaches? "Probably not," said Canter. Still, all that information gets reported to doctors and patients on the label.

"Part of drug development is to have a very high level of suspicion, looking for the first hint of something," said Canter. Side effects occurring in individual volunteers "helped define the proper dose range for Lipitor that is used by prescribing doctors to this day," he added. Clinical trial volunteers in effect "protected other patients from us going too far" with dosing recommendations.

"The accuracy of data gathered from that original group of 3,520 has stood the test of time," said Canter. "We did not have to modify the label for information that was missing for several years." Large-scale trials conducted after Lipitor's approval by the FDA found that the drug, in addition to lowering cholesterol, also helped prevent strokes and heart attacks and the need for coronary artery bypass surgery.

"Study volunteers contributed to learning in a variety of important ways. Healthy volunteers, the first-time users of Lipitor, helped Pfizer demonstrate the drug's ability to lower bad cholesterol in precisely the same manner that was subsequently seen with people with elevated cholesterol," said Canter. Volunteers in early trials of Lipitor also helped researcher learn that it "made no difference at all" if the drug was taken once rather than twice a day. So, for the sake of patient convenience and compliance, it was decided that Lipitor would be administered once a day. Similarly, volunteers helped researchers determine that Lipitor could be taken at any time of the day, either with or without food.

A likely dose range had already been established by the time Lipitor was given to study volunteers diagnosed with high cholesterol. Initially, study patients were treated for six weeks, to confirm the positive response seen in the healthy volunteers, said Canter. "This was the first really important study, because it gave us an idea of how well tolerated Lipitor was across a wide range of dosages [from 2.5mg to 80mg], and included a placebo group." Confirmatory studies placed volunteers on the drug in narrower dose categories for a 12-week period. All this taught researchers that "10mg is a great place to start because, at that dose, side effects were no different than a placebo and the benefit of lowering LDL cholesterol was about the same [40%] as competing products [at their highest dose]. It was our feeling that Lipitor started where other drugs left off and we were happy about the safety we had seen to date."

In 1993, a third major group of trials got underway that was designed to compare the safety of Lipitor to a half dozen standard therapies available in the U.S. and Europe—including the statin drugs Zocor, Mevacor, and Pravachol. Patients in these 52-week trials all got either Lipitor or standard therapy. "Lipitor appeared to have the same safety profile but offered possibly greater benefit," said Canter. Appearances proved correct, and the FDA approved Lipitor as an all-purpose cholesterol-lowering drug. It also, for the first time ever, allowed the label to include comparative information about competing products. "The differences were all significant at the starting dose." In parallel with the big studies, researchers conducted a series of smaller, specialized studies to answer some additional concerns, including use of the drug in patients with liver or kidney disease. "We learned that both groups of patients could take the drug, but that extra caution and safety monitoring is required in the case of those with liver disease," said Canter.

FDA approval of Lipitor only "invited us to the party," said Canter. Managed care payers, who control patient access to prescription drugs via "formularies," also had to be convinced that the drug had advantages over other treatment alternatives. To that end, further comparative studies have been ongoing since the drug gained FDA approval. "The big idea is to show the value of a drug like Lipitor and how it might alter clinical practice including being an alternative to medical procedures like stents and angioplasty," said Canter. Researchers have been both exploring Lipitor's ability to improve clinical outcomes and its potential to help patients with non-cardiac medical conditions.

Among the 26 "pivotal studies" conducted since Lipitor's marketing approval have been the landmark Anglo-Scandinavian Cardiac Outcomes Trial (ASCOT), involving more than 19,342 patients with high blood pressure. The study was designed to determine if newer blood pressure medications produced greater benefits than older ones. Half of the 10,305 patients enrolled in the lipid-lowering arm received either Lipitor or a placebo to determine whether cholesterol-lowering therapy could provide additional cardiovascular benefits. It is estimated that between 35% and 50% of patients with high blood pressure suffer from high cholesterol.

Participants in ASCOT helped further support Lipitor's outstanding efficacy. The study found that patients with normal or mildly elevated cholesterol levels who took Lipitor had 36% fewer fatal coronary events and non-fatal heart attacks than patients treated with placebo. Lipitor-treated patients also experienced a 27% reduction in fatal and non-fatal strokes, as well as 21% fewer cardiovascular events and procedures. More than 16 million adults in the United States who have high blood pressure and normal to mildly elevated cholesterol levels stand to benefit from the finding, said cardiologist John Tsai, MD, the Lipitor medical team leader.

A second landmark Lipitor trial, called the Collaborative Atorvastatin Diabetes Study (CARDS), involved more than 2,800 patients with type-II diabetes. Among the findings were that Lipitor significantly reduced heart attacks and strokes in patients with diabetes, said Tsai. Specifically, trial participants who took Lipitor rather than a placebo had 37% fewer major cardiovascular events, including chest pain that required hospitalization, cardiac resuscitation, and coronary revascularization procedures. They also had 48% fewer strokes and were 27% less likely to die. The findings came as welcome news to the 65% of diabetics (estimated at more than 110 million worldwide) who were expected to suffer a heart attack or stroke—four times higher than in adults without diabetes. The American Diabetes Association now recommends that adults with type-II diabetes be treated with statin therapy regardless of their LDL levels.

Recent epidemiological evidence has also shown that statins may well have some value for patients with other non-cardiac medical conditions, such as Alzheimer's disease and the prevention of colon cancer. Lipitor clinical trials suggest statins are not beneficial in reducing the symptoms of osteoporosis and prostate enlargement.

There have been a total of over 300 clinical trials of Lipitor done to date, involving over 80,000 patients. Lipitor's proven cholesterol-lowering properties alone make it a true "blockbuster" drug. "The link between cholesterol and heart disease is very strong," said Canter. "The end result appears to show that, too. This country has the same level of heart disease that existed in 1900. The situation had seriously gone awry in the 1960s and 1970s. Heart disease was rising rapidly." The heart disease rate stabilized in subsequent years due to a combination of factors, including the development of Lipitor. The Framingham Heart Study remains the "cornerstone" of public health policy when it comes to heart disease, and provided clues about what types of interventions needed testing.

"Study volunteers are very much a part of the story," said Canter. "Individual patients in the Lipitor trials made a major contribution to public health, helping prolong the lives of tens of thousands of people across the world."

Gleevec Trials: Brightening the Outlook for Cancer

For many patients who enrolled in a clinical trial for Gleevec, it was literally a matter of survival. Once diagnosed with Philadelphia chromosome-positive chronic myeloid leukemia (CML), doctors gave them only about five years to live. A bone marrow transplant offers a potential cure, but only a fraction of patients make appropriate candidates for such a risky procedure. The standard therapy for most patients was a cocktail of interferon and chemotherapy, which helped maintain them in the "chronic phase" of CML before their inevitable slide toward death.

In one of the more important trials of Gleevec, developed by Novartis Pharmaceuticals, the drug was compared with the standard therapy in newly diagnosed CML patients. By the time Gleevec was approved in May 2001, many patients randomized into the interferon/chemotherapy arm of the trial had already quit the study and switched over on their own to Gleevec, said Laurie Letvak, MD, who heads up medical affairs for the blockbuster drug. "Seven months after that, a data monitoring committee looked at the data and found that on almost every efficacy point, Gleevec was better."

At that point, participants were free to cross over to Gleevec without abandoning the study. "Of those who were originally in the interferon plus chemotherapy group, only 3% are still on it [as of December 2005]," said Letvak. In contrast, 72% of those who started on Gleevec continue taking it. Most impressively, more than 90% of the patients who went into the Gleevec arm were still alive nearly five years later and only 7% had gone into advanced disease. "The exciting news at the [2005] American Society of Hematology meeting was that, for chronic phase patients, the annual percentage that went into advanced disease . . . was lower than the percentage in prior years."

"All the experts in this disease say Gleevec has changed what it means to have CML," said Letvak. "Patients have a different conversation with their doctor. They talk about long-term survival . . . possibly 20 years or longer. Because this was a new therapy, people were reserving judgment and waiting for the other shoe to drop. But so far, it hasn't happened." Some experts have started talking about how CML will not be such a rare disease anymore "because patients are not progressing and dying with the pace previously seen. It's changing into a truly chronic disease."

Of the more than 10,000 patients who have participated in over 200 pre- and post-marketing trials of Gleevec, the majority have CML—one of the major forms of leukemia afflicting adults, said Letvak. A fair number also have gastrointestinal stromal tumors (GIST), a very rare form of cancer that is associated with a different molecular abnormality targeted by Gleevec. In February 2002, Gleevec was specifically approved for treatment of GIST. "Patients with advanced GIST usually died fairly quickly," said Letvak. If the disease was progressive and spreading, it was not unusual for patients to die in less than a year. "With GIST, we literally had people in hospice who responded and were still doing well about five years later." Patients like these "drive further interest and awareness of rare cancers and support for clinical trials—[sponsored] by all pharmaceutical companies, not just Novartis. A lot is being done on a global scale and on the Internet."

Gleevec was originally approved in May 2001 as an oral therapy for treatment of CML among patients in the advanced phase of the disease, or in the chronic phase after failure with the standard medical therapy. "The vast majority of patients entered [a Gleevec study] not to help register the drug, but under an expanded access program," said Letvak. "It had such fantastic efficacy that we had to make it available to patients before it became commercially available."

Most patients in Gleevec's phase I trials started to show some improvement at very low dose levels. "Traditionally in most phase I cancer studies, patients don't personally get a benefit," said Letvak. "If 10% of patients do, that would be considered good." The first improvement seen was a reduction in patients' white blood cell count. At a dose of 300mg–400mg, abnormal chromosomes associated with the disease began to disappear. "Researchers were surprised and delighted. It was almost like disbelief." Unlike those newly diagnosed with CML, a fair number of these sicker patients later had a relapse.

Today, an estimated 80,000 people worldwide are taking Gleevec. The drug has received government approval for sale in more than 90 countries, said Letvak.

Participants in some of the more recent Gleevec trials have helped shed light on the drug's potential in other subsets of patients. At the end of 2005, Novartis filed for approval in the U.S. and Europe for use of Gleevec in the treatment of Ph+ acute lymphocytic leukemia (ALL). "A number of studies around the world have found consistently good results," said Letvak. "The filing is a bit unconventional because we're relying mostly on published data in combination with data from our own studies." Approval is also being sought for use of Gleevec in treating a handful of other cancers, including some so rare that they exist only "anecdotally." Meanwhile, researchers in several laboratories have unraveled the underlying pathology of a rare blood disorder that physicians discovered responds well to treatment with Gleevec even at 50mg-100mg doses given three times weekly.

Beyond the personal benefit derived by study participants, the Gleevec trials furthered science in many noteworthy ways. Trials targeting GIST, for instance, prompted doctors to start looking for that particular sarcoma in the clinical practice setting, said Letvak. Consequently, far more cases of GIST are being diagnosed.

The Gleevec trials spurred a lot of research about genetic mutations that happen in the advanced stages of CML. Researchers also were motivated to start looking at the body's response to Gleevec at the molecular level. A specialized blood test is used to measure the amount of an abnormal protein in the blood that is associated with CML, explained Letvak. "Of the patients in our study who have had a major molecular response [to the drug], none have gone on to advanced disease." The scientific community is now concerning itself with how to make the specialized blood test for this molecular response more widely available, "so when we talk about 'results' we're talking about the same thing."

In terms of the long-term impact Gleevec has had on the lifestyle of patients, "the biggest change is that they generally feel well," said Letvak. "Today, many patients treated with Gleevec are able to travel, go to work, and even lift weights at the gym—often with no or only mild physical complaints."

These are but a few examples of the profound gift that clinical trial participation bestows on public health. The next chapter will consider why clinical trials are necessary to evaluate the safety and effectiveness of medical therapies.

CHAPTER TWO

Why Clinical Trials Are Conducted

People want and expect their doctors to use treatments that work well and to stop using those that do not. Long ago, trial and error was the primary way that physicians and medical care providers learned how to recognize treatment alternatives. Later, through rigorous approaches that use clinical trials, physicians and researchers have been able to gather far more meaningful information about diseases and how to best treat them.

For thousands of years, healers, shamans, and medical care providers have been administering treatments and remedies. One of the earliest known medical treatments dates back more than 3,500 years to ancient Egypt. Some ancient remedies, such as those used for simple fractures and minor injuries, are effective even today. However, many ancient medical treatments did not work and were actually harmful and even fatal. Two hundred years ago, cutting open a vein to drain a pint or more of blood and giving toxic substances to force vomiting or diarrhea were common remedies. And only a century ago, along with mention of some useful drugs such as aspirin and digitalis, the Merck Manual—one of the most respected sources for information on medical treatments then as well as now—mentioned cocaine as a treatment for alcoholism; arsenic and tobacco smoke as treatments for asthma; and sulfuric acid nasal spray as a treatment for the common cold. Today these approaches are known to be very dangerous.

There are many reasons that doctors recommended ineffective and harmful treatments and that people accepted them. In many cases there were no alternatives. Doctors and patients usually prefer doing something to doing nothing. Patients also find comfort in sharing their problems and ailments with an authority figure. And doctors feel compelled to provide attention, support, and reassurance.

The primary reason doctors recommended ineffective and harmful treatments is that doctors couldn't tell what worked from what didn't. Doctors relied on cause-and-effect to identify potential treatments. For example, if an ill person's fever broke after the doctor drained a pint of blood or after the shaman chanted a certain spell, then people naturally assumed those actions must have been what caused the fever to break. To the person desperately seeking relief, getting better was all the proof necessary. Unfortunately, these apparent cause-and-effect relationships observed in early medicine were rarely correct. Still, they were enough to promulgate centuries of ineffective remedies.

Of course, people had to be getting better in order to reassure doctors that a given treatment was working. Indeed, this is exactly what often happens. People do get better spontaneously. Sick people often get well on their own—and despite their doctor's care—when the body heals itself or the disease runs its course. Colds are gone in a week; stomach flu passes within hours; migraine headaches typically last a day or two; and food poisoning symptoms may end in 12 hours. Many people even recover from life-threatening disorders, such as a heart attack or pneumonia, without treatment. Symptoms of chronic diseases (such as asthma or sickle-cell disease) come and go. Many treatments may seem to be effective if given enough time. And any treatment given near the time of spontaneous recovery may seem dramatically effective.

Belief in the power of a treatment or remedy is often enough to make people feel better. Belief cannot cause an underlying disorder—such as a broken bone, heart disease, or diabetes— to disappear. But people who believe they are receiving a strong, effective treatment very often feel better. Pain, nausea, fatigue, and many other symptoms can diminish. This happens even when the drug contains no active ingredients and can be of no possible benefit, such as a sugar pill or an inactive substance called a placebo. An ineffective (or even harmful) treatment prescribed by a confident doctor to a trusting, hopeful person often results in remarkable improvement of symptoms. This improvement is termed the placebo effect. People may see an actual (not simply misperceived) benefit from a treatment that has no real effect on the disease itself.

Some people argue that the only matter of importance is whether a treatment or remedy makes people feel better. Whether it works or not is of little consequence. This argument may be reasonable when the symptom is the problem, such as in many day-to-day aches and pains, or in illnesses such as colds, which always go away on their own. In such cases, doctors do sometimes prescribe treatments for their placebo effect. However, in any dangerous or potentially serious disorder, or when the treatment itself may cause side effects, it is critically important for doctors not to miss an opportunity to prescribe a treatment that really does work.

The Concept of Clinical Trials

Because doctors realized long ago that people can get better on their own, they naturally tried to compare how different people with the same disease fared with or without treatment. But until the middle of the nineteenth century, it was very difficult to make this comparison. Diseases were so poorly understood that it was difficult to tell when two or more people had the "same" disease. In addition, doctors using common terminology were often talking about different diseases entirely. For example, in the eighteenth and nineteenth centuries, a diagnosis of "dropsy" was given to people whose legs were swollen. It is now known that swelling can result from heart failure, kidney failure, or severe liver disease—quite different diseases that do not respond to the same treatments. Similarly, numerous people who had fever and who were also vomiting were diagnosed with "bilious fever." It is now known that many different diseases cause fever and vomiting, such as typhoid, malaria, and hepatitis. Only when accurate scientifically-based diagnoses became common, about 100 years ago, were doctors able to effectively evaluate treatments.

Even when doctors could reliably diagnose diseases, they still had to determine how to best evaluate whether treatments were safe and effective.

It wasn't until the mid-twentieth century when the concept of doing carefully designed trials held as a framework for determining safety and efficacy and ensuring that the observed effects were real and not due to chance. The first randomized, controlled clinical trial in modern medicine began in the late 1940s. Clinical trials are based on a number of key principles and methods. For example, observing treatment effects among a large enough group of people reduces the likelihood of chance occurrences. Doctors and researchers typically compare results between a group of people who receives an experimental treatment (treatment group) and a group who receives an older treatment or no treatment at all (control group). Studies that involve a control group are called "controlled" studies.

Initially, doctors and researchers simply gave all their patients with a certain illness a new treatment and then compared their results to those of people with the illness treated at an earlier time (either by the same or different doctors). For example, if doctors found that 80% of their patients survived malaria after receiving a new treatment, whereas previously only 60% survived, then they would conclude that the newer treatment was more effective. Studies that compare current treatment results to past results are called retrospective or historical studies.

A problem with historical studies is that the treatment group also has the benefit of other advances in medical care that had since been developed. It doesn't make sense to compare the treatment results of people receiving a therapy in 2006 with those who received a therapy in 1966. Medical advances during the intervening period may be responsible for any improvement in outcome. To avoid this problem with historical studies, doctors and researchers try to create treatment groups and control groups at the same time. Such studies are called prospective studies.

The biggest concern with all types of medical studies, including historical studies, is that similar groups of people should be compared. In the previous example, if the group of people who received the new treatment (the treatment group) for malaria was made up of mostly young people who had mild disease, and the previously treated (control) group was made up of older people who had severe disease, it might well be that people in the treatment group fared better simply because they were younger and healthier. As a result, a new treatment could falsely appear to work better. Many other factors besides age and severity of illness also must be taken into account including the overall health of people being studied (people with chronic diseases such as diabetes or kidney failure tend to fare worse than healthier people); the specific doctor and hospital providing care (some may be more skilled and have better facilities than others); the percentages of men and women that comprise the study groups (men and women may respond differently to treatment); and the socioeconomic status of the people involved (people with more resources to help support themselves tend to fare better).

Doctors and researchers have tried many different methods to ensure that the groups being compared are as similar as possible. It might seem sensible to specifically choose people for treatment groups and control groups by matching them on various characteristics. For example, if a doctor was studying a new treatment for high blood pressure (hypertension), and one person in the treatment group was 42 years old and had diabetes, then the doctor would try to ensure the placement of a person near 40 years of age with hypertension and diabetes in the control group. These types of studies are called case-control studies. However, there are so many differences among people, including differences that are often not even considered, that it is nearly impossible to ensure an exact match.

Instead, doctors and researchers take advantage of the laws of probability and randomly assign—typically with the assistance of a computer application—people who have the same disease to different study groups. If a large enough group of people is divided up randomly, the odds are that people in each group will have similar characteristics. Studies that use these methods are called "randomized." Prospective, randomized studies are the best way to make sure that a treatment or test is being compared between equivalent groups.

Once doctors and researchers have created equivalent groups, they must make sure that the only difference they allow is the experimental treatment itself. That way, they can be sure that any difference in outcome is due to the specific treatment under investigation, and not to some other factor, such as the quality or frequency of follow-up care.

Doctors and researchers must also account for the placebo effect. People who know they are receiving an active experimental treatment rather than no treatment (or an older, presumably less effective treatment) often expect to feel better. Some people, on the other hand, may expect to experience more side effects from a new, experimental treatment. In either case, these expectations can exaggerate the effects of treatment, causing it to seem more effective or to have more complications than it really does.

To avoid the problems of the placebo effect, people in a study are "blinded"—they do not know whether they are receiving the active experimental treatment. Blinding is usually accomplished by giving people in the control group a pill or substance that is identical in appearance to the experimental treatment. However, when an effective treatment for a disease already exists, it is not ethical to give the control group a placebo. In those situations, the control group is given the standard or established treatment.

But whether a placebo or an established drug is used, the substance must appear identical to the study drug, except for the active ingredient. That is necessary so that people cannot tell whether they are taking the study drug. If the treatment group receives a red, bitter liquid, then the control group should also receive a red, bitter liquid. If the treatment group receives a clear solution given by injection, then the control group should receive a similar injection.

Because the doctor or nurse might accidentally let a person know what treatment they are receiving, it is better if all healthcare practitioners involved in a clinical trial remain unaware of what is being given. This type of blinding is called "double-blinding." Double-blinding usually requires a person separate from the study, such as a pharmacist, to prepare identical-appearing substances that are labeled only by a special number code. The number code is broken only after the study is completed.

An additional reason for double-blinding is that the placebo effect can even affect the doctor, who may unconsciously think a person receiving treatment is doing better than a person receiving no treatment, even if both are faring exactly the same. Not all medical studies can be double-blinded. For example, surgeons studying two different procedures obviously know which procedure they are performing (although the people undergoing the procedures can be kept unaware). In such cases, doctors at least make sure that the people evaluating the outcome of treatment are blinded as to what has been done so they cannot unconsciously bias the results.

The best-known approach to gathering information on the real effects of a new treatment is a prospective, randomized, placebo-controlled, and double-blinded clinical trial. This design allows for the clearest determination of the effectiveness and safety of a treatment. In some situations, this trial design may not be possible. For example, with very rare diseases, it is often hard to find enough people for a randomized trial. In those cases, retrospective case-control trials are often conducted.

Jennie, breast cancer survivor in a relapse prevention trial

When my doctor mentioned the trial to me, I was skeptical. I had heard of the drug because it was already FDA-approved for the treatment of arthritis, only in this study it was going to be given in higher dosages. My doctor said if it didn't help keep the cancer away, at least my knees wouldn't hurt. It's a double-blind study and I think I'm getting the actual drug because, when I take it, the arthritis pain goes away. The study was supposed to end after one year, but I did so well that the pharmaceutical company decided to continue it for at least another year.

Clinical Trial Phases

There are four clinical trial phases, each with a different set of objectives and requirements—from simple outpatient studies requiring only a couple of hours a month to situations requiring overnight or extended stays at medical facilities.

During phase I studies, a drug is tested for the first time in small numbers (20 to 100) of healthy volunteers, often college students.

Phase I trials typically last from several months up to one year. The goal of these trials is to learn about safe dosage ranges in which a drug can be administered, the method of absorption and distribution in the body, and the possible toxicity of a new treatment. Researchers start by giving volunteers a single dose of the drug. Then they gradually increase the dosage level until minor side effects like nausea or headaches start to occur. That's how researchers learn about the more common side effects that limit the treatment dosage levels. Payment to participants in this phase of the process is also common because it's often the only way to get enough volunteers.

Only certain new, very toxic treatments for cancer and infectious diseases are tested on actual patients in phase I trials. And only in terminally ill cancer patients—where there are often no other options available—is the dosage amount increased until it is literally intolerable. For these cancer patients, the greatest hope of survival lies in destroying the highest possible number of cancer cells in the body just short of death. Researchers are usually leading experts in their field.

Until 1993, mostly males were enrolled as study subjects in phase I clinical trials because researchers were concerned that women might become pregnant during a clinical trial and put both the subject and her child at risk. Today, however, more women are allowed to make that decision for themselves. But they must not get pregnant while participating in a clinical trial. During the trial, female study subjects are typically expected to use some form of birth control, usually contraception or abstinence.

Phase I studies are conducted in numerous locations—frequently in academic settings or in private, specialty centers. Participants are often confined for 24-hour periods to a special inpatient unit complete with kitchen and recreational facilities, where they may undergo frequent blood and urine tests. These tests help researchers understand how the investigational drug is absorbed, distributed, metabolized, and excreted by the human body. This will assist researchers in determining if a new drug will have to be given one, two, three, or more times a day. But how safe the drug truly is remains a mystery because so few people have taken it. Due to safety and toxicity problems, many investigational drugs are abandoned during phase I testing. According to the FDA, approximately 70% of new medical treatments pass this testing stage.

In phase II studies, researchers begin to understand how safe and effective an investigational drug will be for patients for whom the drug is intended. Similar to phase I, safety is still the primary goal. Phase II studies are usually conducted on a relatively small number of volunteers—approximately 100 to 300 patients—who have the disease or condition targeted by the new medical therapy. Clinical trials in this phase take between one and three years to complete. Phase II studies look to answer such basic questions as "Do patients improve?" and "What are the usual side effects?" Researchers also learn if the treatment dosage needs to be lowered or raised.

Success rates by phase for investigational drugs

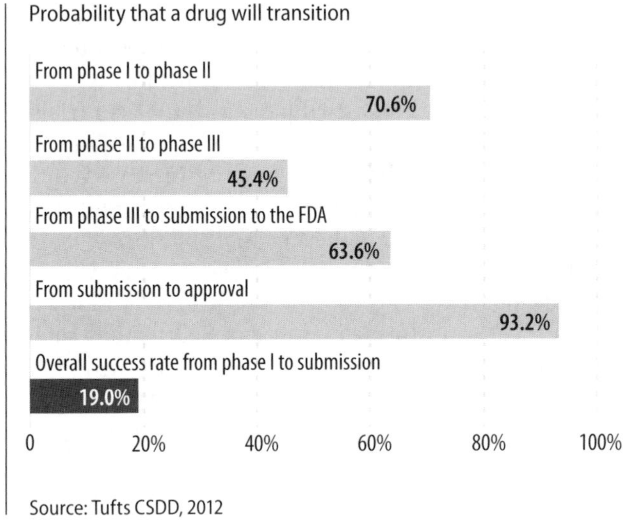

Probability that a drug will transition

From phase I to phase II
70.6%

From phase II to phase III
45.4%

From phase III to submission to the FDA
63.6%

From submission to approval
93.2%

Overall success rate from phase I to submission
19.0%

0 20% 40% 60% 80% 100%

Source: Tufts CSDD, 2012

Eligibility requirements tend to be strict in phase II trials. These scientifically demanding studies are usually "randomized," meaning that volunteers are assigned to different groups, of which only a subset will receive the investigational drug. The control group will get another standard treatment or a placebo for part of, or perhaps throughout, the entire study. This method helps take the bias out of study results due to human choices or other factors unrelated to the treatments being tested. Typically, the study is double-blinded, meaning that neither the patient nor the researcher knows who is getting the investigational drug and who is getting the placebo or standard treatment.

A phase II study may measure something that isn't the drug's ultimate clinical value, such as improving survival after a heart attack. It would instead look at how well the drug opens blood vessels after a heart attack. Overall, it's shorter than a phase III study and involves a smaller population of people. Phase II trials are also the period when researchers look at the body's response to different doses of a drug.

Less than half of drugs that enter clinical testing ever successfully complete phase II and progress to larger-scale phase III studies. This stage provides hard, statistical facts about a drug. Phase III clinical trials involve extensive testing to assess safety, efficacy, and dosage levels in a large group of patients facing a specific illness. The study drug is tested on as many as several thousand people over a period of two to five years. Often, "real-world" results—such as how long a person can sit at a basketball game, write a letter, or hike up and down stairs—are seen as equally important as clinical findings (lower blood pressure or higher white cell count, for example) in measuring a drug's usefulness. Phase III trials are most often conducted in a doctor's office.

The goal in this research phase is often to have an investigational treatment evaluated by practicing physicians who might one day prescribe it. These trials often involve a more diverse patient group for whom the treatment is initially intended. The number of volunteers needed for a phase III study depends on how many people have the targeted disease. Compared to studies of medications designed to prevent heart attacks, those for asthma would be smaller because researchers can learn something from every single participant, and every enrollee will actually have the disease.

Phase III studies almost always involve a relatively large number of participants with similar demographic characteristics. At this stage, researchers may also look to compare the drug's safety and effectiveness in different subsets of patients—men versus women, blacks versus whites, elderly versus young—and how well the treatment works in mild, moderate, and severe forms of the same disease. Researchers are also able to test different dosage levels of the drug so that they know, quite precisely, how much of it most people need to get the good effects with as few bad effects as possible.

Drugs tested in phase III clinical trials may include remedies already approved by the FDA to treat a different medical condition—such as a study of a multipurpose antimicrobial to treat a specific opportunistic infection in AIDS patients. Phase III studies usually test a new drug in comparison with a placebo or an existing treatment.

Therapies that have reached phase III have already passed toxicity testing and have proved to be at least somewhat effective. But subjects in phase III trials still usually have no better than a 50% chance of getting the investigational treatment versus a placebo or standard therapy. About 65% of drugs that enter phase III will successfully complete this stage.

* * *

Once clinical trials are completed and the results are analyzed, the company sponsoring the research may submit a New Drug Application (NDA) to the Food and Drug Administration if there is enough positive information about the safety and effectiveness of the treatment. The NDA is given to one of two groups within the FDA: either the Center for Drug Evaluation and Research (CDER), or the Center for Biologics Evaluation and Research (CBER). The former review group is responsible for evaluating prescription and over-the-counter drugs. The latter group is responsible for evaluating blood and blood products, vaccines, allergenics, and medical treatments made from living organisms. The FDA will also look to advisory committees made up of medical experts to assist in determining whether a treatment should be approved for sale on the market. Applications for new medical devices are submitted to the Center for Devices and Radiological Health.

How long does it take for a drug to complete clinical research?

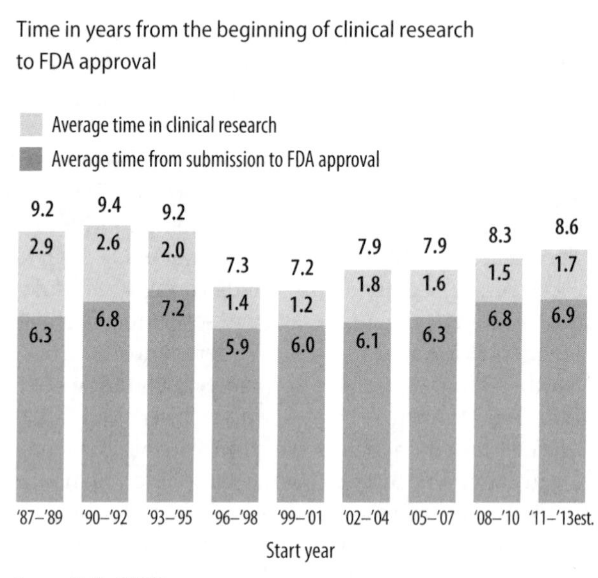

The FDA review period usually takes 12–18 months for most NDAs. The FDA also has an expedited review process for priority drugs—usually lasting under six months. Priority drugs are those that represent a notable treatment benefit for critical and severe illnesses. FDA review and approval doesn't always happen as quickly as pharmaceutical and biotechnology companies would like. The FDA withheld its approval for an effective nasal flu vaccine aimed at toddlers, for example. The agency asked the company to conduct more studies looking at how well the new treatment combined with other vaccines and whether there was a rare risk of pneumonia or asthma among certain children.

The FDA would also be skeptical, for example, if a high-blood-pressure medication caused a higher-than-expected rate of facial swelling among a minority population. It wouldn't matter if researchers believed they could fix the problem by changing the dose. To demonstrate to the FDA that a lower dose did not produce a higher-than expected rate of facial swelling, the pharmaceutical company would have to conduct a large-scale study of the drug specifically targeting that population.

After pharmaceutical companies receive FDA approval to market a drug, they will sometimes conduct phase IV studies. These clinical trials are performed to uncover additional information about a new treatment. What is the long-term safety and effectiveness of a drug? What impact does it have on improving patients' day-to-day lives? When do physicians decide to prescribe the new treatment relative to others in the market? How does the new treatment compare with other similar treatments available to patients? Phase IV clinical trials typically involve large numbers of patients who are routinely taking the medical treatment under investigation. Although these types of studies often have happened at the FDA's urging, recent drug safety concerns surrounding popular painkillers and antidepressants have left many companies wanting to invest resources to better understand potential risks. In some cases, phase IV studies are conducted to see if a drug causes unique problems for a certain patient subgroup. The results of these studies may be used to revise product labeling or to further support claims and comparisons that pharmaceutical companies make in package inserts and product advertisements. The offices of community-based physicians are particularly well suited for phase IV studies because they provide routine care for patients and they administer prescriptions regularly.

If you or a loved one is looking to gain access to a novel, investigational treatment not yet available on the market, then you should primarily consider phase II and III studies; however, your participation in any clinical trial is dependent upon your meeting strict inclusion and exclusion criteria, as described in the protocol. Not only are you looking for trials that are right for you, but you must also be the right subject for the trial.

Outside of clinical trials, there are unique situations where desperately ill patients may gain access to medical therapies yet to be approved by the FDA. A treatment IND may be issued if an investigational drug has provided enough data to suggest that the drug may be effective without posing unreasonable risk. Under a treatment IND, seriously ill patients—not participating in clinical trials—can begin to receive a drug from their physician before the drug receives FDA approval. Investigational drugs can also be administered in an urgent situation in which there isn't enough time for the sponsor company to submit an IND. In these instances, the FDA may authorize shipment of the drug to health providers for a specific emergency use. There are occasions when clinical trials have ended and patients are allowed to continue taking the investigational medication while awaiting FDA approval. The FDA may grant Compassionate Use when a study drug is already being marketed in another country and when the drug is the only reasonable treatment available.

In the next chapter, we'll look at the reasons that people volunteer to participate, or choose not to participate, in clinical research studies.

CHAPTER THREE

Why People Choose to Participate

"I didn't enter the studies for relief, because there were other things I could take. Even if I found something better, it wouldn't be approved for public consumption right away. The main reason I did this was because I had several friends who died from prostate involvement—in their case, cancer. Any trial with 300 people is just a small step and being one part of 300 is an even smaller step, but it's necessary. It's the way the system works in this country, and it protects people. I saw it as an opportunity to do something for science."

Robert, a volunteer in three enlarged-prostate clinical trials

"I know what I went through with chemotherapy treatment. If I can in any way help someone else not go through that, it can't be anything but good. The trial I'm in is for a possible new treatment for breast cancer and could help millions of people down the road. That in itself outweighs any possible chances of major side effects [for me]."

Jennie, a volunteer in a breast-cancer relapse prevention trial

"I was interested in this trial, among the several others presented to me, because I did not want to go off of my current maintenance treatment or the infusions I was already receiving. I also did not have to undergo another colonoscopy. I had a 33% chance of receiving a placebo only, and the opportunity to participate in an open-label trial and automatically receive the product upon completion of the 12-week study. I was paid $25 per

Paula, a volunteer in a phase II Crohn's disease trial

visit. There were no other 'special perks' other than the feeling of receiving a potentially helpful treatment and good healthcare during that time."

Patty, a volunteer in a trial for primary progressive multiple sclerosis

"The trial drug was approved by the FDA years earlier, so I wasn't worried about side effects and had no other options anyway. Since there was no drug approved for my condition, I was eager to see if this drug would help stop [its] endless progression. With a chronic, incurable illness, one has to have hope of a cure, or at least slowing down the progression."

It is a common misconception that receiving treatment in clinical trials is the same as receiving regular treatment as a patient. The hard reality of a clinical trial is that it is designed to answer a scientific question, not to provide medical treatment. Someone thinking about participating in a clinical trial needs to understand the difference between research and medical treatment. When you're a study volunteer, you often feel like a patient. You usually make visits to a doctor's office where you're examined by a doctor, undergo lab tests, and receive a medication. In many ways participating in a clinical trial seems just like visiting with your doctor to receive medical care. But the difference is that a doctor's primary goal is to help you feel better, whereas in a clinical trial, the principal investigator's primary goal is to see how you will react to a new drug, and to determine whether that drug will be medically useful.

This truth doesn't change the fact that many people feel better while on an investigational drug. Many investigational products prove to be far superior to the older drugs they will one day replace. Some drugs administered during clinical trials have not only improved, but also have saved, thousands of lives. The opposite is also true: some drugs administered during clinical trials have worsened people's conditions and have caused death.

Patients in clinical trials are treated with drugs for everything from ulcers to strokes years before the FDA approves them. Even people with common illnesses, such as sinusitis or sore throat, are often very motivated to enroll in a clinical trial when other drugs have failed to relieve their suffering. People with AIDS and certain cancers are particularly anxious to sign up for a trial because it gives them access to investigational drugs that may offer their only hope of survival. About 95% of children with leukemia are in clinical trials.

The kinds of benefits people may receive depend not only on the specific study in which they participate, but also into which part of the study they are randomized. Subjects who get randomized into the control group will, at best, get a standard treatment that is already available at pharmacies and drugstores. But they may also get free screenings and exams, the camaraderie of people dealing with the same medical condition, the opportunity to be an active player in their own healthcare, and the knowledge that they're helping to answer questions that can improve the healthcare of future generations.

A surprising number of people participate in clinical trials even when they personally have little, if anything, to gain by doing so. Some volunteers get involved because they want to contribute to the advancement of medical knowledge or to help people suffering from an illness. A few do it out of simple curiosity or because they believe study volunteers get better medical care. An altruistic spirit offers no special protections or guarantees. Altruism—unless it's balanced with a healthy dose of skepticism—can leave people vulnerable. Smart patients ask questions and get second and third opinions, even if they expect little or no medical gain for themselves.

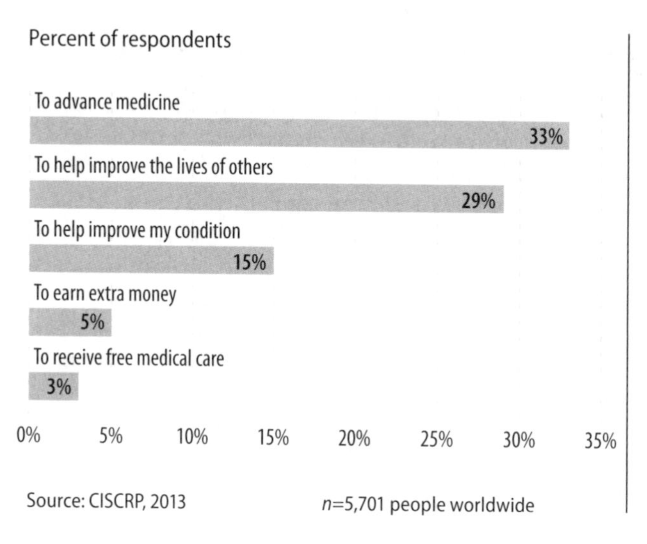

Top reasons people choose to participate in clinical trials

This was the case for Christopher, who had expected to die years ago from an aneurysm on the tip of his heart. Despite being successfully treated with a standard therapy for his high blood pressure, he volunteered himself for a five-year hypertension study. He was well aware that he had nothing to gain, clinically, by participating:

> *"My doctor checked with the study's investigator, to be sure the medication they'd be putting me on would be okay. There were two different drugs being used in the study and he said either one would take care of my hypertension. I felt fine during the whole trial, and since the trial ended. The study nurse still calls me every six months to see how I'm doing, and whenever there's another study she thinks I might be interested in. That's a nice little side benefit. I wouldn't hesitate to enter another study, if the right one came along. I think anyone who has the time and is in a situation where they can do it should. It's kind of like picking up trash left out on the street or in your yard—if you don't do it, you're asking someone else to. That's not fair. We all stand to benefit from research if something happens to us."*

People who participate in clinical trials often learn a great deal more about their illness and about other conditions (including underlying heart disease and diabetes) they may not have known about. Study-related x-rays, lab tests, and physical exams have picked up unsuspected cases of many types of cancers early enough to be successfully treated by specialists. For some participants, the best end result of a clinical trial is that they start taking better care of their own health.

Another common benefit of volunteering for clinical trials is that participants get to meet research professionals who can help introduce them to other patients suffering from similar illnesses. Volunteers also may meet scientists and professionals who can help them better understand their illness and can tell them about new treatment options under development. The many people whom you meet in a clinical trial can greatly enrich your knowledge.

For individuals diagnosed with a severe and possibly life-threatening illness, the greatest benefit of clinical trials is that they offer hope. At its best, a clinical trial is an enlargement of—not a substitution for—a patient's regular medical-care team and support circle.

Fred has been bouncing from trial to trial since he was diagnosed with gastrointestinal cancer at age 49. His treatment options have been relatively limited:

> *"In 1999, I woke up with a tumor that burst. When I got to the hospital, I was operated on immediately and told I had cancer. I went on a modified treatment for cancer, but the tumor started growing back." Six months later, when four new tumors were discovered, Fred opted to*

enter his first clinical trial, which involved being continuously infused with an experimental drug. After two months, CT scans showed the drug hadn't helped. So he entered a second trial, using the drug Gleevac (already FDA approved as a leukemia treatment), which worked out "semi-miraculously." It virtually annihilated all 40 tumors he had by then developed. When the tumors came back two and a half years later, he tried a drug that was thought to break down the metabolism of tumors. It didn't work. Neither did the next two study drugs he tried. One of them caused him to hallucinate.

"It was horrible," said Fred. "I had a lot of mental anguish." So he went back on the Gleevac, which at least killed some of the biggest tumors. But after six months, the drug started to lose its effectiveness and the tumors slowly began to reappear. During the "extremely grueling" eight months that followed, he was put on yet another experimental drug regimen. "I finally dropped out. I was getting no results and feeling sad. I was living at the hospital." The study required Fred to get a series of six EKGs over a 12-hour period once and sometimes twice a week. "It was one of the most tedious trials I have ever been in, he said. I just lay in bed."

Fred is "cautiously" optimistic that the latest drug he's on will at least buy him more time. "It's unbelievable," he said. "I only have to go in once a month. My doctor says there's a slew of stuff coming down the highway, so there's no reason to pin my hopes on this one drug. We'll see if this drug helps and then decide what to do. I was told that if my attitude is good enough and I participate in enough of these trials, my cancer can be treated as a chronic condition. So far, that approach has worked for me. Clinical trials have given me hope that there can be a happy ending to all of this."

Some people participate in clinical trials because they don't have health insurance and need help covering medical treatment costs. Drugs for cancer and AIDS can run upwards of $1,500 a month. Volunteers in clinical trials almost always get free medication, as well as physical exams and other medical services like blood tests and EKGs (a tracing of the heart's electrical activity) that help researchers monitor the drug's effects. Often, they also get treated at no charge for other minor illnesses that happen to develop during the clinical trial. The free drugs and medical care are primarily provided to ensure compliance with the study protocol and to help the volunteer remain in the study.

Some study volunteers participate primarily to earn extra money. Payment is most often used as an incentive to recruit healthy volunteers who derive no direct benefit from the research, such as in most phase I studies. Depending on the clinical trial, testing phase and the company sponsoring the research, this can be a significant amount—from $100 to more than $2,500.

There are even some people who make a profession out of being a clinical trial volunteer. They may only earn several thousand dollars a year, but their participation doesn't involve hard labor and it doesn't require much mental work. Professional volunteers feel that they are treated well and that they are needed. But along with the common risks in clinical trials, professional volunteers also face another risk: the long-term, cumulative effect of consuming investigational drugs. Professional patients tend to be young and to feel invincible.

The volunteer compensation on most clinical trials primarily covers the costs of participation. These costs might include time, transportation, a babysitter, and/or lunch. Some studies simply hand out money to pay for parking. For other types of trials, a flat fee of between $40 and $60 per visit to the study site is pretty typical. But payments can vary considerably from city to city and from study to study. Research institutions may also have their own unique payment policy. Some institutions limit how much a person can earn during a given time period.

Other factors can influence the amount of compensation that a volunteer will receive. Clinical trials that require numerous procedures and visits, or involve some discomfort—such as wearing a 24-hour blood pressure monitoring device or involving an invasive procedure—often pay higher compensation. Compensation would be higher for a phase III vaccine trial requiring a five-night inpatient stay, for example.

A few other examples: In Georgia, a recent placebo-controlled study of an oral drug for menopause-related symptoms involving six visits, an EKG, blood work, and a vaginal exam was paying $150 per visit. The same per-visit fee was being paid to adults with certain cardiac conditions to run on a treadmill. And in Florida, a two month study of an investigational medication for GERD (gastroesophageal reflux disease) was paying a total of $1,700. But it involved having an endoscopy—an inspection of the digestive tract using a tube-like viewing instrument fed through the mouth—on three different visits.

And a clinical trial in Kentucky that involved taking an IV analgesic and pain response test four times over a two-week period paid

$275 to each volunteer who completed the trial. So did an eight-week, placebo-controlled psoriasis trial in Arizona that involved regularly applying ointment to the skin and keeping a journal of any observed changes.

Most people who participate in a clinical trial have a positive experience. In exit interviews with volunteers, the majority report that they received high-quality care, experienced high levels of professionalism, and would participate again.

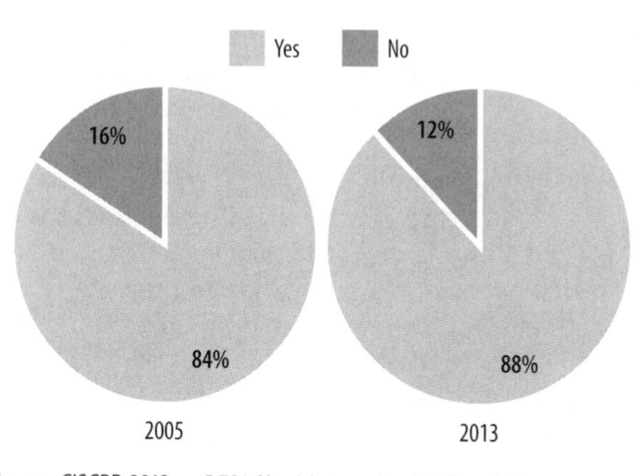

Source: CISCRP, 2013 *n*=5,701; HarrisInteractive, 2005 *n*=2,261

Majority of volunteers would participate in a clinical trial again

Wesley, who enrolled in a two-month, placebo-controlled psoriasis trial, was one such volunteer:

"My experience was very good. The study staff was very professional and very compassionate. Nothing went wrong. The best thing was that the medication worked. I have had psoriasis for approximately ten years and have tried many 'cures,' as well as countless doctor visits through these years." When the trial ended, Wesley said, the principal investigator consulted with his regular physician so that he could get a "follow-up prescription" for the treatment.

Rose, who participated in a six-month trial of an experimental drug for the treatment of hot flashes, also had a positive experience:

"I was very happy, both with the benefit I received from the medication and the way the study was conducted," she said. "The study involved a placebo and a low dose

and high dose of the study drug. I think I got the higher dose. It didn't totally eliminate my symptoms, but it decreased the frequency of the hot flashes." Rose was a little worried initially about the study drug potentially raising her already high cholesterol, but relieved to learn she wouldn't have to discontinue taking her cholesterol-lowering medication to participate in the trial. She was also very pleased with the coordinator and investigator. They were easy to work with, pleasant, careful about how they conducted the study, and accurate in recording the details. She ought to know. She makes her living as a research site manager and has served as a clinical research coordinator.

The reason people initially enroll in a clinical trial is not always the same reason they remain in a clinical trial. The experience is an ever-changing one and, unfortunately, the changes aren't always for the better. When that happens, the temptation to drop out of the study can be very strong. Waning interest in a clinical trial—or sudden, mixed feelings about the whole ordeal—is understandable and completely natural. These feelings should not be disregarded. There may be good reasons to drop out of a clinical trial. There may also be good reasons to stick with it.

Less than one third of all people who come in for a screening end up completing a clinical trial. Some participants never pass the eligibility criteria. Others drop out because the drug isn't helping them or the side effects are too unpleasant. Some volunteers get too busy to make visits to the research center or they grow tired of the study procedures and having to complete a detailed diary. Some volunteers may move out of the area. Some simply don't like the location of the research center or they don't like the study staff. Some volunteers find another clinical trial.

Estimated total volunteers completing clinical trials in 2013

Number of Study Volunteers

Government-funded clinical trials
700,000

Industry-funded phase I–III clinical trials
875,000

Industry-funded phase IV clinical trials
750,000

0 200,000 400,000 600,000 800,000 100,000

Source: CISCRP, 2013

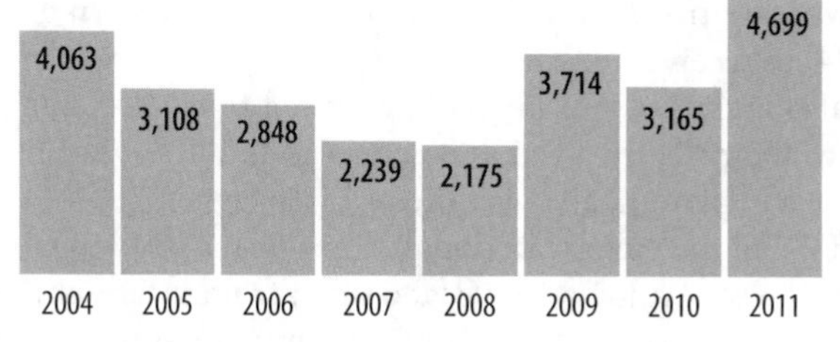

Source: PAREXEL, 2013

Average number of study volunteers per new drug application

When you have conflicting and ambivalent feelings, you might begin by talking with the investigator or study coordinator at the research center to find out if other study volunteers are feeling the same way. You may also want to speak with your primary-care or specialty-care physician or nurse.

Dropping out of a study—at any point and for any reason—is always an option. But it should not be a decision based solely on a bad mood or misinformation. The mood will pass, and answers to questions and problems may be forthcoming.

A clinical trial is a partnership between study staff and study volunteer, and it's based on informed trust. Dropping out on a whim betrays that trust. Study staff deserves the courtesy of being approached if something feels wrong.

If there are serious problems that can't be corrected or evidence that the investigator or study staff can no longer be trusted, you should most certainly drop out. You have the right to quit a trial at any time, for any reason—or no reason at all. Researchers may not like it if you drop out of a study for seemingly trivial reasons, like a headache, because investigational drugs must be tested in volunteers who remain in a clinical trial to the end. A research doctor, however, may well make the first move to drop participants from a clinical trial if a drug appears to be endangering their health.

No ethical investigator would ever try to penalize study subjects—however subtly—for making the decision to quit on their own. But study dropouts should be aware that their financial compensation, if offered, will probably be lower than that had they stayed in the study until the end.

Factors to Consider Before Participating

The reasons people choose to participate in clinical trials are compelling: (1) to gain access to new therapies; (2) to advance science and help others who are trying to cope with illnesses; (3) to earn extra money; and (4) to receive free medical care.

There are also many reasons people choose not to participate, including fear of the risks involved and concerns about the inconvenience of having to periodically visit the research center.

Only about 2% of the American population gets involved in clinical research each year. Among people who suffer from severe, chronic illnesses, only 6% participate. As a result, an increasing number of clinical trials are delayed because too few people are willing—or even knew they had the opportunity—to get involved.

Most people appreciate the value of clinical research and say they are likely to participate in a study. Yet no more than a third of those who identify and qualify for a clinical trial choose to enroll. There are a number of reasons for their reluctance. You may share some of these concerns:

They don't want a placebo

They want a guarantee that they'll receive a drug meant to treat their disease, not an inactive pill. For medical conditions for which there is already an effective, FDA-approved drug, such as high blood pressure, this may not be a concern. The investigational drug may be compared to a standard one for the entire study. In other cases, a "crossover" study may be done that rotates study subjects through equal periods on the new drug, the standard one, and a placebo. The best (and sometimes only) way to figure out how well some medications work is to compare people who take them with people who don't. The problem is that patients receiving a placebo are not being treated. Therefore, they may have increased pain and discomfort. Their condition may worsen, making it more difficult to treat later. However, some subjects do improve with a placebo because they believe they are being treated.

That is why a placebo component is included in some protocols—to study how effective the investigational drug is, compared with how effective the placebo is.

They worry about side effects and potential risks

Previous testing, on animals and other people, never completely rules out new, unexpected reactions to a drug. Side effects, also called adverse events, can be minor, such as those associated with drugs already on the market. Volunteers are told of new side effects identified during a clinical trial. Serious side effects, also called serious adverse events, such as anaphylactic shock or liver failure, would require immediate investigation and could stop a study. The research center would cover the cost of any ensuing medical bills for study-related illnesses, but the center may not cover all the bills that might pile up during a participant's recovery.

Fred, for example, said he has always worried about complications that might develop while taking an experimental drug. He has experienced many unpleasant side effects already:

"I've had depression, cataracts develop out of nowhere, and I've lost my night vision. I also have a lot more trouble hearing and paying attention. I love reciting long quotations and I've memorized every country and capital in the world. I can't do that anymore. I get through five or six countries and I get all tongue-tied. Other times I wonder if this stomach pain will ever go away. It comes and goes.

Less bothersome have been side effects, like a craving for sweets, that don't necessarily get documented as potential 'risks.'"

They're concerned about losing access to the drug when the trial ends

Very little of a drug is made until a pharmaceutical company has approval from the FDA to sell it. But volunteers with serious or life-threatening illnesses who have completed a phase III study may be rolled into an "open-label" study, allowing study subjects to take the investigational drug, for free, until the FDA approves it.

On rare occasions, a life-saving drug will be so popular among study participants that the pharmaceutical company literally can't make enough of it and has to divvy up what it can produce by means of a "lottery." This didn't quite work out as planned for the AIDS drug AZT. Because half of the subjects requesting the drug from every research site were randomly given a placebo, patients ended up putting their pills together and sharing from a common supply. That way, they figured, everyone at least had some chance of getting the actual drug. Drugs that effectively treat a serious or life-threatening condition and have the potential to address an unmet need are now put on a "fast-tracked" FDA approval process, limiting the wait for the product outside the clinical trial environment.

A standard therapy is already available

Some people would rather not take a chance on a new drug if treatments offering even small benefits are already available. Often it is simply inconvenient to change treatments. And the small benefits of a standard therapy are better known than those of a novel therapy. Patients who are on a helpful medication run the risk of relapse in their illness because testing a new drug requires that study volunteers withdraw from their current treatments. If study participants become too ill, researchers may shorten the "washout" period, which is the period of time when a study participant cannot take any medication in order to "wash out" any drug effects. But there's still the possibility that they they'll receive a placebo. FDA-approved "rescue medications" (Tylenol, for example) might also be used to reduce discomfort.

They're inconvenient

The requirements to participate in some trials might also be viewed as unreasonably burdensome. Some people can't be paid enough to endure repetitive blood draws, rectal exams, needles, or even to temporarily quit smoking, drinking beer, or having sex. Some people do not have the time to fill out a diary of their symptoms and experiences several times a day or week.

Some potential volunteers cannot make numerous visits to research centers that are far away or travel tens of miles to perform a test procedure.

They can't afford unexpected costs

There is rarely a cost to the patient for the experimental drug, unless the FDA has given the study sponsor special approval to charge for it. In fact, most of the "direct" costs of care are paid for by the study sponsor. However, the FDA does not prohibit charging participants for treatment or services in a trial. It is also important to consider any "indirect" costs for clinical trial participation, such as travel, lodging, and lost time from work—for you and anyone else who plans to accompany you to study visits.

Many health insurers and Medicare now pay for the costs of routine care given in a clinical trial, including doctor visits, hospital stays, and blood tests. Only a handful of states actually require commercial health insurance plans to cover even part of the cost of care during a clinical trial. These costs include services that would otherwise have been provided under the contract for standard therapy. Generally, the state laws specify the type of trial insurers are required to cover—often, cancer clinical trials only. Health insurers often make their decision about what trial costs to pay for on a case-by-case basis. You would be wise to ask up front what will be covered, including the costs of treatment for any complications or side effects caused by trial participation.

In Florida, a volunteer in a phase III antibiotic study was stunned to receive a hospital bill for thousands of dollars simply because of her treatment choice for a severe hand infection. Her insurance company wouldn't pay because the treatment was "experimental." And the study sponsor wouldn't pay because the study medicine is what healed her wound—not what landed her in the hospital.

Health maintenance organizations (HMOs) and other insurers that embrace clinical research generally limit patients' options to phase III and IV trials, which best fits their philosophy of covering only treatments that are scientifically proven as both safe and effective.

So—Are You Ready to Consider a Clinical Trial?

Before volunteering for any clinical trial, there are two essential questions that you need to ask:

1. "Do I have all of the information that I need to make an informed choice?"

2. "How far am I willing to go?"

For patients and their families facing a serious, life-threatening illness, these questions are often easy to answer. But for less severe though unpleasant illnesses, these questions may be more difficult to answer. Your answers to these questions dictate how hard you will push yourself to gather as much information as possible about the clinical trials actively seeking volunteers with your illness.

Clinical trials are not only time-consuming, but also require an unprecedented commitment from you to intelligently and carefully pursue appropriate trials and the professionals conducting them, to possibly forego using medications with known benefits, and to have potentially uncomfortable procedures performed. And, in the end, you may receive a placebo.

The research center isn't the only—and may not even be the best—source of information about a particular clinical trial. Research centers recommend specific clinical trials for a variety of reasons—scientific, political, and even economic factors are all influences. Some clinical trials bestow professional prestige and monetary rewards, for example, on researchers and research centers. Often these rewards may cloud otherwise sound medical decisions. Some research centers may overpromote clinical trials that are having trouble finding study volunteers.

It's a good idea to seek second opinions—medical or otherwise. Doctors and health professionals should not discourage you from seeking clinical trials when appropriate and should provide you with the information you need to make an informed decision.

Each person's experience in a clinical trial is unique. Two people with similar conditions—the same diagnosis, the same stage of disease and complicating factors, receiving the same active drug at the same place and time—will not always react the same way to an investigational drug. The human body responds differently to illnesses and illness-fighting drugs due to many factors. The best that researchers can do is seek to do what is best for most people most of the time based on the best available knowledge.

CHAPTER FOUR

A Very Human Enterprise

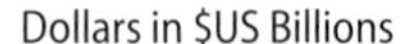

For every conceivable health condition, there is probably a clinical trial being done on it somewhere. Most trials test either a new drug or new uses for or forms of an existing drug, such as a painkiller given through a skin patch rather than by mouth. Other research studies simply measure the benefits of one drug over another. Many thousands of clinical trials focus on preventing, or more efficiently treating, chronic health conditions like osteoporosis, Parkinson's disease, depression, and diabetes. Even for cosmetic conditions like male-pattern baldness and acne, research scientists across the country are busily testing treatments that could be next year's medical breakthroughs. Some of these treatments may only be available to you through clinical trials.

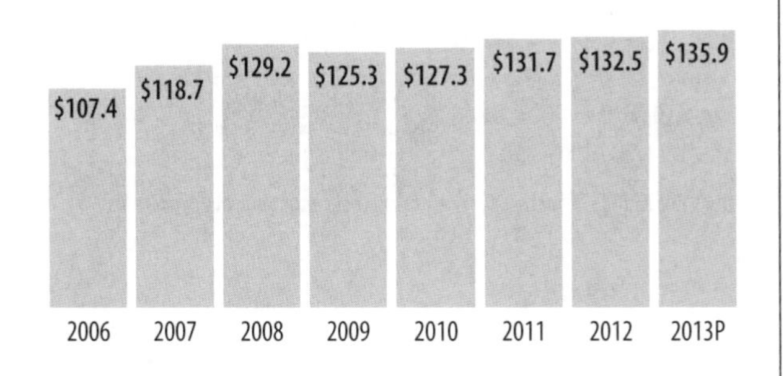

Total spending on biopharmaceutical research and development

Pharmaceutical and biotechnology companies and US government agencies spent more than $180 billion on research and development in 2013. Approximately $13 billion was specifically spent by the industry and the National Institutes of Health (NIH) on clinical trial grants to research centers. Pharmaceutical and biotechnology companies sponsor 75% of research on new medical treatments and interventions, and the NIH and other foundations sponsor 25%.

Total US government spending on health related research

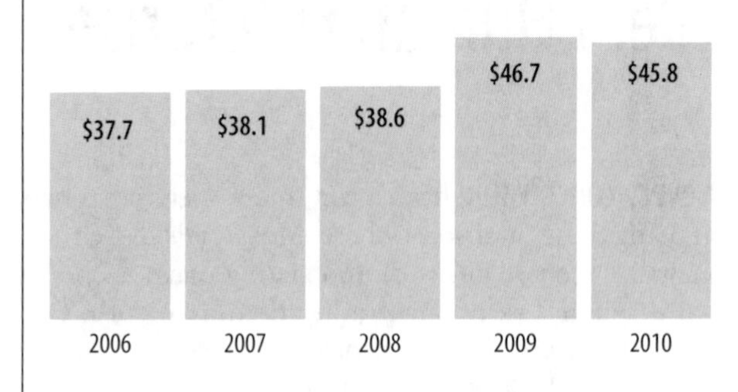

Source: Research!America

US clinical trial grant spending

Dollars in $US Billions

	NIH/Other federal spending	Industry*	TOTAL
2000	$1.6	$3.8	$5.4
2004	$2.5	$6.1	$8.6
2008	$3.0	$8.3	$11.3
2012	$3.2	$9.6	$12.8
Annual Growth	6.0%	8.0%	7.5%

* Does not include global study monitoring costs and medical device trials

Source: Tufts CSDD

Many of the largest pharmaceutical companies have hundreds of new drugs in development and many of these drugs are being actively studied among participants in clinical trials. In 2012, for example, GlaxoSmithKline had 259 active drugs in R&D and Pfizer had 243 active drugs.

Here is a sampling of the many types of clinical trials that have actively sought volunteers in recent years:

- Experimental vaccine for urinary tract infection
- Oral insulin for controlling blood sugar in diabetics
- Treatments to prevent restenosis following cardiac surgery
- Topical cream for early-stage skin cancer
- Oral drugs to improve sexual performance
- Cancer screening tests for smokers and people with emphysema and bronchitis
- Non-stimulant drugs for treating attention-deficit hyperactivity disorder
- Drugs to prevent joint deterioration in people with rheumatoid arthritis
- Comparisons of treatment options for heart failure patients
- New medications to treat age-related memory loss

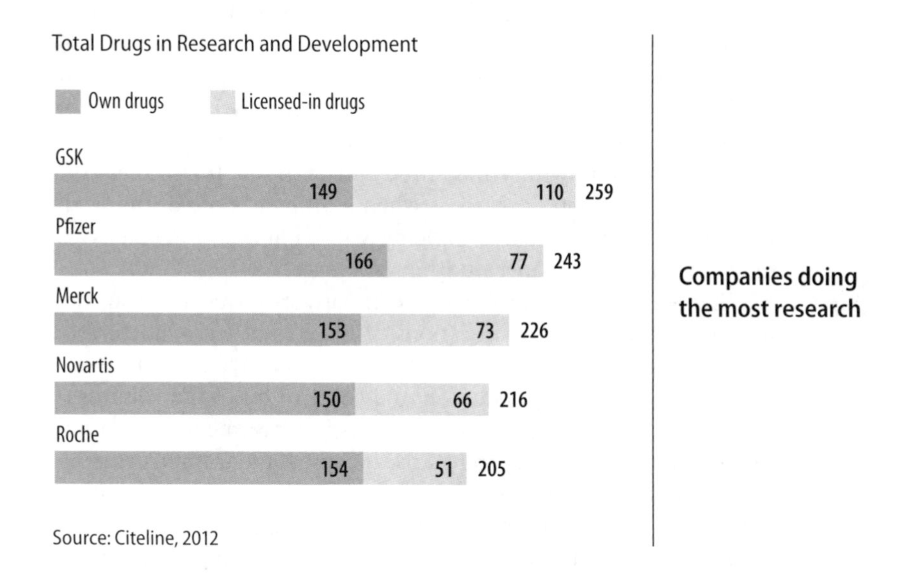

Regardless of the disease condition under investigation, no medical therapy is tested in a clinical trial without the approval of the Food and Drug Administration (FDA)—the chief agency in the United States overseeing research and development by the pharmaceutical and medical device industries. No new medical therapy is allowed by the FDA to be sold unless it is properly tested according to strict guidelines designed to ensure that the drug works and does no unexpected harm. One of the FDA's top concerns is the safety and ethical treatment of human subjects, or volunteers in clinical trials.

In the United States, pharmaceutical and biotechnology companies sponsor the majority of clinical trials of medical treatments. In total, these companies will spend nearly $40 billion on clinical research in 2014. This money is used to pay for the research professionals managing the projects, for equipment and facilities, for research supplies, and for study grants to research centers conducting the projects.

In 2013, the industry spent more than $10 billion on grants to investigators within these research centers. Investigators are primarily physicians who agree to carry out clinical trials according to a very detailed plan known as the study protocol. The protocol safeguards human subject protection and provides direction for research professionals to follow in order to ensure that the study is conducted properly.

The study protocol builds on what is already known about an investigational drug based on results from lab and animal testing and from what is later learned in studies on humans. The protocol establishes the purpose and goals of the clinical trial; who will be included in the trial and who will be excluded from enrolling in it; and what variables will be measured and analyzed. It also spells out other important details, such as when a different dose of the study drug might be tried and how patients will be followed and taken care of while participating in a study.

When developing a protocol, a company or government agency has to consider dozens of questions. What is to be learned from the study? What outcomes will be measured? How long should the trial last? Who will participate? Should some or all of the volunteers receive the study drug? Is there an existing treatment to compare to the new one? What, currently, is the best standard of treatment? Should some subjects be given a placebo? What procedures will be done during research visits? How can the study optimize the potential benefits of a novel treatment while minimizing the potential harm? Under what conditions will the protocol be changed or the study stopped?

Clinical trial results will not be taken seriously by the FDA unless the protocol follows accepted principles of scientific research. When comparing drug treatments, for example, patient groups must be alike in all important aspects, such as stage and character of disease and age range, and must only differ by the drug that each group receives. Clinical trials must also study different ethnic groups who will eventually be taking a new drug or medical treatment.

The protocol must make sense for the type of trial and condition under study. If the standard medication for an illness is usually ineffective, for example, early clinical trials may involve only the new investigational drug. Worldwide, there are an estimated 14,000 investigational drugs being studied from the discovery phase through the clinical phase.

The number of people allowed to participate in a trial will depend on a host of factors including: the number of people with the condition in question; the availability of other treatments; the number of people willing to volunteer; and how much is known about the therapy being studied. This sample size is also arrived at by doing statistical calculations that ensure there are enough participants in studies to answer the research question.

The age, health, and gender of participants to be recruited also have a big effect on how the study protocol is written. Pediatric clinical trials, for instance, need to consider changing body size and drug absorption rates as children age—and even whether it is appropriate to use healthy youngsters as volunteers. Trials designed for women have to take into account gender differences in behavior and aging and the possibility of pregnancy. Clinical trials designed specifically for pregnant women—and there aren't many—must give careful thought to how patients' vital signs are taken and how medications are given. They must also include a thorough check of the baby after delivery to look for any unintended effects, good or bad. Trials for life-threatening diseases require rules for stopping the study earlier than planned so that a particularly promising product can quickly be made available to the desperately ill, even before any real clinical benefit has been confirmed.

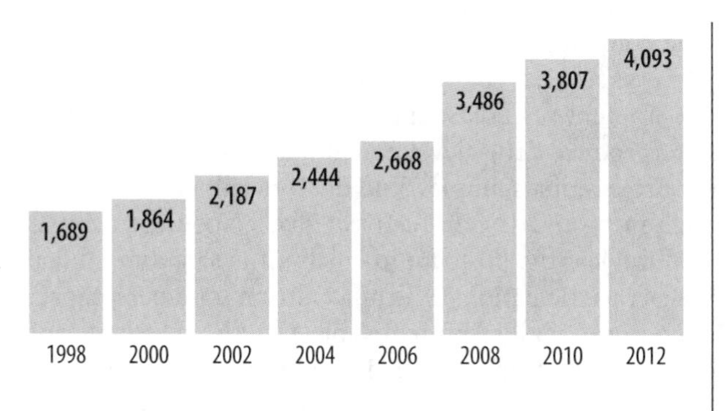

Source: Citeline, 2012

Number of drugs in clinical development phases I–III worldwide

These criteria also serve to identify serious toxicities or poisonous substances that would cause the trial to be terminated early. A clinical trial is sometimes called a clinical research study or a research protocol. But a clinical trial primarily refers to the location where a study protocol is being tested. In other words, a single protocol involves multiple locations across a variety of cities, states, and even countries where clinical trials are conducted. The government and the pharmaceuticual industry together sponsor more than 80,000 trials in the United States each year, representing 4,000 to 5,000 drugs in clinical phases I–III. The majority of drugs in clinical development are in early-stage clinical trials.

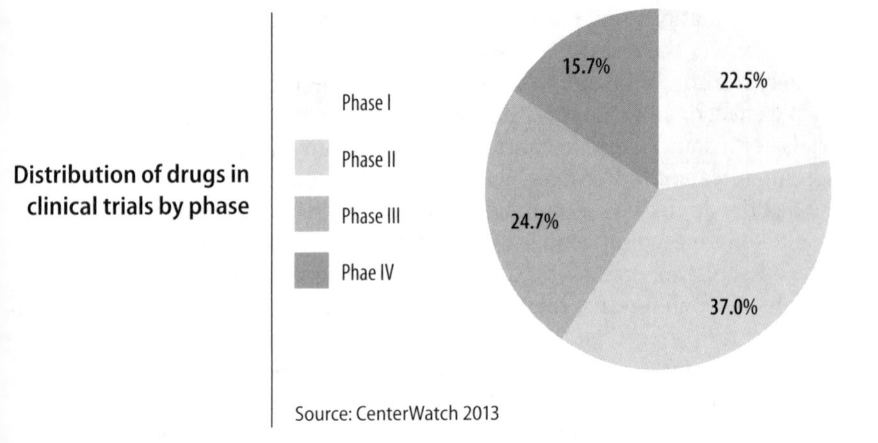

Distribution of drugs in clinical trials by phase

Clinical trials are a very human enterprise. Each year, more than 150,000 research professionals will manage and conduct clinical trials in the United States. And more than two million volunteers will complete clinical trials annually.

Many people come together to make a clinical trial happen long before the first person even volunteers to participate. The collective brainpower of eminent scientists, operating managers, and statisticians is used to produce drug-development plans and study protocols. Research professionals, nurses, and doctors will be involved in clinical-trial planning and design. Teams of physicians and scientists at the FDA will review the protocol to ensure it is safe and ethical for human subject participation. (The official term for a person participating in a clinical trial is "human subject," although the terms "Participant" and "Volunteer" are used increasingly to recognize the participant as an active partner in the clinical research process.) Local and national review committees—called Institutional or Ethical Review Boards (IRBs)—must review and approve study protocols. IRBs are made up of doctors, nurses, and other community members who are responsible for determining if a study is safe, sensible, and in keeping with the local standards of healthcare quality.

Once a clinical trial is underway, many more people get involved. Research sponsors dispatch study monitors to assure that research sites are collecting data and making sure that study volunteers are following and complying with the protocol. The IRB oversees advertisements to make sure that they aren't misleading people who may be considering volunteering. The IRB also follows the study's progress, intervening on the subject's behalf if questions or problems arise. The FDA inspects research sites to be sure its rules about trial conduct are followed. It immediately handles any serious safety concerns involving the investigational drug or the conduct of researchers.

In recent years, a growing number of clinical trials involve genetic tests—usually based on blood samples—that look for changes in chromosomes, genes, or proteins inside a person's body. There are several hundred different types of genetic tests currently in use. A positive result means a greater likelihood of developing or passing on an inherited disorder, such as type 2 diabetes or some forms of cancer. Many new therapies are now under development that target defective, disease-causing genes. Some use drugs to block the action of the protein controlling a particular gene. Others involve inserting genes into the body that produce healthy copies of the protein in question.

Genetic testing is not a routine procedure. Most doctors' offices don't have an in-house laboratory or an affiliated laboratory that offers tests for genetic disorders. Even commercial laboratories that do genetic testing look for only common gene mutations. For people with very rare disorders who are willing to undergo genetic testing, a research laboratory may be the only option. Though the tests are often free, test results may not be available for months or years. A person's regular physician may not even be contacted if no change is found in the gene being tested.

There are a number of social and emotional issues that discourage some people from getting tested for either personal or research purposes. Understanding the risks and benefits of genetic tests, and the potential consequences of testing, is of utmost importance. Rules about what constitutes proper "informed consent" for genetic testing vary from state to state.

FDA rules and regulations help eliminate the temptation of pharmaceutical companies to cut corners in their zeal to get a product to market. They also help ensure that physician researchers, for whom clinical trials can mean prestige as well as income, follow sound scientific practices. Pharmaceutical companies and physician researchers tend to vigorously defend the FDA's watchdog role, even if they feel the agency can sometimes be overly cautious. Some doctors and patient advocates argue that, in this age of genetic research, even more human subject protections are needed.

With every new drug, the mission of the pharmaceutical company is to determine if a product's promising performance in the lab and during animal testing can be replicated in people. The challenge then becomes determining the best ways to administer a new treatment—by pill, liquid, injection, inhaler, or patch—and at precisely what dose. Any unintended reactions to the drug during testing must be recorded. If unintended reactions are severe and frequent enough, these serious adverse events (SAEs) could immediately end a clinical trial. But if the adverse events (AEs) are minor (in relation to the drug's benefits) and the FDA later approves the drug for sale in the market, the information will appear on the drug's label and package insert as possible side effects.

You have probably seen these package inserts in many of the medications that you buy from the retail pharmacy. The wording contained in the package insert—including product warnings and a description of side effects—are reported results from numerous clinical trials that have been conducted on that drug.

Building a Support Network

Another important part of the human side of clinical trials is the support network that you create. Study volunteers are not alone in their clinical trial participation. Your decision to participate in a clinical trial is best made with input from the people you know and trust. Your network should include your family physician or specialist who has previously been treating your disease or condition. Your primary-care and specialty nurses may be very helpful in sorting out your identification of a clinical trial and the risks and benefits of participating in one.

Perhaps no one has a greater interest in your well-being as a potential study subject than your family and friends. They will want to be actively involved in the decision-making process. Young children rely on their parents or guardians for support and guidance. Parents in their later years may well depend on their adult children. Whatever your support network, you need to draw comfort, assistance, and resolve from your family, friends, and advocates in order to determine if a clinical trial is right for you. And once you've enrolled in a trial, you may need to tap that support network for aid, all the way from ongoing encouragement and advice down to transportation to and from the research center.

Many medical conditions have special support groups and communities that can help assist in evaluating clinical trials as treatment options. In the appendix of this book, we have provided information about helpful national health associations and patient-advocacy groups. You can also find information about local support groups in the Yellow Pages, your primary-care centers, hospitals, the Internet and even your public library. There are also a growing number of online self-help groups that provide up-to-the-minute information on new drugs and treatments, as well as electronic bulletin boards and chat rooms where patients can share their personal stories and experiences with both standard and investigational therapies.

From Discovery to Market

For many patients, a clinical trial is an opportunity to gain access to a drug—albeit, generally short-term—as much as five or six years before it becomes commercially available through retail, mail-order, or health-system pharmacies. Clinical trials are part of the final leg of a new medical treatment's journey from the laboratory to your medicine cabinet. In all, it may take as much as twenty years and an estimated $1.2 billion dollars to bring a single new drug treatment from its initial discovery through to the market. The chance of a promising drug candidate even reaching the clinical trial stage is very low.

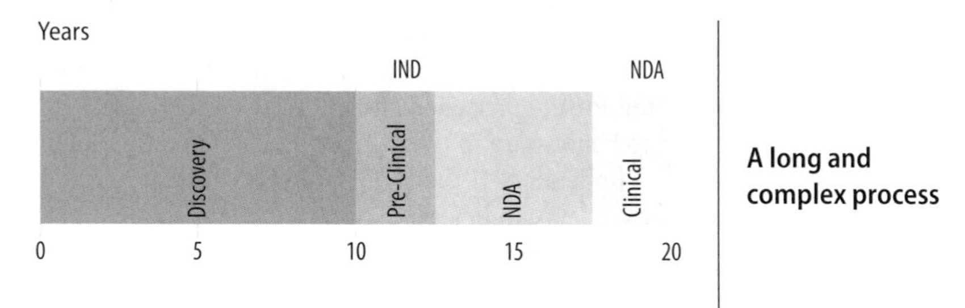

Source: Food and Drug Administration

A drug making its debut in a clinical trial begins as a molecule discovered by scientists in the research laboratory. It takes approximately 10 years of study in test tubes and laboratory mice to reach the point where a treatment might be tested for its safety and effectiveness in humans.

During the discovery phase, scientists find new molecular entities (NMEs) that can be tested for their usefulness as drugs. NMEs are typically extracted from plants or are created by modifying known molecules. Researchers conduct extensive test-tube experiments on NMEs to learn about their effects on human cells. These tests help scientists determine the molecule's role in altering biological processes and may also reveal whether a molecule, when administered as a drug, will be toxic. Scientists at pharmaceutical companies evaluate hundreds of thousands of molecules in order to find a few that have the potential to become a safe and effective treatment. Those few NMEs then advance to testing in animal models.

Testing in animals marks the beginning of pre-clinical testing and is a critical step in the process. Animal testing reveals important information about how a drug will behave in a living organism. During pre-clinical studies, researchers will be able to observe how a drug affects the animal's organs (such as the brain, liver, kidneys, and reproductive organs) and how it is absorbed and excreted from the animal's body. Scientists set out to answer two fundamental questions during animal studies: first, is the drug likely to be safe when administered in humans?; and second, is the drug likely to have a desirable therapeutic effect? For example, does the drug lower the animals' blood pressure or does it fight infection? If the answer to both questions is yes, then researchers may decide to begin the process of testing a new drug in humans.

Approximately one in 50 drugs that enter pre-clinical testing prove safe enough and effective enough to be tested in people. And animal studies can only help researchers approximate a drug's safety and effectiveness in humans. But before researchers can begin testing a drug in people, they must submit an application to the FDA that provides the results of the laboratory and animal studies along with a detailed plan for the proposed clinical trials. This request for FDA permission to begin human testing is called an Investigational New Drug (IND) application. If the IND application is not rejected by the FDA, clinical trials can begin.

Clinical trials are designed to answer five basic questions about an investigational new drug or device:

- Is it safe?
- Is it effective?
- What side effects does it produce?

- What dosage is most effective?
- Is it more effective than or equally as effective as other treatments already on the market?

Only one in five drugs that enter clinical trials will prove safe and effective enough to receive FDA approval. And some of these drugs end up being most effective for patients with different diseases than those that they were originally created to treat.

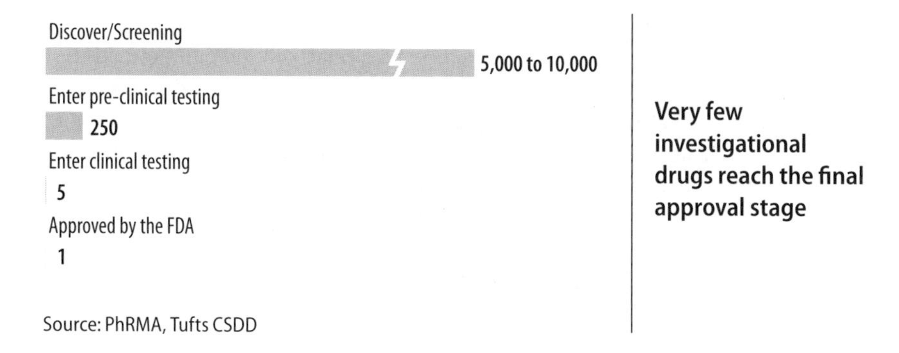

Very few investigational drugs reach the final approval stage

It is this long, costly, and exhaustive process of clinical research that has brought so many scientific advances and has ultimately saved immeasurable numbers of human lives. Clinical research brought the world vaccines for polio and diphtheria, antibiotics for tuberculosis and pneumonia, and medicines to lower cholesterol and control asthma attacks. Today, new drugs continue to be discovered and developed at an ever increasing pace. During the past decade, the FDA has approved an average of 26 novel treatments annually. In 2012, 39 new drugs were approved—one of the highest years for new drug approvals in recent memory.

In addition to the examples presented in Chapter 1, clinical trials have led to a vast number of new treatments for a wide variety of illnesses. Clinical trials, for example, led to an approved drug for preventing the progression of joint damage in rheumatoid arthritis; brought to market an antibody engineered to target and kill cancer cells in patients all but given up for dead; provided victims of cancer and AIDS with a medicine that mimics the pain-blocking abilities of a marine snail; and offered patients with advanced Parkinson's disease an injection to reduce the loss of control of body movements. Clinical trials have also given us a treatment for hospital patients with serious bacterial infections resistant to other antibiotics, as well as another cancer drug that blocks the growth of the most common type of lung tumor. Treatment for virtually every disease category has achieved progress as a result of clinical trials.

Even relatively small improvements to existing drugs, which represent over 40% of new drugs approved by the FDA each year, provide important health benefits to patients. Newer drugs often have fewer side effects, are safer and more effective, and are taken more easily and conveniently. Not surprisingly, these top the list of drugs physicians mostly commonly prescribe. A new drug form—tablets instead of liquids or a pill taken once a day versus two or four times a day—can be a major benefit to individuals who have trouble chewing, swallowing, or remembering to take their medications. If you or someone you care about is taking a relatively safe and effective—yet inconvenient or invasive—treatment, there is a good chance that better treatments are being tested.

Behind every drug that has been tested and approved are thousands of people who have volunteered to give the gift of their participation. The table below shows examples of well-known medical treatments that were approved by the FDA, the number of years they were in clinical development, and the total number of volunteers who participated in clinical trials.

Examples of the duration and size of drugs successfully completing clinical trials

Drug name	Treatment for	Years in Clinical Trials	Number of study volunteers
Allegra	Seasonal allergy relief	2	3,600
Celebrex	Rheumatoid arthritis	3	13,000
Lipitor	High cholesterol	2.5	20,000
Prilosec	Ulcers, GERO	4	4,000
Viagra	Erectile dysfunction	2.5	3,000
Vibativ	Skin infection	7.2	1,794
Vioxx	Osteoarthritis	4	10,000
Zocor	High cholesterol	2.5	20,000
Zytiga	Prostate cancer	5.3	1,195

Source: CISCRP, 2013

Importance of Diversity in Clinical Trials

Fifteen to twenty years ago, pharmaceutical research was limited primarily to 30- to 40-year old white males. These days, virtually everyone—men, women, children, the elderly, and minorities—has the right and the opportunity to participate in clinical trials. This is largely a result of regulatory pressure from the FDA to spread the benefits and burdens of research participation equitably. It has also become clear that drugs behave differently in people, depending on their gender, age, and ethnic group.

The National Institutes of Health (NIH)—one of the government's largest sponsors of clinical research—specifically requires that its clinical studies include women and minorities. The FDA, through regulation and regulatory guidelines, expects the same.

Study sponsors are now voluntarily submitting data to the FDA that will help the agency track participation rates of women, men, children, the elderly, and various minority populations.

The FDA also has the authority to require that children participate in clinical trials for new medications that will be or could be used to treat conditions or diseases in children. And the FDA provides incentives for drug companies to conduct similar studies on certain marketed drugs now used to treat pediatric conditions.

Medicare eliminated a key barrier to participation by the elderly several years ago. The federal program now covers care required during clinical trials. This includes payment for all services normally covered in conventional care settings and for services provided during clinical trials that wouldn't otherwise be provided free of charge. The chief requirement is that the clinical trials involve a study drug that intends to treat a specific condition such as high blood pressure, diabetes, or migraines.

Women in clinical trials

Gender mix in clinical trials, overall, appears to be relatively balanced. Recent research conducted by the Center for the Study of Drug Development at the Tufts University School of Medicine found that in clinical trials conducted in support of drugs submitted to the FDA between 2001 and 2011, on average 52% of all patients that participated were men and 48% were women.

There is no question, however, that protocol designs have historically addressed disease as it manifests in adult males. Beginning in the early 1990s, public pressures fueled stricter government requirements for the presentation of data by gender in market applications to the FDA and valid analysis by gender at the NIH. In 2000, the

FDA further specified that a clinical trial excluding persons having reproductive potential could be placed "on hold," preventing further product development. This requirement helped ensure that women of childbearing potential were included in studies.

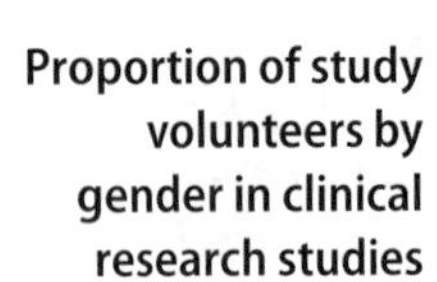

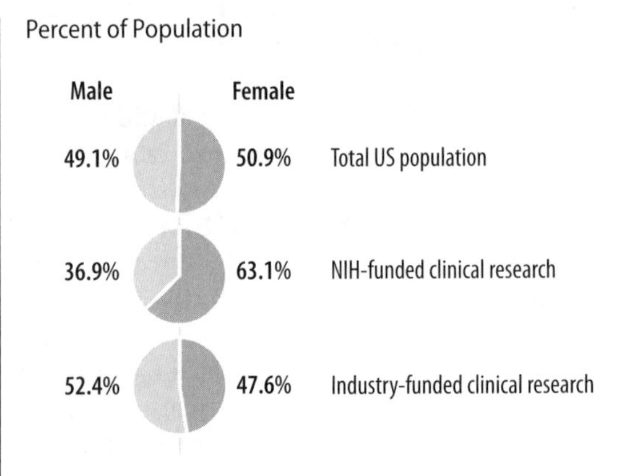

Pharmaceutical and biotechnology companies have also sought ways to increase the market potential for new and existing drugs by gathering clinical data to make specific claims about drug safety and effectiveness among women. As a result, clinical trials are increasingly being designed to assess the safety and efficacy of gender-specific medical treatment, and medical treatments are being "personalized" for gender differences in response.

Many diseases behave differently in women than in men. Risk factors, symptoms, the clinical course, and response to treatment can all be gender-specific. Among a long list of differences, men and women vary by:

- body size, composition, and metabolism
- the ways their bodies change during the aging process, e.g., puberty and midlife
- endogenous hormones
- exogenous hormones

Due to these differences and to other factors researchers have discovered that:

- Lung cancer kills more women than any other cancer.
- Alzheimer's disease is twice as prevalent in women.

- Men and women experience pain differently.
- Women are two to three times more likely to experience depression, due to less serotonin uptake in the brain.
- About 75% of autoimmune diseases occur in women, most frequently during childbearing years.
- Urinary incontinence and dysfunction are more common in women and often are an entirely different cause than the same conditions in men.
- Cardiovascular disease kills approximately 250,000 more women each year than all forms of cancer combined, accounting for 58% of all deaths. Within a year of the first myocardial infarction, 44% of women die, compared to 27% of men. Hormone-replacement therapy does not prevent heart disease, as was previously assumed.
- The initial HIV viral load may be significantly lower in women, who represent an estimated 30% of new infections, but both sexes develop AIDS at the same rate.

Although the FDA recommended in 1993 that clinical studies include enough women to understand the unique ways in which their bodies respond to drugs, women are still underrepresented in small, phase I trials. And when eligibility is restricted by age, older women are disproportionately excluded from studies of diseases that are more common in women at older ages. Although regulations prohibit the explicit exclusion of women of childbearing potential, the possibility of becoming pregnant can result in women in their childbearing years not being included in studies.

Generally, a woman capable of conceiving a child won't be considered for a clinical trial unless she's not pregnant and agrees to use birth control. Some studies require that women of childbearing age use two forms of contraception to participate in a study. Pharmaceutical companies don't want their drugs tested among women who are—or might get—pregnant, mostly because the risk of exposure or a lawsuit by the mother is too high. Even in normal pregnancies, 1% to 2% end with an abnormal birth. Many parents are quick to blame poor birth outcomes on drugs. Some doctors erroneously believe that certain drugs cause fetal abnormalities. But genes and chromosomes are the primary culprits, according to Marilynn C. Frederiksen, M.D., associate professor of obstetrics and gynecology at Northwestern University Medical School.

"All of this presents a major barrier to clinical trial participation by women who don't want, can't afford, or are religiously opposed to contraception," says Frederiksen. Things aren't bound to change unless the NIH comes up with the funds to conduct special dosing studies in pregnant women. And that probably won't happen quickly or easily. The NIH has an Office of Research on Women's Health to help strengthen policies requiring inclusion of women in clinical research and to help translate new knowledge into clinical practice, but it doesn't have any institutes that devote research dollars specifically to female health issues.

As a direct result of the 1993 NIH Revitalization Act, NIH-sponsored clinical research now routinely includes sufficient numbers of non-pregnant women. In 2001, additional protections were given to pregnant women (as well as human fetuses and neonates) that spell out the conditions under which they can be involved in federally funded research—if earlier studies provide data on the potential risks, for example, and the risk to the fetus is caused solely by interventions that could directly benefit either the women or the fetus. Participation of women in NIH-funded studies, overall, is proportional to the percentage of women in the general population when sex-specific studies are excluded.

The FDA recommended back in 1977 that women of childbearing potential be excluded from many early drug trials. At that time, the level of participation of women in all phases of clinical trials was affected. The FDA's current stance—that a "reasonable" number of women be included in all clinical trials—hasn't fully addressed all participation inequities. This is especially evident in the early phases of clinical development when a drug is introduced for the first time into humans and doses are escalated until toxic levels have been reached.

In clinical trials where women are included, the Government Accounting Office has reported that about one third of FDA reviews do not present gender-specific safety and efficacy analyses. It is difficult to know whether these analyses have been done and no identifiable differences were identified, or if the assessments were simply not conducted. A gender analysis (or any other demographic analysis, such as race or age) must be presented to the FDA when there are observable differences. Pharmaceutical companies are required to submit in investigational new drug (IND) annual reports tabulations of the number of study participants by gender, age, and race, as required by the FDA in 1998. A pair of surveys by the FDA's Office of Special Health Issues found growing compliance with the requirement between 1999 and 2003, when 70% of INDs included tabulations by gender.

The participation of women in clinical trials is essential. The exclusion of women from early-phase studies, in particular, delays the discovery of sex-specific dosing requirements and the identification of gender-specific side effects, limiting the identification of drugs that are useful just for women. The problem is compounded by the fact that animal studies, when scientists learn about many of a drug's potential adverse reactions, also tend to exclude females. Limiting studies to a single gender requires fewer study subjects (animal or human) and, thus, shorter and less costly studies.

There are many hopeful signs of change. Pharmaceutical companies are devoting a tremendous amount of money to trials focusing on diseases and conditions that only affect women. The Pharmaceutical Research and Manufacturers Association (PhRMA), the industry's primary lobbying group, reports that in 2012 there were 851 drugs in development targeting diseases that disproportionately affect women. That total number of drugs is more than double the number in 2002.

Among the 851 drugs targeting diseases that disproportionally affect women

- 139 drugs are for cancers affecting women, including 91 for breast cancer, 49 for ovarian cancer, and 9 for cervical cancer.
- 114 drugs are for arthritis/musculoskeletal disorders.
- 64 drugs are for obstetric/gynecologic conditions.
- 110 drugs are for autoimmune diseases, which strike women three times more than men.
- 72 drugs are for depression and anxiety; almost twice as many women as men suffer from these disorders.
- 83 drugs are for Alzheimer's disease; two-thirds of the 5.4 million Americans living with Alzheimer's today are women.

Source: PhRMA, 2012

Pharmaceutical companies are also pushing for more representative patient populations in their non-sex-specific studies. But women can be tough to attract to trials because the protocols written for them tend to involve many time-consuming tests. In some cases, women—like minorities—are not included in trials because they're stereotyped as "difficult to reach," "noncompliant," "unreliable," and "unwilling," according to a December 2002 NIH Outreach Notebook aimed at principal investigators.

There are many ethical issues to consider when conducting clinical trials among women, especially when a woman is pregnant. Does a mother have the right to expose her unborn child to investigational substances whose side effects are not yet fully understood? And what, if anything, does the father have to say about it? What if the couple is no longer married, or the father of the baby is not her husband? Will babies born to these women later sue their mothers for allowing them to be exposed to a drug while in the womb?

Many of the same types of questions have been raised when children are enrolled in studies by the consent of a parent. Children, like pregnant women, are considered a "vulnerable population" and have therefore been given special protections by research regulators.

"In a very real sense, what is good for a mom is good for her unborn child," said Frederiksen. Treating pregnant women with investigational AIDS drugs, for instance, helps prevent prenatal transmission of the virus. Pregnant women who take antibiotics for sinusitis also lower the odds their baby will develop nasal allergies and asthma and, by heading off fever, reduce the likelihood of a preterm birth. Some conditions are pregnancy-related and can only be treated during pregnancy. "If we don't test drugs then, we'll never know if they're effective."

Minorities in Clinical Trials

During the past ten years, the number of drugs targeting diseases that disproportionately affect minority patients has increased dramatically. At the present time, for example, more than 600 drugs are being developed for diseases that disproportionately affect Hispanic Americans, up from 245 in 2001. And more than 750 new drugs are being developed for diseases that disproportionately afflict African Americans up from 156 drugs in 1999.

Certain minority populations are more likely to suffer from specific diseases, such as diabetes and hypertension, and respond to medications differently. Asthma, for example, is very prevalent among African Americans and Hispanics; osteoporosis is more prevalent among Asian and Caucasian women. Certain drugs and interventions also affect ethnic groups differently. Statins, for example, are more potent among Asians putting them at higher risk for side effects associated with this class of drugs (e.g., muscle breakdown [Rhabdomylosis]). Among African Americans, there is a higher incidence of breast and prostate cancers.

There are documented racial differences in the way people respond to a long list of drugs from ACE inhibitors to antidepressants. Drug responses depend on a wide variety of factors—many of them related to an individual's racial and ethnic background.

Consequently, the government has made minority inclusion mandatory for trials that it sponsors. Pharmaceutical and biotechnology companies are following suit. They realize that it is in their best interest to study drugs in the specific populations that will use them most frequently.

The government directly funds many clinical trials. The NIH Revitalization Act of 1993 requires that all studies funded by the National Institutes of Health have representation from different minority groups unless there's a good reason to exclude them. The NIH believes data from these groups needs to be analyzed separately in case gender, race, or ethnic origin has some bearing on the research results.

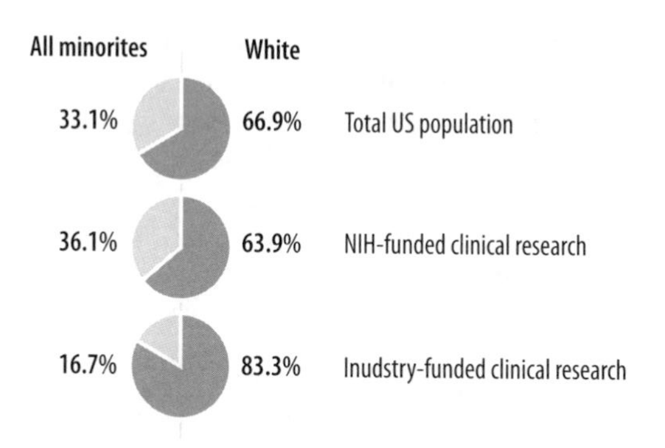

Proportion of study volunteers by race and ethnicity in clinical research studies

According to data provided by the NIH, at the present time the proportion of minority volunteers participating in clinical research studies is comparable to the proportion of minorities in the general population. The same cannot be said for industry-funded clinical trials where a substantial disparity exists. Whereas minorities represent approximately one-third of the overall population in the United States, only one in six study volunteers completing clinical trials are minorities.

Research professionals have long claimed that minority patients are not as willing to participate in clinical research. This claim assumes they don't trust the scientific community due to historic failures to protect minority patient safety (such as the infamous 1932–1972 Tuskegee syphilis study). A 2006 study by Wendler and colleagues does not substantiate this claim. In a review of a large number of clinical research studies, Wendler found that minority patients consistently demonstrate an equal or higher willingness to participate in clinical research studies than do their white counterparts. Instead, the authors identified the lack of access to clinical research studies as the primary explanation for poor minority representation in clinical trials.

In a subsequent study (2008), the Tufts Center for the Study of Drug Development (Tufts CSDD) confirmed Wendler's explanation. Tufts CSDD quantified the incidence of physician involvement in clinical research studies and found that whereas 10% of all board-certified white physicians participated, less than 4% of minority physicians participated as clinical research investigators.

A number of medical societies and professional associations have established initiatives designed to encourage minority physician involvement in clinical trials. Several nonprofit organizations have also been established to address minority disparities among clinical research volunteers and professionals:

1. ENNACT
Bethesda, MD
http://www.ennact.org

Stated Mission: To improve minority patient access to cancer clinical trials through education and collaboration with communities, health care providers, and researchers.

Programs: Training services, technical assistance and educational programming nationwide including: Webinar series, The National Cancer Clinical Trials Collaborative Learning Network (NCCTCLN), e-learning courses.

2. Enhancing Minority Participation in Clinical Trials (EMPACT)
Minneapolis, MN (at the University of Minnesota)
http://www.empactconsortium.com

Stated Mission: To increase recruitment and retention of racial and ethnic minority study volunteers with the ultimate goal of reducing cancer-related health disparities

Resources: Offers training courses for healthcare professionals on minority recruitment, cultural competency, increasing awareness of opportunities for trial participation among potential minority participants, and assessing effectiveness of minority recruitment efforts.

3. National Minority Clinical Research Association (NMCRA)
Fairfield, NJ
http://www.nmcra.org

Stated Mission: To reduce racial and ethnic disparities in health-care prevention, clinical treatment, and health-related research outcomes among minority populations.

Resources: Free membership includes a journal, current information about active clinical trials, conferences, and research papers

4. National Minority Quality Forum's National Clinical Trial Network (NCTN)
Washington, DC
http://www.nctrialnetwork.com

Stated Mission: To improve diversity within clinical trials by encouraging greater participation of racial and ethnic minority patients.

Resources: National Clinical Trials Research Atlas (a national database of clinical trials actively recruiting volunteers), physician registry

5. Project I.M.P.A.C.T.
Washington, DC
http://impact.nmanet.org

Stated Mission: To encourage greater participation of African Americans in all aspects of biomedical research and clinical trials.

Resources: Project I.M.P.A.C.T. is a program of the National Medical Association and provides educational materials, multimedia materials, physician education and training.

As the overall number and size of clinical trials continue to grow, government agencies and pharmaceutical and biotechnology companies are making greater efforts to ensure that clinical trials see higher levels of participation from racial and ethnic minority groups.

Participation of a representative group of volunteers helps researchers understand the different ways that people respond to medical treatments. Clinical research scientists typically conduct "Subset Analyses" of clinical trial data in order to draw conclusions about specific racial and ethnic responses to investigational drugs.

Under the NIH Revitalization Act of 1993, no phase III study will receive government funding without the inclusion of minorities such that a "valid subset analysis" of potential racial differences can be conducted.

Subset analysis requires statisticians to collect data on as many non-white patients as are needed to draw meaningful conclusions. The FDA has issued guidelines that emphasize the need for new drug applications (NDAs) to describe the number of people of various racial/ethnic groups that were given the study drug during clinical trials and how well the data were analyzed for differences between them. As part of this rule, FDA is evaluating demographic subgroups that take part in clinical trials. This allows them to determine whether information specific to these groups needs to be put on the labels for new medical products.

It is essential that diverse communities are adequately represented in clinical trials in order to understand disease and how to treat it among these special populations. Public, patient, and professional community awareness of this issue is a critical first step.

Let's now move to the next chapter and look at the information you need to gather, and the questions you need to ask, to make an informed decision about whether to participate in a clinical research study.

CHAPTER FIVE

Education Before Participation: Do Your Homework

"Every visit took a long time. I'd eat lunch, read a couple of chapters in a book and fill out surveys. We had to go to different places on the campus, and it's a huge place and my mom didn't walk very well. It would take us a half-hour to walk from neuropsychiatry to the neurology lab. Our days there were a three- to four-hour affair. After two years in the study, it finally got to be too much. We dropped out of the study. My daughter had just been born and I had no time."

Karen, daughter of a subject in an Alzheimer's disease clinical trial

"Following a 12-week, placebo-controlled study, I continued in an open-label study because of the benefit I received from the product. At the end of that two-year trial, the product was reported to be associated with a rare and often fatal disorder. This prevented me from entering yet another trial for possible continuation. It also involved entering into a new 'study' for safety evaluation, having additional blood work taken, visiting a neurologist, and having an MRI. It also involved a lot of concern and anxiety for me and my family!"

Paula, subject in a series of Crohn's disease clinical trials

Patty, subject of a trial for primary progressive multiple sclerosis

"The trial required daily self-injections of the drug for three years. Study visits took about three hours, plus lab work time. I had to go to the [research] office every three months to repeat the tests and get a full neurological exam. I also had to do a timed walk, as well as tests of my memory and attention and upper extremity function. Brain MRIs were done yearly. I was given a calendar to mark down any adverse events or problems. There were no unanticipated holdups or expenses during the trial and the staff went out of its way to make appointments at my convenience, midday, since I'm not a morning person. I really liked the office staff, doctors, and lab techs, as they were all very caring people. They even had a Christmas party for all the patients to attend!"

Your decision to participate in a clinical trial is a major decision—one that must be taken very seriously and one that requires that you do your homework. You, your family, and your friends need to play the role of dogged detectives to learn as much as you can. In order for you to evaluate whether a given clinical trial is—or is not—right for you, you need to gather objective answers to the following questions:

What is known about my specific disease or medical condition?

Even well-educated people usually have at least a few misconceptions about their particular illness. Purging these misconceptions from your mind involves a lot of reading and a lot of listening. Among the most trusted sources of information are your primary-care and specialty-care physicians and nurses, current medical encyclopedias and reference books, top medical journals, professional medical societies and associations, other board-certified medical doctors, pharmacists, and other allied health professionals. Hospitals frequently choose some of the top medical minds in a community to lead lecture series on different health topics. It may be worthwhile for you to attend a medical conference. Local and national support and advocacy groups may be excellent sources of information about your illness. Often there are useful articles published by your health provider, major health magazines, and reputable newspapers.

There's also a great deal of information available on the Internet, but the quality of the content is mixed. You might do best to stick with major, well-known web sites like the National Library of Medicine, CenterWatch, WebMD, and disease-specific web portals. Listings and directories of valuable and reputable resources are available in the appendix of this book.

You might even consider contacting research centers directly and asking if they can help you understand more about your illness or if they can refer you to someone who can. You can compile listings of investigative sites organized by disease condition by reviewing listings on the NIH web site at www.clinical trials.gov and the CenterWatch web site at www.centerwatch.com. Contact information is provided in these web sites for you to phone or email research center professionals. The Center for Information and Study on Clinical Research Participation (CISCRP) also performs searches of clinical trial listings and of research centers on behalf of patients and their families. The service is provided free of charge. Contact information is available at www.ciscrp.org.

A number of social-media communities and online disease-advocacy communities have also become valuable places to find information about disease and how to treat it. Entering the name of a disease in a major search engine (e.g., Google, Yahoo, Bing) or in Facebook will help you easily identify these online communities.

What are ways that people like me are currently being treated?

Medical knowledge is not distributed equally around the country, or the world. Reputable medical journals, health references, and Internet sites may do a good job of keeping up with common knowledge, but there is a lot of information that has not been published. Your primary-care and specialty-care physicians and nurses may have information for you. They may also know medical experts and thought leaders—across town, out of state, or in another country—who specialize in researching and treating specific illnesses.

Chances are very good that someone belonging to your local support group or frequenting an online chat room or social-media community dedicated to your disease will have already gathered some information. They will willingly share their experiences with you. And it never hurts for you to ask.

Once you've learned about current treatments for your illness, you need to determine if these treatments have any significant drawbacks. Many medications may be only marginally effective and may have bad side effects, such as nausea, drowsiness, and diarrhea. Depending on the medical condition, people will search for something—maybe anything—that will bring better relief. Some treatments may be too expensive, or may be administered in an unpleasant or uncomfortable way (e.g., by injection or taken several times each day).

You may find an available treatment that works well, is reasonably priced, and is easy and convenient to take. In this case, you will have to think seriously about what, if any, reason exists to try an investigational treatment. Perhaps you have a genuine desire to volunteer solely to help advance science. But you need to recognize that you are trading a known treatment for an unknown treatment, and you may gain no personal health benefit from participating in a clinical trial.

Will You Receive a Placebo?

A clinical trial, like any scientific experiment, needs one or more "control groups" or "comparison groups" to help researchers tease out results—good or bad—caused by something *other than* the investigational treatment.

Patients in a control group may receive a different treatment known to be effective, if one is available. Or they may receive a look-alike pill, called a placebo, which contains no medication. This "dummy treatment" usually looks identical to the investigational treatment in terms of its color, weight, taste, and smell. Neither the investigator nor patient knows which is which. If different doses of the investigational treatment are being studied, or another actual treatment is being used, more than one placebo may be used.

Studies that use a placebo are widely regarded as the most efficient, cost-effective, and decisive means of testing the safety and effectiveness of a therapy when no other known treatment exists. They have also been a hotly debated topic in and outside the U.S. There are scientifically sound reasons for comparing a placebo against an experimental drug. It can minimize bias caused by the mere *expectation* that a drug will bring relief—the so-called "placebo effect" described in Chapter 2.

Placebos also control for other potential influences, including the natural history of the disease and the use of another therapy. The more practical issue, for drug companies and investigators, is that trials controlled by a placebo rather than a standard therapy generally require fewer study subjects to demonstrate the value of the test treatment.

However, the Center for the Study of Drug Development at the Tufts University Medical School estimates that less than one-third of phase II and III clinical trials used a placebo in 2012. Placebo-controlled trials pose no problems when the study drug is aimed at a condition for which there is no known treatment. But serious issues are raised when an effective remedy is already available, particularly if it prevents serious harm or death. For example, it would be considered unethical to do a placebo-controlled trial of a new treatment for heart attack. Some argue that it is difficult to justify the use of placebos in trials of new medications for treating depression, given that so many proven treatments exist. Even Alzheimer's disease now has a treatment that slows the decline of many patients. For them, a placebo-controlled trial not only carries the possible risk of their disease worsening but also that of their inability to consent to participating at all.

The FDA hasn't taken a stand on placebo-controlled trials, other than to issue a document discussing the pros and cons of the approach and alternatives like an "active control-arm" (which includes both standard treatment and placebo groups), "add-on studies" (where participants all receive standard treatment in addition to the study drug or placebo), and limiting the time participants are potentially exposed to a placebo. However, it has defended the use of placebos in studies of treatable, life-threatening conditions in poorer countries across Asia and Africa where access to standard therapies is limited.

The FDA's position on placebo use in clinical trials is in stark contrast to the position taken by regulatory agencies in other parts of the world. These agencies—including the European Medicines Agency—follow the Declaration of Helsinki, an international medical research ethics document guiding clinical-trial conduct. The latest revision of the Declaration states that using placebos is unethical in nearly all experiments involving diseases that already have good treatments.

Doctors in the US generally accept the use of placebos under certain circumstances, such as when there is no other therapeutic alternative. They also tend to consider placebo-controlled trials acceptable in cases where a currently available treatment doesn't work well or has side effects that patients find unpleasant.

As a rule, doctors are more tolerant of placebos when the clinical trial targets diseases that only modestly affect the well-being of patients, or that have symptoms which stop and go unpredictably.

Compared to treatments available, are clinical trials an option for me?

Some clinical trials will offer you potential therapeutic benefit for your illness. But all clinical trials will carry a degree of risk. In considering a clinical trial, you have to weigh the benefits and shortcomings of known treatments with the inherent risk and potential benefit of an investigational treatment—including the possibility that you won't be getting treated at all.

Your primary-care and specialty-care physicians and nurses may be helpful sounding boards in thinking through the pros and cons of clinical trials relative to those of other treatment options. Should participation in a clinical trial be considered? You will want to include your physicians and nurses in the early stages of your decision-making process. They may have, or may know professionals who have, some specific information about drugs being tested in clinical trials.

Your family and friends can also be good advisors. If they're not convinced that a clinical trial is an appropriate and reasonably safe treatment option, they may be right. It also makes sense to talk over the particulars of the trial with them because they may well be involved in the process. If the study drug causes nausea, will a family member be there to assist you? If you can't drive to the research center, will a friend be able to take time off from work to drive you? If the trial becomes hard for you to endure, who will be listening to your complaints and providing needed comfort and encouragement?

Narrowing the List of Prospects

With 5,000 to 6,000 different study protocols and approximately 80,000 government- and industry-sponsored clinical trials conducted in the United States every year, there will likely be many trials to choose from. But choosing the "best" clinical trials require a lot of homework. Some trials may involve a new drug to treat a specific illness, while others may be testing a novel drug taken in combination with other therapies already available. Some clinical trials may be evaluating new therapies that help patients cope with disease symptoms. Other clinical trials may be testing new medications that prevent disease or slow its progression.

If a clinical trial sounds like it might be a good option, you need to identify specific trials that are best suited for you. In Chapter 6, I'll describe in detail the many approaches that you can use to identify clinical trials that target your disease. Sometimes clinical trials will find you—often when you first receive a diagnosis. If you're dealing with a serious, life-threatening illness, you may not have much time to evaluate clinical trials. Depending on the time you have available, some of the factors that you'll need to weigh include:

Study phase

Both phase I and phase II drugs focus primarily on safety testing. Later-stage clinical trials—phase III studies—have many more patients. Appropriate doses and uses of drugs are generally established, and common side effects are known.

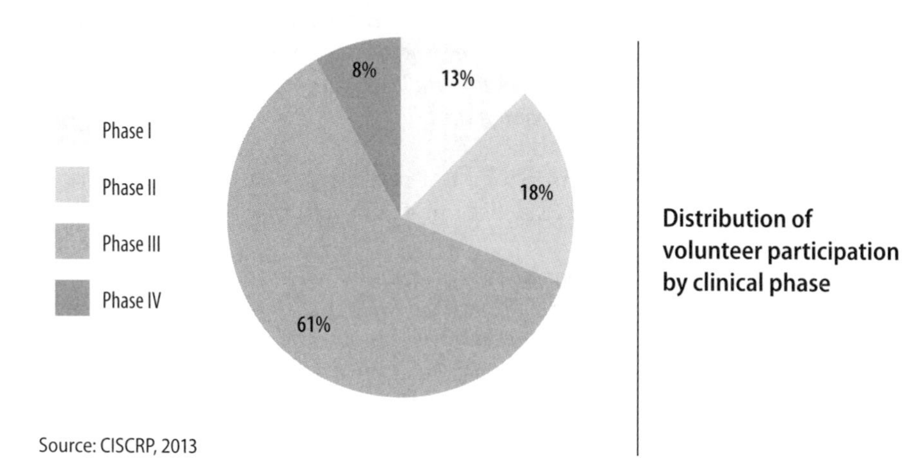

Distribution of volunteer participation by clinical phase

Source: CISCRP, 2013

Time commitment

Clinical trials can last a month or continue indefinitely. The typical clinical trials lasts 175 days, approximately 6 months. It's important that you decide up front how long you're willing to be a study subject, and under what terms. How often will you be expected to visit the study site? How long will each visit take? What kind of procedures will you have to undergo? Can the visits be scheduled for any time of the day or night? What about weekends? What study-related activities will you be required to do at home? When will the study end?

You should be aware that there are sometimes holdups in the beginning of a study that can't be foreseen. You may be screened over the telephone and be scheduled for your first visit, only to have it rescheduled because the sponsor failed to manufacture enough of the experimental drug. Study visits when you have to see the investigator in addition to the coordinator may also involve lengthier waits—particularly if the doctor is also juggling time between research and full-time office practice.

For Rose, a participant in a six-month trial of an experimental menopause drug, the time commitment was the worst part of an otherwise pleasant experience:

> *"I had to drive to get to the doctor's office, several cities away, for study visits. There were a total of six. The first two visits were a couple of weeks apart, and the rest were weekly. I work full-time at home, but my time is not entirely flexible. Keeping a daily written diary of my symptoms also became wearisome," Rose said. "I made entries in the morning about the day before. I had to carry a pad with me all of the time to keep track of when I had hot flashes. I did that for the whole length of the study. It got to be a pain by about the fifth or sixth week."*

During her open-label study, Paula spent a considerable amount of time at the doctor's office but took it in stride:

> *"I went for monthly infusions. After checking in, waiting for the staff, and waiting for the pharmacist to come prepare the infusion, I was prepared for the actual infusion through an injection in my arm. Infusions lasted one hour and I was monitored for one hour. Total visit time was about 3 to 4 hours each month. Initially, I kept daily journals between study visits; then they were less frequent."*

For Jennie, in a multi-year trial of a breast cancer relapse prevention drug, participation put few demands on her time:

> *"I have to go to the doctor's office every month for routine blood work and to go over any problems I might be*

having. I'm usually there for only about 15 minutes. Every three months, a bone and CT scan is required, but I think that's particular to my case. My cancer spread to just under my collar bone and close to my pelvic bone."

The only issue that Jennie ever brought up for discussion was a bout with nausea and diarrhea, which was never connected to the drug:

"I think the problem was that I wasn't eating enough. Since the chemotherapy, I haven't felt hungry. At home, I chart on a calendar that I'm taking my pills twice a day as instructed. It helps me remember to eat twice a day, because I have to take my drug with food."

Overnight stays

Depending on your underlying medical condition, you may be required to stay overnight in a hospital or special research facility. Drugs targeting serious conditions like cancer and heart failure frequently involve patients already in the hospital. Many phase I studies also require an overnight stay, regardless of the condition being targeted. Overnight stays can pose a problem for single parents or anyone who has trouble taking time off from work.

Location and access

You need to think about how convenient it will be to get to the research center on a regular basis. What's the drive time? Is it located in a safe neighborhood? Will parking be a hassle? Does public transportation cover this part of town? If a spouse is coming along, are there things for him or her to do (eat, shop, visit a museum, etc.) while waiting? Are office hours convenient?

Research center reputation

Research centers earn a reputation, good or bad, over time. Newspaper articles—not advertisements—can be good sources of objective information about certain centers. Friends and acquaintances may have had experience with a specific center. Your physician or nurse, and a variety of community health organizations, may also have an informed opinion about research centers to consider and to avoid.

For his latest cancer clinical trial, Frederick sought out a reputable research center. The experience exceeded his expectations:

"I've sometimes had to call the research center at 1 or 2 a.m. I'm so embarrassed that my wife has to place the call and get me on the phone. I talk to the doctors and they do more than I could have expected. I have a lot of faith in them; they treat me like family. I felt comfortable from the very beginning because the [lead investigator] seemed so well informed. I found out later that he was really the focal point, nationally, for research on this disease."

His only regret is the toll all of this has taken on his wife. "She has been there to help me absolutely every minute. At times, I wish there were more transportation services available so she wouldn't always have to bring me in."

The FDA audits research centers and clinical investigators from time to time—especially if there is cause for concern. This audit information is available online at the FDA web site (www.fda.gov). If you visit this web site, look for the Investigational Human Drugs Clinical Investigator Inspection List, a large database of names, addresses, and other information gathered from research center inspections since 1977. Also available on the FDA web site is a list of investigators who have been blacklisted for repeatedly or intentionally disobeying federal regulations or submitting false information to study sponsors. Other investigators are named because of special research restrictions placed on them. If you don't have a personal computer, you should log on at your local public library. Printed versions of the FDA's audit information are available through the Freedom of Information Act. But obtaining a printed copy of the audit is likely to be a long and slow process.

Social-media communities, discussion forums, and chat groups may also be good ways to learn about volunteer experiences with specific research centers. You may also find blogs and other comments about research centers online.

Research environment

Are you comfortable and confident with the center and its staff? Your answer to this question may require that you visit the research center. The following checklist of questions may assist you in evaluating the research environment:

Are the receptionist and research staff friendly and professional?

- Is the waiting room clean and comfortable?
- Are exam rooms and consultation areas clean and well equipped for the research that is taking place there?
- Are check-in procedures private and confidential?

- If a child is to participate in the study, are there people on staff with experience and skill in dealing with their special concerns?
- Is the center experienced in conducting trials among elderly and physically or mentally disabled volunteers?
- Are there accommodations for family members to accompany you?
- Do the research doctor and staff invite your questions?
- Do they seem to genuinely care about the welfare of their volunteers?
- Do they treat volunteers in a culturally appropriate manner?
- Are researchers involved in educating the community about the impact of disease on patients and options other than clinical trials?
- Do they offer literature about their clinical trials and the rights of study volunteers? Is the literature professional and understandable?

Are you eligible to participate?

All clinical trials have certain eligibility requirements that may prevent some volunteers from participating. Potential volunteers on certain medications, with history of an uncontrollable disorder, or who are pregnant or breast-feeding, may be excluded from a trial. A recently advertised study on a heartburn treatment, for instance, would only accept people between the ages of 18 to 65 years old who are having symptoms at least two days per week. There are a number of eligibility requirements that often exclude volunteers from participating in most clinical trials, including:

- Participation in another clinical trial within the last 30 days
- Drug use or alcohol abuse
- Elevated liver function enzymes
- Serious disease processes, such as renal (kidney) failure or coronary heart disease
- Cancer (excepting clinical trials targeting cancer-related illnesses)
- Pregnancy
- Refusal to use any form of standard birth control (females only)
- Known allergy to ingredients in the study drug

Preexisting health conditions and current medications being used may—or may not—disqualify you from a particular study. It all depends on the clinical trial—its objectives and requirements.

Many people are deemed ineligible for one reason or another during a brief "pre-screening" over the telephone. The remaining potential volunteers may need to have an EKG, a blood or urine test, their blood pressure checked, or a combination of tests before they can be formally accepted into a clinical trial. Test results can also be useful as a "baseline" measure against reactions to a study medication. Some clinical trials require would-be volunteers to track the frequency of their symptoms in a diary before determining if they would make suitable candidates for a particular trial.

The criteria for being enrolled in some studies can be hard to meet. Some trials, for example, may require that volunteers have no prior treatment—even if certain drugs are readily available. Coming close to meeting the eligibility criteria isn't good enough to get you into a clinical trial. After all, the purpose of a clinical trial is to determine if an investigational drug works while protecting study participants from harm.

It's important to try not to get discouraged if you fail to qualify for a clinical trial. Keep looking. There is a good chance that you will find other clinical trials that may be appropriate at another research center or, in some cases, at the same center if it is participating in a large number of studies.

Sadly, according to a recent study conducted by CISCRP, only about one-third of people who are deemed ineligible continue searching for other clinical trials for which they may qualify. Two-thirds did nothing or consciously decided to give up their search. You may even become eligible for clinical trials that were originally too restrictive. In some instances, research professionals may modify the eligibility requirements after a trial is under way. If you were originally ineligible, you may want to periodically check with a research center to determine if you might later qualify.

Most volunteers who are ineligible for a clinical trial don't search for another

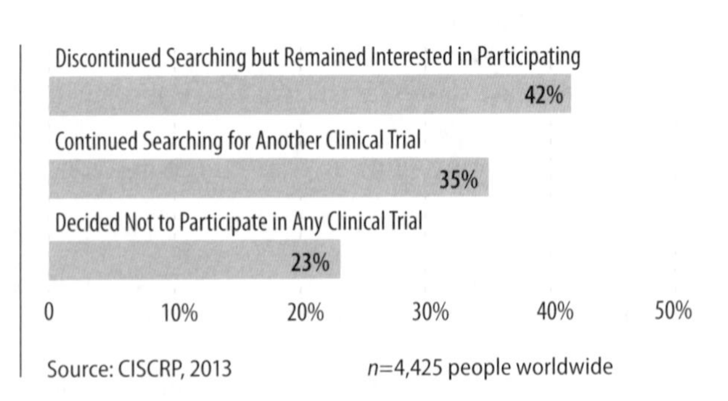

The amount of time it takes to screen for study volunteers—to determine volunteer eligibility—varies a lot. In clinical trials for "acute" conditions that come on quickly the enrollment process may be less than a one-hour affair that happens on the day a patient shows up at the doctor's office for treatment. For more chronic, long-standing diseases—like migraines, high blood pressure, or heart disease—the enrollment process can last hours, days, or even weeks. Trials occasionally get canceled before enrollment even gets under way for a variety of reasons. For example, there may be new findings about an investigational drug's safety, or too few people may be interested in participating.

The study staff

Principal investigators, the people who supervise clinical trials, may only meet with you briefly to do a physical exam and required medical procedures. With the exception of dental studies, principal investigators are usually medical doctors. Research visits with physicians can seem like a routine doctor visit with added paperwork. But principal investigators do a great deal of behind-the-scenes work that study participants rarely see, including trial design and monitoring of results. Protocols that pharmaceutical companies and research consultants develop can be hard to qualify for and grueling to be in. Some principal investigators spend a significant amount of time reworking these trials to be more patient-friendly. Sub-investigators—including other doctors, graduate students, residents, and lab staff—may conduct study-related procedures under the supervision of the principal investigator.

With few exceptions, the professional with whom you will interact directly and frequently is the research nurse—called a study coordinator. Study coordinators are frequently registered nurses. They essentially run the clinical trial. Among their long list of duties are recruiting and screening patients, obtaining your written consent to participate in a study, monitoring your progress at home, and reporting any adverse drug reactions. Study coordinators are the individuals with whom you likely will first meet to discuss what you can expect during a clinical trial and the potential risks and benefits of the investigational therapy. Coordinators can, in many ways, make or break the clinical trial experience for you.

Both study investigators and coordinators usually make themselves available 24 hours a day to answer questions about the study and any unexpected reaction—or non-reaction—to the investigational medication. This also allows them to respond quickly to any adverse event that occurs.

Many research centers will go to great lengths to assist you in feeling comfortable and well-cared-for. A number of studies have shown that the vast majority of study volunteers highly rate the level of professionalism and the quality of care that they received during their participation. The center may provide transportation services, on-site day care, after-hour appointment times, waiting rooms stocked with refreshments, friendly administrative staff, special dinners, and birthday cards. Some research centers even offer valet parking. Patients who repeatedly volunteer for drug trials targeting their particular illness are sometimes even supplied with free medications and treatments between studies.

Study volunteer ratings of clinical research staff professionalism

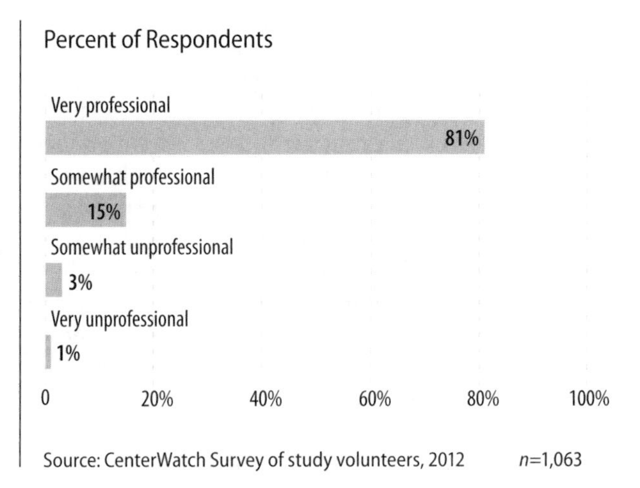

Study volunteer ratings of the quality of care that they received in a clinical trial

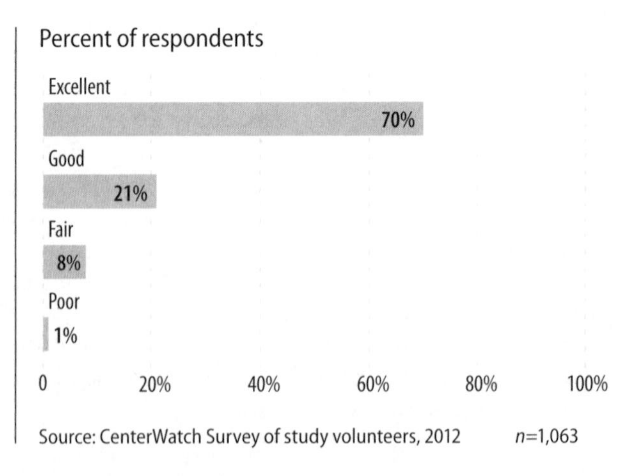

What you should expect from study staff

You should expect that the clinical trial will be conducted in a safe environment

If a trial involves the administration of an intravenous medication, there may be a higher risk of an allergic reaction to the drug. Therefore, the research center should have the necessary medications and emergency equipment on hand to be able to manage serious allergic reactions. The doctors and other personnel at the site should be trained in handling such emergencies. If the study involves any invasive procedure, or if anesthesia is required, it should be performed in a hospital or clinic setting that is fully equipped to manage complications.

You should expect that you will not be charged for any study medication or for study visits

It should not cost you anything to participate in a clinical trial. During a clinical trial, study-related medications and office visits are paid for by the study sponsor. These costs should never be passed along to you.

You should expect to be notified of any safety issues that arise during the trial

Occasionally, during the course of a clinical trial, new information may be learned about a drug's safety. For example, a study drug may be found to cause an unexpected side effect such as drowsiness. If this happens, the study staff is required to inform you because it may change the risk/benefit balance of the study. After you receive the new information, you may wish to continue in the study. In this case, you will be asked to sign an amendment to your consent form indicating that you understand the new information and have consented to continue in the study. If serious safety problems are discovered, however, the study may be suspended until the problem can be better understood.

You should expect to be able to withdraw from the study at any time without any negative impact on your care

If for any reason you decide that you want to drop out of a clinical trial, you should feel entirely free to do so. If you elect to withdraw from a trial, the researcher may want to discuss the situation with you to see of there are any problems that can be addressed which would make it acceptable for you to remain in the study. However the study staff should not pressure you in any way to remain in a study if you still wish to withdraw.

If a clinical trial involves an investigational medication for a disease or condition that required you to take a prescribed medication, your doctor will probably ask you to stop taking your medication before starting the trial. After you've completed the trial or if you're withdrawn from the study, your doctor may ask you to start taking your original prescription again.

It is helpful to discuss alternative treatment options before you agree to participate in a clinical trial. That way you will know in advance what treatment options will be available should you decide to withdraw from the study.

You should expect that your confidentiality will be maintained

No one beyond the medical personnel directly involved in your care should have access to your medical records without your knowledge and consent. There are two exceptions to this rule: Your insurance company may have limited access to your medical records so that they can verify the treatment that you received and determine whether it is covered under your insurance plan. And inspectors from regulatory agencies that monitor the care provided by doctors and hospitals may be permitted to view your medical records to ensure that the care being provided is appropriate. Other outside parties cannot obtain your medical records, and cannot be given any information from them without your knowledge and consent. Your employer, for example, cannot call your doctor's office or hospital to find out if you are taking medication for depression.

As part of any clinical trial that you may participate in, detailed personal information about you and your illness will be collected and maintained in written study records that are very similar to your medical records. Just as you would expect a doctor or hospital to treat this information as confidential, you should expect the researchers conducting the study to do the same.

In addition to the researchers who are directly involved in the clinical trial, your records may be reviewed by the Institutional Review Board, which may conduct periodic reviews to ensure the safety and ethical conduct of the research studies it oversees. In some cases outside agencies such as the Food and Drug Administration or the National Cancer Institute may conduct similar reviews for regulatory purposes. The sponsor also has access to the medical records and study files. While the results of the clinical trial may be published in a medical journal, your identity will never be revealed in these published reports.

You should expect to have any questions or concerns addressed promptly at any time during the study

Your ability to obtain information about a clinical trial—and to have your concerns addressed—is one of the fundamental rights that you have as a study volunteer. Your questions should be answered in everyday language, and not in scientific or medical terms that you can't understand. You should always feel completely comfortable asking questions before and during the study.

You should expect to make a time commitment

On one end of the spectrum, there are clinical trials that require no tests and only one brief visit. On the other end are clinical trials that require hourly checks of vital signs, diary entries, uncomfortable tests and procedures over the course of many visits, and overnight stays in a hospital or research lab. Trials for life-threatening conditions, such as AIDS, often have no finite end. Some volunteers may take a life-lengthening drug their entire lifetime as part of an informal, open-label study. Most clinical trials fall somewhere in the middle, often requiring a handful of study visits.

Frank enrolled in a 12-week double-blinded, placebo-controlled study for his Irritable Bowel Syndrome:

"I had to call in once a day and answer multiple choice questions over an automated telephone setup. There were maybe 15 questions, like 'Have you had a bowel movement today? How often? Have you had any cramping? If so, was it mild, moderate, or severe?' It was the same questions each time. At the end, I could get through it in about two minutes." Frank only had to go to the research center about once a month to repeat the same tests he had during his initial screening—blood, urine, and stool—as well as checks on his blood pressure and weight. The study coordinator also asked if he had experienced any side effects. "The visits weren't long, maybe 25 minutes," he said.

HIPAA and your privacy

The layers of privacy protection that exist for medical records —including state laws and the standards of professional and quality-monitoring organizations—are generally absent for research records. Likewise, the federal Health Insurance Portability and Accountability Act (HIPAA) does not regulate the practice of research, according to Gary L. Chadwick, PharmD, MPH, CIP, director of the Office for Human Subject Protection at the University of Rochester. "In most clinical trials, the 'source records' are, in fact, the medical records and the research records are transcribed case report forms. In this instance, the medical records would be protected under medical record rules and regulations, but the case report forms would not necessarily have the same protection."

Likewise, under HIPAA, subjects can read, get copies, and request changes in their medical records. This access does not extend to research records, said Chadwick. But because research records are not provided to insurance companies and other health care providers, "the information in them is really only accessible to the research team, sponsors [usually not readily identified data], and regulators [again, usually in an anonymous form], so the potential for breaches is minimal."

In terms of the confidentiality of study volunteers' medical records, most researchers view HIPAA as an "added burden" that negatively affects the informed consent process, said Chadwick. Complying with the regulations means extra paperwork and time for explanation with little, if any, actual increase in privacy protection for subjects. During the consent process, subjects often don't even bother reading the section on confidentiality. "They don't understand it if they do, and generally don't care when it is explained to them."

Perhaps most troubling is that HIPAA is having some unintended, negative consequences—especially in epidemiology and public health research. "Some clinical sites, such as doctors' offices, have misinterpreted the regulations as preventing collaboration in research efforts." Others won't risk violating the regulations, which are almost universally viewed as confusing and contradictory, because the penalties for doing so include steep fines and criminal prosecution. "Even in clinical trials, researchers sometimes have difficulty obtaining past records of treatment." HIPAA may be slowing the speed of research, and as a result the development of new treatments may be taking longer.

Not all research visits are short and routine. Some clinical trials involve regular trips between a research center and a doctor's office, where required tests—such as endoscopies—may be performed.

Martha, suffering from melanoma, had to make the 500-mile trip to Bethesda 18 times over two years, running between tests at the National Cancer Institute campus and doctor visits at Bethesda Naval Hospital. Then she would rest at a nearby motel room for several days at a stretch. The investigational vaccine was delivered, by injection, to alternating spots on her thighs and right arm once a month during the first year. Thereafter, Martha returned every few months for follow-up visits when the principal investigator reviewed a copy of her latest CT scan taken back home. The first few times she got the vaccine, she had to stick around for several days in case she had a bad reaction.

"You were supposed to swell up like a huge bee sting and have a lot of redness," said Martha. "I had to measure that every day with a tape measure, as well as keep a diary of any other effects," she said. Every so often researchers had to draw some of her blood, remove selected components, and then re-infuse it to see how the vaccine was behaving. It was an all-day procedure, two hours of which was spent weighed down by sandbags to stop the bleeding. I just got tired of lying in bed," said Martha.

Downtime in a study is not necessarily unpleasant. Volunteers generally aren't required to lie flat on their back at any point. For some people, participation can bring some relaxation.

Jill, 41 and self-employed, had to stay at a research center for several 24-hour observation periods as a participant in a three-month arthritis study. After receiving an injection of the study drug, researchers drew blood from her every three hours.

"It really wasn't bad," she said. "They fed me well and had a TV and tapes. It was a relaxing day." She also had to make shorter outpatient visits to the center every two weeks, as well as a follow-up visit a day or two after the study ended. "The best part was that it helped my arthritis. I had no pain whatsoever for six months."

Visits during a clinical trial take on additional challenges when the visits require the involvement of a parent or spouse. Disability, in particular, can make every research visit a tiring one for the driver and caretaker. Simply navigating from test to test can take enormous effort and a great deal of patience. Patient and caregiver experiences are bound to change as a result of new technologies being introduced for volunteers to use.

Use of electronics (e.g., smartphones and tablets) rather than paper diaries may ultimately make participation more convenient and may reduce the number of in-person visits volunteers need to make in order to deliver self-reported data. New handheld devices, for example, now use beeps and on-screen messages to remind study volunteers to answer questions when prompted and will then send responses to a central repository.

Smartphones and other mobile technologies now measure and relay vital signs. Some devices pick up on inconsistencies and double-check responses, much like a human researcher would do. The next several years will see major new developments in the application of technology solutions designed to make patient participation in clinical trials easier and more convenient while at the same time delivering better data quality and higher levels of efficiency for clinical research professionals.

CHAPTER SIX

Where to Find Clinical Trials

"When I was diagnosed with progressive primary multiple sclerosis in 1999, my neurologist said 'There's no cure or treatment . . . so join a support group and live with it.' I told him I had to do something to help myself. After much research on the Internet, I told him I found a clinical drug trial and wanted to sign up. He said he couldn't stop me, so go for it. I did well physically during the trial, but it was stopped after three years because . . . statistically, not enough people were helped by the drug. I await new trials in my area and I have also encouraged others to look into drug trials for their medical conditions. If nothing else, it guarantees a more thorough exam than is possible during a 15-minute, HMO-style appointment."

Patty, participant in a double-blind, industry-sponsored study

Only 10 years ago, it was very difficult for patients to actively identify clinical trials. The vast majority of clinical trials were done in academic medical centers—many of them within major metropolitan areas. Unless your physician was close in proximity and affiliated with an academic medical center, it is unlikely that you would have found a clinical trial opportunity.

Today, there are numerous resources in print and online for professionals and patients to use. And with more clinical trials being conducted by independent, community-based physicians, there is a far greater chance that your own primary- and specialty-care physicians and nurses will be able to assist you in identifying clinical trials that you may be right for. Your family and friends may be able to assist you both in conducting a broad search and in narrowing down your options to a few targeted opportunities.

Remember that when you begin your search, your goal is to be as thorough and comprehensive as possible. Every piece of information that you collect and every individual you speak with may assist you in tracking down a clinical trial that could hold some potential for you. Once you have isolated a few clinical trials whose posted inclusion and exclusion criteria you meet, then you and your support network can begin to scrutinize which, if any, of these trials might be a good match for you.

Search Strategies for Finding Trials

Currently, a large number of people refer themselves to clinical trials. Accordingly, you're in the driver seat. Different sources may point you in certain directions, but it is up to you to identify all of your options and to thoroughly review and evaluate them. Never assume that one source will have all of the information that you're looking for.

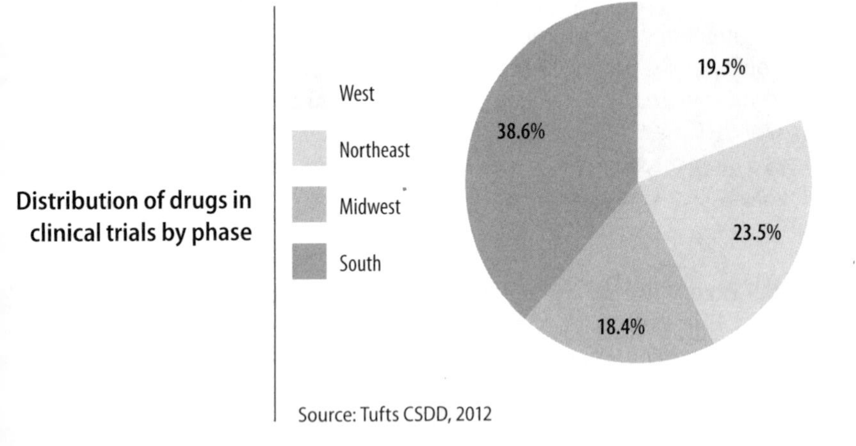

Distribution of drugs in clinical trials by phase

There are essentially two ways for you to find clinical trials, which are being conducted all over the country. One is to search for the trials themselves. The other, perhaps easier, approach is to search for investigational drugs and then determine where they are being tested.

Regardless of your approach, there are numerous people, organizations, and publications available to assist you. But you have to know whom to ask and where to look. Here are a few good bets:

Health professionals

Primary- and specialty-care physicians and nurses, in particular, may have access to some specialized (and expensive) medical journals and online databases where clinical trials and study drugs are routinely-discussed topics. These professionals are also worth consulting after you've found some initial sources of information. Not all medical publications and web sites provide accurate information. Health professionals can generally help you narrow down your list. They're also invaluable when it comes to translating medical jargon into everyday language and to finding sources that may assist in extending your search.

Libraries

Public libraries, college and university libraries, pharmacy libraries, and hospital medical libraries are all terrific sources of information on trials and investigational drugs. Many libraries subscribe to the "Gale Group's Health & Wellness Resource Center" database, which has journal articles on study drugs and how they're faring in clinical trials. University libraries often subscribe to Dialog, a leading provider of online health information. The libraries of hospitals and universities with an affiliated medical center are both particularly good sources. They subscribe to medical journals, which carry news of drugs under development and the latest study results. Hospital libraries tend also to have trial-listing pamphlets for big research centers like the Mayo Clinic and Johns Hopkins.

Medical libraries aren't always accessible to the public. If they are, they may be open at odd hours and staffed by volunteers rather than a trained medical librarian. To order full-text medical articles from services like Medline may involve a charge or require a subscription, depending on the publisher. For anyone without a home computer, public libraries generally provide free access to all sorts of helpful online databases, medical journals, major newspapers, and web sites. Those that have a research librarian on staff may even do the search for you, but there may be a fee.

Online databases

Some great databases, such as those offered by the Dialog Corporation, Informa Health Care, and the Gale Group, are available only by subscription and are out of the price range of most home computer users. But there are many others available for free over the Internet. These include online databases offered by CenterWatch: the Drug

Intelligence Service and the Clinical Trials Listing Service (www.centerwatch.com), and the National Library of Medicine's (www.clinicaltrials.gov), pharmaceutical companies, professional societies, and disease-specific associations.

Web sites

The Internet has become the most popular approach to finding information about clinical trials. Today, there are literally hundreds of web sites sponsored by pharmaceutical companies, professional associations, for-profit and nonprofit organizations, and research institutes that provide information about investigational drugs and ongoing clinical trials that are open and recruiting patients. Many general-health web sites also periodically run articles about drugs in development, though the content is of mixed quality and reliability. Several dozen web sites exclusively list clinical trials including web sites managed by the pharmaceutical companies sponsoring the study.

Top ways that people report finding out about clinical trials

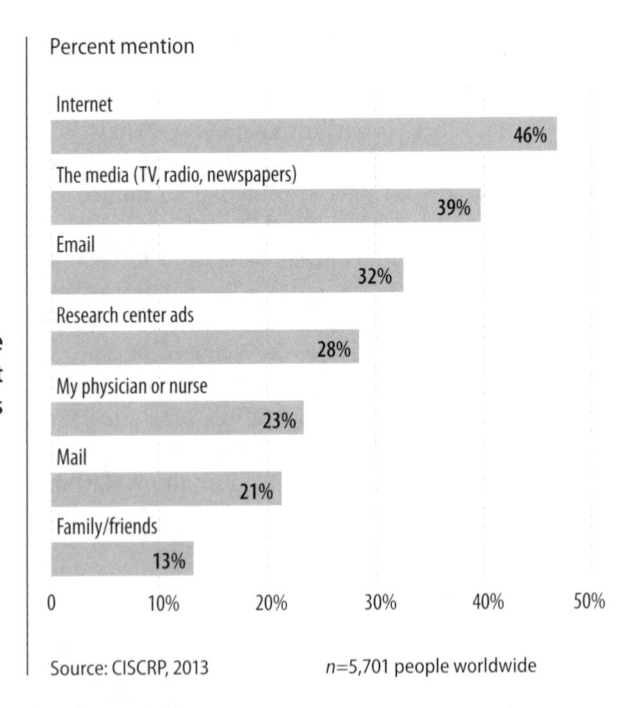

Over the past few years, mounting pressure from medical journal publishers, the public, and politicians has also spawned a growing number of clinical-study results databases designed to improve "information transparency" and bolster the American public's waning trust in clinical research. Study results, both positive and negative, are now voluntarily being made public on the web sites of many major pharmaceutical companies. However, the information in these databases is highly scientific in nature and directed toward those with medical and health backgrounds.

CenterWatch—an independent publishing company that provides information about the clinical-trials industry—maintains an online database of clinical trial results associated with drugs that have been recently approved by the FDA at www.centerwatch.com. The CenterWatch web site also lists industry-funded clinical trials actively recruiting volunteers.

The National Library of Medicine, on behalf of the National Institutes of Health—www.clinicaltrials.gov—provides a database of clinical research study results. All clinical studies that test the effectiveness of drugs for serious or life-threatening conditions are, by law, listed here. Clinical studies are now voluntarily listed at www.clinicaltrials.gov because they are required by medical journal editors as a condition for publication.

What follows is a brief review of some of the many web sites listing searchable information, which helps patients and their support network to identify clinical trials actively enrolling volunteers. In addition to clinical trial listings, many of these web sites also provide general educational resources that may be useful for patients and their support network, as well as notifications and alerts of upcoming clinical research studies. Many web site hosts disclose very little information about themselves and their information sources, making it difficult to determine the quality and accuracy of their information.

Searchable Databases of Clinical Trial Listings

There are many web sites providing listings and registries of clinical trials. Some of these web sites only list clinical trials for which the provider receives compensation. Plan to conduct your search on more than one web site in order to ensure that you have a more complete list of relevant clinical trials.

Clinicaltrials.gov—www.clinicaltrials.gov

Maintained by the National Library of Medicine at the NIH, provides patients, researchers and institutions with searchable information on more than 100,000 active clinical research studies targeting a range of diseases and conditions now underway in 50 states and more than 150 countries. In addition to listing all of the clinical research studies funded by the NIH, pharmaceutical and biotechnology companies are required by law to list certain clinical trials here.

CenterWatch
http://www.centerwatch.com

CenterWatch, an independent publishing company, provides the oldest and largest online database of international FDA-regulated pharmaceutical and biotechnology-funded new drug and device clinical trials. The Clinical Trial Listing Service contains a searchable list of 60,000 clinical trials, from a wide variety of diseases and conditions, actively enrolling study volunteers. The Listing Service provides notification when new trials are added. The CenterWatch web site also provides clinical research news, market intelligence, a service that tracks the progress of drugs in the pharmaceutical R&D pipeline, and a directory of investigative sites actively participating in clinical trials.

Clinical Research
http://www.clinicalresearch.com

Clinicalresearch.com is sponsored by Quintiles, a leading global contract research organization. The site lists clinical trials that are actively recruiting patients for Quintiles's client companies.

Clinical Connection
http://www.clinicalconnection.com

Clinical Connection provides a searchable database of clinical trials on behalf of its client companies and clinical research studies drawn from the National Library of Medicine's clinicaltrials.gov.

Clinical Trials Search
http://www.clinicaltrialssearch.org

Clinical Trials Search.org provides a clinical trials search service.

ClinicalTrialsIfpma
http://clinicaltrials.ifpma.org/

This web site is hosted by the International Federation of Pharmaceutical Manufacturers & Associations (IFPMA)—a global non-profit organization representing research-based pharmaceutical and biotech companies. The web site provides a searchable international database of open clinical trials and an email notification service.

Current Controlled Trials
http://www.controlled-trials.com

Current Controlled Trials is a searchable database of clinical trials maintained by BioMed Central, a publisher of life-science journals and books.

TrialReach
http://www.trialreach.com

TrialReach provides a searchable database of clinical trials sponsored by client companies. TrialReach also draws clinical trial search results from other web listings including the National Library of Medicine.

WHO International Clinical Trials Registry Platform Search Portal
http://apps.who.int/trialsearch/

The Clinical Trials Search Portal, sponsored by the World Health Organization (WHO), provides a searchable clinical research database that draws information from registries around the world.

The Coalition of Cancer Cooperative Groups
http://www.cancertrialshelp.org/cancer-trial-search/

TrialCheck, operated by the non-profit organization Coalition of Cancer Cooperative Groups, is an online search engine for patients seeking information about enrolling in international and US-based cancer clinical trials at hospitals, cancer centers, and oncology practices.

AIDSinfo HIV/AIDS Clinical Trials
http://aidsinfo.nih.gov/clinical-trials

AIDSinfo is a government-funded clinical trial search engine created to improve public access to clinical trials under the Health Omnibus Programs Extension Act of 1988. The site provides a searchable database of clinical trials and study results.

ClinicalTrials.com
http://www.clinicaltrials.com

ClinicalTrials.com is sponsored by PPD, a leading global contract research organization. The site lists clinical trials that are actively recruiting patients for PPD's client companies.

National Cancer Institute
http://www.cancer.gov/clinicaltrials

The National Cancer Institute, part of the National Institutes of Health (NIH), is the federal agency sponsoring cancer clinical research studies. This web site provides a searchable database of 30,000 cancer studies funded by the government, pharmaceutical companies, medical centers, foundations, and other international organizations.

Search NIH Clinical Research Studies
http://clinicalstudies.info.nih.gov/

The NIH Clinical Research Studies searches through all the clinical studies in the National Institutes of Health's database.

CISCRP's Search Clinical Trials Service

CISCRP conducts custom searches on behalf of patients (and their family, friends, and advocates) overwhelmed by the process of finding relevant clinical trials. Patients and members of their support network can contact CISCRP by telephone (617-725-2750) or online (www.ciscrp.org) to request a search. CISCRP will conduct a thorough search—usually within 2–3 days—and then compile the results and mail or email them.

At this time, CISCRP conducts 75–100 custom searches each month. The service is offered to patients free of charge.

Organizations Sponsoring or Hosting Clinical Trials

Pharmaceutical, Biotechnology, and Medical-Device Company Clinical-Trial Listings

Most pharmaceutical, biotech, and medical-device companies provide listings of their open clinical trials by disease and location. Larger sponsors even provide search engines on their web sites for patients and researchers to use. Some companies—including Novartis, Sanofi, Merck, and Johnson & Johnson—prefer to link over to their specific listings posted on www.clinicaltrials.gov.

Hundreds of pharmaceutical and biotechnology companies have at least one active investigational drug in clinical trials at any given time. When conducting your search, it's important not to look at only the largest companies, but to make sure that your search includes mid-size and smaller companies that may be sponsoring studies on their own or under a co-development arrangement with other companies. Appendix I in this book lists the web URLs for hundreds of pharmaceutical and biotechnology companies. Here is a list of web sites containing searchable clinical trial databases for some of the largest companies:

- **Bayer HealthCare Trial Finder**
  http://healthcare.bayer.com/scripts/pages/en/research_development/clinical_trials/trial_finder/index.php

- **Pfizer**
  http://www.pfizerpro.com/clinicaltrials

- **Roche**
  http://www.roche-trials.com/main.action

- **GlaxoSmithKline**
  http://www.gsk-clinicalstudyregister.com/

- **AstraZeneca**
  http://www.astrazenecaclinicaltrials.com/

- **Eli Lilly**
  http://www.lillytrials.com/

- **Bristol-Myers Squibb**
  http://www.bms.com/clinical_trials/Pages/home.aspx

Universities

In their mission to educate the community, many universities make research a priority and provide ample opportunities for students and the community to get involved in research studies. Some schools have a complete listing of studies while others advertise only those studies—by department—that are actively recruiting. Depending on whether the university has a hospital, the types of studies may range from simple surveys and behavioral studies requiring a few hours to clinical studies looking at specific diseases and conditions.

Examples:

- **Stanford School of Medicine**
  http://med.stanford.edu/clinicaltrials/

- **University of Chicago Medicine**
  http://www.uchospitals.edu/clinical-trials/index.html

- **University of Miami**
  http://uhealthsystem.com/clinical-trials

- **Temple University**
  http://www.temple.edu/medicine/research/CLINICAL_TRIALS/index.htm

- **Rush University Medical Center**
  http://www.rush.edu/rumc/page-R10021.html

- **University of Virginia**
  http://www.healthsystem.virginia.edu/pub/ct

- **Columbia University**
  http://sklad.cumc.columbia.edu/psychiatry/clinical_trials/search.php?type=simple

Hospitals & Cancer Centers

Most top-tier hospitals and cancer centers provide listings of clinical research opportunities organized by therapeutic criteria or condition. These listings are usually easy to find on each center's main website, and a search engine is often provided. A few examples are listed below.

- **Partners HealthCare (MassGeneral, Brigham's, McLean, Spaulding)**
  http://clinicaltrials.partners.org/

- **Boston Children's Hospital**
  http://www.childrenshospital.org/research/clinical/Search.cfm

- **Dana Farber**
  http://www.dana-farber.org/research/clinical-trials.aspx

- **Memorial Sloan-Kettering Cancer Center**
  http://www.mskcc.org/cancer-care/clinical-trials/clinical-trial

- **University Hospitals**
  http://www.uhhospitals.org/clinical-research/clinical-trials

- **Brooks Rehabilitation Clinical Research Center**
  http://www.brookshealth.org/brooks-uf/our-research/clinical-trials/

- **Hospital for Special Surgery**
  http://www.hss.edu/clinical-trials-directory.asp

- **Northwestern Memorial Hospital**
  http://www.nmh.org/nm/clinical-trials

- **Lombardi Comprehensive Cancer Center**
  http://lombardi.georgetown.edu/clinicalprotocols/

- **Cincinnati Children's Hospital**
  http://www.cincinnatichildrens.org/service/c/clinical-trials/search-studies/default/

- **University of Colorado Hospital**
  http://www.uch.edu/conditions/cancer/research/research_trials/

- **Siteman Cancer Center**
  http://www.siteman.wustl.edu/FindProtocol.aspx

Clinical Research Centers

As part of your search, plan to contact local clinical research centers with expertise in your medical condition. Some of these centers may be advertising online, on television, the radio, or in the newspaper for trials that are currently recruiting volunteers. But even research centers that are not actively recruiting for their own trials may know about those going on at other locations near you. Some centers, however, may not be comfortable referring you to their competitors.

You can identify research centers in a variety of ways. Your physician or nurse, and even friends and family, may know of reputable centers. The phone book may also contain listings. Many research centers actively advertise in the media and in newspapers. They may have their own web sites and they may be linked to academic health centers if they are an affiliate.

The CenterWatch web site (www.centerwatch.com) provides a large directory of nearly one thousand research centers actively seeking study volunteers. These centers are often listed in connection with clinical trials also listed on the CenterWatch web site. The NIH's site (www.clinicaltrials.gov) and other listing services also provide the name and contact information of research centers. CISCRP (www.searchclinicaltrials.org) can also be used to identify research centers.

Clinical Trial Matching Services (Services that match patients to actively recruiting clinical trials)

Matching services provide a useful option by actively pairing patients with relevant clinical trials. For some patients, a matching service offers real peace of mind over conducting multiple searches simultaneously. It's important to remember, however, that matching services typically only match patients to trials for which the service provider is receiving compensation. As a result, matching services are only looking to match patients to a limited number of trials and not all of the options available.

Some patients engage multiple matching services to increase their options. In addition, patients and their advocates should also compile their own list of clinical trials found on various listings and registries to ensure that they are aware of, and considering, a more complete set of options.

Acurian
http://www.acuriantrials.com

Acurian is one of the largest global patient recruitment services companies. They offer a matching service for patients through the use of an online questionnaire. Acurian is owned by PPD—one of the largest global contract-research organizations.

EmergingMed Navigator
http://www.emergingmed.com/

EmergingMed.com offers a matching service for patients searching specifically for cancer-related clinical trials. Patients complete a profile and are matched to cancer clinical trials in EmergingMed's database. EmergingMed's process for matching patients is also offered on the web sites of many non-profit organizations and hospitals including:

- **Alzheimer's Association TrialMatch**
  http://www.alz.org/research/clinical_trials/find_clinical_trials_trialmatch.asp
- **OncoLink Clinical Trials Matching Service**
  http://www.oncolink.org/treatment/trials.cfm
- **Ovarian Cancer National Alliance Clinical Trial Matching Service**
  http://www.emergingmed.com/networks/ocna/
- **American Association for Cancer Research Clinical Trials Finder**
  http://www.emergingmed.com/networks/aacr-su2c/
- **The Melanoma Research Foundation Clinical Trial Finder**
  http://www.emergingmed.com/networks/mrf/
- **National Lung Cancer Partnership**
  http://www.emergingmed.com/networks/NationalLungCancerPartnership/
- **Colon Cancer Alliance Clinical Trial Matching Service**
  http://www.emergingmed.com/partners/CCA/

CureLauncher
http://curelauncher.com/

CureLauncher provides summaries of clinical trials that match patient profiles.

Researchmatch
http://www.researchmatch.org

Researchmatch, partly funded by NIH, is a site that matches potential clinical research volunteers with research scientists. Patients register and answer certain questions about their condition. Research scientists initiate contact if they feel a patient is a good match for an upcoming study.

American Cancer Society Clinical Trials Matching Service
http://www.cancer.org/treatment/treatmentsandsideeffects/clinicaltrials/app/clinical-trials-matching-service

The American Cancer Society Clinical Trials Matching Service, in partnership with eviti, Inc., is free, and assists patients and their advocates in finding cancer clinical trials.

FoxTrial Finder
https://foxtrialfinder.michaeljfox.org/

FoxTrial Finder, developed by the Michael J. Fox Foundation, helps match patients and their advocates with clinical trials targeting Parkinson's disease.

Corengi
https://www.corengi.com/

Corengi matches patients with clinical trials targeting type-2 diabetes.

TrialX
http://www.trialx.com

TrialX, created by Applied Informatic Inc, is a search and matching tool used by hospitals and medical centers to match patients to relevant clinical trials based on personal health records and other criteria.

Breast Cancer Trials
http://www.breastcancertrials.org

BreastCancerTrials.org (BCT) is a non-profit organization that encourages patients to share their online health histories. BreastCancerTrials will then alert patients of recent and relevant clinical trials targeting breast cancer.

Social-Media Clinical-Trial Communities

Social-media communities provide opportunities to share information and interact with other patients and their advocates. Some social-media communities invite feedback into clinical-trial designs and volunteer requirements. Generally, however, social-media communities may make it difficult for patients to maintain privacy and confidentiality. As a result, these communities are not for everyone.

And like other services, social-media communities need a viable business model. Many communities sell their membership lists, allow targeted advertisement, and receive fees for promoting specific clinical trials. As part of a thorough search for clinical trial options, social-media communities may represent a useful option but should be included among other approaches discussed in this chapter.

Patients Like Me
http://www.patientslikeme.com/

PatientsLikeMe is an online community of patients sharing their histories and experiences dealing with their illness and available treatments. For a fee, PatientsLikeMe provides this data to pharmaceutical companies and organizations providing and supporting patient care. PatientsLikeMe also provides data on select clinical trials that are actively seeking volunteers.

Craigslist
http://www.craigslist.org

Research investigators and study coordinators often post their clinical trials on Craigslist. These posts can be found in the "volunteer" section under "Community" on the main Craigslist website for your state. Studies posted range from those looking for healthy individuals to others seeking people with specific diseases or conditions. One benefit of finding clinical trials on Craigslist is that these are often smaller studies requiring little time and commitment. As with anything on Craigslist, take precaution and inquire as to the authenticity of the posting and clinical trial before agreeing to participate.

Inspire
https://www.inspire.com/search/

Inspire designs and powers social-media communities for a variety of health associations. Inspire posts information about select clinical trials that are actively recruiting study volunteers.

Genomera
http://genomera.com/

Genomera gives patients an opportunity—as part of a social-media community—to provide input into the design of clinical trials. It also encourages these patients to participate in clinical trials.

Transparency Life Sciences
http://transparencyls.com/

Transparency Life Sciences also encourages patient input into the design of clinical trials through a social-media community and extends opportunities for these patients to participate in clinical trials.

Social-media outlets such as those listed below are also often used to provide information in the form of advertisements to prospective clinical research volunteers.

- **Google+**
  www.plus.google.com

- **Facebook**
  www.facebook.com

- **Twitter**
  www.twitter.com

- **LinkedIn**
  www.linkedin.com

- **YouTube**
  www.youtube.com

Other Listing Services Resources

CISCRP's Search Clinical Trials
http://searchclinicaltrials.org/

In 2006, patients and their advocates feeling overwhelmed with the process of searching for clinical trials began contacting CISCRP for assistance. At that time, CISCRP started conducting custom searches and mailing or emailing the results of the search back to patients and their advocates. Since then, CISCRP has conducted nearly 15,000 searches and averages nearly 100 custom searches each week. This service is offered free of charge to patients and their advocates—healthy individuals and those suffering from specific diseases. Patients and their advocates can also contact CISCRP by telephone to begin a search: 617-725-2750.

Tips for Conducting a Search

One of the best ways to look for information online is to do a keyword search. Simply enter a search term, like "clinical trial" or "clinical research study" to single out documents and materials that contain these specific words. Putting them in quotation marks turns up only entries where two words are found together in a phrase.

Try several different forms, and combination, of words—such as "clinical trials," "clinical research," "experimental drug," and "study drugs"—because each search may turn up considerably different results. If you find an article that seems to provide what you're looking for, cross-reference the researchers listed or drugs used to find other relevant articles. You can also search for drugs and trials by typing in the name of a particular disease, like "mesothelioma" (an incurable cancer).

Gathering Drug Intelligence

You may have read about a particular investigational drug in clinical trials or you may identify one during your search. Once you learn the name of a specific investigational drug (or its number, if it's very new), you might try calling the pharmaceutical company that manufactures it for more information—or an outside pharmacologist with some expertise in the therapeutic area it targets. Some pharmaceutical companies offer toll-free information lines for patients. When perusing through medical journals and newspaper articles about an investigational drug, you should jot down the names of scientists who authored the papers or offered commentary on the drug's prospects and limitations.

Consider tapping into your support network to help cover all the bases. It also wouldn't be a bad idea to cultivate a relationship with someone in the media with access to a newswire service.

Announcements about new clinical trials, and recent trial results, are routinely posted. Only a fraction of those announcements make it into the editorial section of most local newspapers.

If you are starting your search by first identifying investigational drugs, you will find no shortage of information online. Major newspapers are all available online. The science and technology sections of the *New York Times*, the *Wall Street Journal*, and the *Los Angeles Times* are particularly reputable sources of information on drugs.

The American Society for Pharmacology and Experimental Therapeutics (www.aspet.org), though designed for clinical investigators, provides links to dozens of pharmacology-related web sites. The most useful links include the American Association of Pharmaceutical Scientists, Bio, and Drug Discovery Today. The site also offers a link to a directory of pharmacology departments worldwide (including names and emails), where you can try to get your drug questions answered directly.

The American Heart Association (www.americanheart.org) has a wealth of information on research under way on treatments for cardiovascular disease and stroke, as well as the full text of several useful online journals.

The American Diabetes Association (www.diabetes.org) offers a free online publication, Diabetes E-News, which contains stories on drugs in clinical trials.

The American Society on Aging (www.asaging.org) sometimes runs helpful articles on developing drugs for conditions like osteoporosis.

BreastLink (www.breastcancercare.org) features lots of helpful drug development news, as well as a list of upcoming breast-cancer conferences.

Imaginis (www.imaginis.com) provides access to a number of general and breast-cancer–related medical journals and offers a free breast-health newsletter with information on newly published medical studies. Check with the health associations for your specific medical condition to see if they publish information on new medical treatments either online or in print form.

Associations and advocacy group web sites are also valuable resources. The Arthritis Foundation (www.arthritis.org) reports on the latest important research advances in rheumatology, including chronic fatigue syndrome, back pain, and osteoporosis. It also provides information on the research it funds, covering eight different conditions.

The National Foundation for Infectious Diseases (www.nfid.org) makes online announcements of annual conferences on vaccine research and provides access to clinical and vaccine updates.

Medscape (www.medscape.com) is a free and authoritative site for news in virtually every therapeutic area. You should go to the specialty home page called "pharmacists" and then click "pharmacists' journals." Once there, you'll have access to the content of Clinical Drug Investigation, which publishes information about drugs in all phases of drug discovery and development.

Doctors pay hundreds of dollars every year for access to a database of medical journals. But many of them—including the venerable New England Journal of Medicine (NEJM) and Drug Topics, which covers new drugs in the pipeline and who's making them—are available at no cost online. The list of free medical journals online continues to grow. These online versions include, in many cases, the full text of articles—not just abstracts. They can be accessed on the web at www.freemedicaljournals.com.

The National Library of Medicine (www.nlm.nih.gov/nlmhome.html) offers some of the largest and best-known databases. These include Medline, which provides citations and abstracts from over 4,600 biomedical journals worldwide, and MedlinePlus, an easier-to-use version that also offers access to top consumer health libraries and organizations. AIDS and HIV information is best sought through the Library's Specialized Information Services.

ScienceDirect (www.sciencedirect.com) offers free access to full-text journal articles. A search engine called Scirus (www.scirus.com/srsapp/) will get you to seemingly inexhaustible information from both journal and web sources.

Articles appearing in top-notch medical journals can also be viewed from NewsDirectory.com (www.newsdirectory.com) by browsing "magazines" under the subject of health. Once there, scroll down and click on "medicine" and/or "pharmacy." You'll find some of the articles appearing in Applied Clinical Trials—otherwise distributed primarily at industry trade shows.

One of the most comprehensive sites is MedBioWorld (www.sciencekomm.at). It is the largest resource for medical and bioscience journals, associations, and databases. Under "medical resources," click "clinical" and then "trials." A number of Internet trial listing services can be found here. The available publications include abstracts and even some full-text articles appearing in the Journal of the American Medical Association (JAMA). You can also do a search for medical conferences.

The CenterWatch Monthly and CenterWatch Weekly newsletters also list drugs about to enter new clinical trials. Many of these publications can be found at pharmaceutical company and institution libraries. You can also contact local research centers to review their copies of these newsletters. CenterWatch newsletters and reports are described in detail at www.centerwatch.com.

A surprising number of patients attend scientific meetings and professional medical conferences where the latest research is being discussed. The fees are sometimes steep—$500 to $1,000—but you may walk away with a wealth of information from hallway conversations with physicians and leading scientists. The conferences aren't all held in large cities. Most major health associations and medical societies list the calendars of conferences and upcoming events in their newsletters and web sites. A list of association web sites is included in the appendix. Contact these associations to learn about their conferences and meetings.

Most nonprofit associations, like the Alzheimer's Association and the American Heart Association, put out annual reports filled with news about promising new drugs in the development pipeline. They're always happy to put interested patients and their caregivers on the mailing list. Online versions of the reports, while often available, may be abbreviated or tough to read using slow computers.

Research Studies Will Find You

Studies aren't hard to find, even for those people not actively looking to participate. Studies are regularly advertised in newspapers and on the radio and TV. They're posted on bulletin boards in community centers and physician waiting rooms. Call centers now routinely contact homes soliciting volunteers. Trials are also detailed in direct-mail brochures, discussed at patient support group meetings and health fairs, and personally offered as treatment options by thousands of investigators across all 50 states.

Major medical centers and doctors doing research part time generally look to patients in their practice for studies. These centers use direct mail, flyers in their offices and even receptionists who quickly schedule patients who happen to call in with a relevant complaint. Some centers look for potential subjects at free screening programs and health fairs. Other research centers rely heavily on referrals from related clinics or offices, or informal word of mouth. Research centers that are dedicated to conducting clinical trials are more apt to employ mass-media approaches to reaching the patient community.

If they're large enough, some centers may have several people on staff who are on the phone night and day trying to solicit patients for studies. Pharmaceutical companies will sometimes hire a patient recruitment company to develop national advertising campaigns to reach health consumers directly, particularly for large clinical trials.

You've Found a Promising Clinical Trial . . . Now What?

There is no set way that discussions with a study site begin. After learning about a clinical trial, most people telephone the research center directly. But you may prefer to contact a center by email, or to show up at the center in person. None of these approaches is inappropriate. It's a matter of preference.

Regardless of your approach, you should plan to deal directly with the study coordinator at the research center. In most centers, coordinators handle the majority of patient recruitment responsibilities, along with the daily research study activities. It pays to get to know the study coordinator early and by name.

Once you've identified several clinical trials, and made initial inquiries into whether those trials are appropriate, you and your support network are now ready to carefully learn about and evaluate the best clinical-trial opportunities for you. This will be the focus of Chapter Seven.

CHAPTER SEVEN

Giving Your Informed Consent

"Unless you've studied medicine, you don't know what you're signing. It was Greek to me. No one ever really explained anything to me. They handed me the papers and gave me a lot of time to look them over. I just asked a few questions, then went ahead and signed it. That was probably a stupid thing to do, but I had suffered with this IBS for so long."

Frank, subject in an Irritable Bowel Syndrome trial

"They wanted to make sure I knew exactly what the terms involved were. They explained everything very well and said what the risks were and side effects might have been. And they were forever reminding me that if I had any problems to call immediately. They also made it clear that I could ask questions at any time."

Robert, subject in three Enlarged Prostate trials

"I was mailed the informed consent document before my first visit. It was nine pages—that's about average these days. It was not so hard to understand, just long. I would have had to read it over two or three times to really grasp what was going on, if I didn't work in this field. I read [the document] in 15 minutes, looking for how many visits there'd be, what would be done at those visits, the risks involved with the drug, and the wording used about the protection of study subjects. All informed consent documents are very similar in the way they're laid out."

Rose, subject in a Menopause trial and manager of a research site

FDA rules require that every adult volunteer must agree to participate—in writing—before he or she can enroll in a clinical trial. This is no small matter. By giving your consent to be in a clinical trial, you are saying that you understand and accept the risks involved. This doesn't take away the responsibility of the principal investigator and the rest of the study staff to protect your safety and to provide ethical and professional care. Your consent doesn't take away your right to file a lawsuit if something goes wrong. But consent does provide a certain degree of protection to investigators, research sites, and drug companies against later accusations of negligence in explaining study risks. And consent ensures that you take the proper steps to fully understand the clinical trial for which you are volunteering to be a subject.

The process of informed consent is not so much about signing a piece of paper as it is about reading brochures, listening to instructions, and asking lots of questions. You can't very well agree to take any medication—available or investigational—until you know what to expect. The consent form is a contract between you and the investigator.

In a very real sense, your informed consent might best be described as your bill of rights. These rights were formally recognized in 1979 in what is well known among research professionals as the Belmont Report. Informed consent, the report stated, demands three basic things:

1. Research subjects are told everything about the study, including risks.

2. The information must be easy to understand.

3. Research subjects who agree to participate must do so voluntarily—they must not be pressured or swayed into it.

How the consent process is handled depends on the individual clinical trial, the volunteer, and the standard operating procedures (SOPs) of the research center. But in no case should investigators simply be handing people a consent form to read and sign. If you are handed a consent form to sign on the spot without discussing its content with the research staff and without having your questions answered, do not participate in that trial. It is often a very complicated document that even well-schooled participants have trouble deciphering unassisted.

Investigators—and more often the study coordinator—review the consent form document with you, line by line, and have you initial every page. For more complex studies, such as those targeting cancer and AIDS, the investigator tends to do most of the explaining.

The initial visit, during which the informed consent form is reviewed with you by the study coordinator and/or principal investigator, can last more than an hour. Screening tests and study procedures are often done on subsequent visits. Patients who do not have a chance to read the informed consent form in advance are asked to give it an initial read-through at the research site. They are often left alone to do so in a waiting area or a private consultation room. If your first chance to read the informed consent form is at your initial visit, you should consider taking it home before signing it. It's important that you think very clearly about your participation in a familiar environment and also give a chance for family and loved ones to raise questions.

Alternatively, if you know you are very interested in a particular trial, you may want to telephone the research center to request that a consent form be mailed to you before your initial visit. That way, you have time to discuss the specifics of the clinical trial with your family and loved ones beforehand. When you go to the center for a face-to-face visit with a research professional, you will have had time to prepare your list of questions and concerns. Having the consent form ahead of time in no way takes away your right to consider it afterward as well. You may want to take home the answers you received to your questions and discuss those with your family and loved ones.

Your principal investigator and study coordinator want you to thoroughly understand what you're signing. Some research professionals will even ask you to verbalize your understanding of the clinical trial's purpose, procedures to be conducted, and the potential risks and benefits before moving forward. The details of a clinical trial can be difficult to recall—even an hour later. You should always keep a copy of the consent form and your notes close at hand. This way, you can refer to them to refresh your memory.

Inside the Consent Form

The consent form spells out the study procedure, how long the study will last, side effects that could happen, and how much (if anything) you will be paid for your participation. The form also states the reasons for various research steps, hoped-for benefits, and other available treatment options. Many other important details are also provided, such as screening tests that you will be expected to take and other medications that you'll be required to stop (or start) taking. Every foreseeable risk—including the remote possibility of infection from a routine blood draw—is covered. Among the many promises made in a consent form is that study volunteers will be told any new information learned about the study drug that could affect their willingness to continue participating. The consent form also gives the name and telephone number of at least one person at the Institutional Review Board (IRB) or a patient advocate. The IRB is made up of professionals and lay people charged with ensuring that the clinical trial follows FDA regulations and protects your safety and ethical treatment. The IRB answers questions about the trial and the rights of study volunteers. The IRB also helps in shaping the specific information to be covered in the consent form.

Research professionals have an ethical obligation to review with you your right to withdraw from a study at any time without penalty, to encourage you to drop out if you do not wish to continue, and to help you access alternative treatments.

A signature on a consent form represents neither an ethical nor a legal obligation from you to participate. It signifies your permission to be a study volunteer for as long as you choose. Some states, such as California, require by law that consenting individuals receive a copy of an "Experimental Subject's Bill of Rights." This document outlines what study subjects can expect to be told, their right to refuse to participate and to change their mind, and their right to a copy of the signed and dated consent form. Federal law requires that all clinical trial participants in every state get a copy of their informed consent form.

For clinical trials involving genetic testing, a section of the informed consent form should address what will happen to any stored biological specimens obtained during the study. Your medical record may have to be reviewed long after the study's completion, if stored biological samples will be used for another study involving genetic testing. You have a right to know whether study samples are likely to be shared with other investigators, or whether you will be informed of the results of future studies. You should also be assured that genetic test results will not be disclosed to any insurance company.

Consent forms can be long and complicated. And unfortunately, they can also be poorly written. Others can be more straightforward and clearly written, such as the one presented later in this chapter. Many experienced clinical-trial participants say researchers make a very big deal out of the process and go to extra lengths to be sure they understand what's in the paperwork before they sign.

Such was the case for Jennie, a volunteer in a breast cancer relapse prevention trial:

"The initial study-related visit was 45 minutes at the most. I was willing to sign the papers before I left because I had already done a lot of research on the drug. But my doctor asked me to take the papers home and read them again before I decided. He wanted to give me a chance to change my mind. Maybe he thought he talked me into it because he had mentioned the trial to me so many times. I was skeptical about taking something that hadn't been used on a daily basis for my particular condition. I have a significant other and he acted as a sounding board for all my questions and doubts and he thought up a few questions that never crossed my mind. It was a couple of months before I said to my doctor that I trusted him and knew he wouldn't give me anything that would bother me or hurt me. I asked him, 'If this was your wife, would you want her to do it?' He said yes and then I said okay."

Elements of the Informed Consent Form

These are the basic elements of informed consent, as determined by the Code of Federal Regulations Title 21, Section 50.25:

- A statement explaining the purpose of the research, the procedures to be followed, the duration of participation, and any investigational treatments or procedures.
- A description of foreseeable risks and discomforts to volunteers.
- A description of benefits that the volunteer can reasonably expect.
- A disclosure of any alternative treatments or procedures that might be advantageous to volunteers.
- A statement about how volunteer confidentiality will be maintained.
- An explanation of compensation and whether medical treatments are available if injury occurs.
- A list of contacts to answer study-related questions and to help with research-related injuries.

- A statement that participation is voluntary and that there is no penalty or loss of benefits for refusing to participate.

These additional elements may be found on informed consent forms if/when appropriate:

- A statement of unforeseeable risks to the volunteer, embryo, or fetus—if the volunteer is or may become pregnant.
- A list of anticipated circumstances under which the investigator may terminate a volunteer's participation.
- A description of additional costs to the volunteer.
- An explanation of the consequences and procedures if a volunteer decides to withdraw.
- A statement about informing volunteers of significant new findings that might affect their willingness to participate.
- A description of the number of volunteers participating in the study.

Evaluating the Consent Form

The consent form contains a lot of information for you to evaluate and understand. Here is an actual consent form used for a clinical trial. This form is more clearly written and intelligible than normal. Most forms will be more difficult to understand. Still, this example will give you an idea of the structure and flow of the informed consent form.

Research Subject Information and Consent Form

Title of Study: An 8-Week, Double-Blind, Placebo-Controlled Trial of Pregabalin (300 mg/day) for Relief of Pain in Patients With Painful Diabetic Peripheral Neuropathy (Protocol 1008-13 1)

Protocol No.: 1008-131-114, WIRB 991249

Sponsor: Parke-Davis Pharmaceutical Research, Ann Arbor, MI 48105

Investigator: James Smith, M.D., (800) 555-1234 (24-hour number)

Site: 2030 Monroe Avenue, Rochester, NY 14618

This consent form may contain words that you do not understand. Please ask the study doctor or the study staff to explain any words or information that you do not clearly understand. Y ou may take home an unsigned copy of this consent form to think about or discuss with family or friends before making your decision.

This section of the consent form provides the title of the study, which is often too technical for most volunteers to understand. The term "placebo-controlled" means that some patients will receive the drug being studied and other patients will receive a placebo, and the findings of the two groups will be compared. "Double-blind" means that neither the research subjects nor the researchers will know which patients will be receiving the active study drug and which patients will be receiving the placebo.

This section also tells you the number assigned to the clinical trial. The first number, 1008-131-114 is the number assigned by the company sponsoring the study. The second number, WIRB 991249, is the number assigned by the institutional review board that reviewed the safety and ethical aspects of the protocol and the consent documents. A reminder that you should ask questions is not always included in a consent form, but your right to do so always applies.

Nature and Purpose of this Study

You have been invited to participate in a medical research study. The purpose of this study is to compare the pain relieving effects and safety of pregabalin (300 mg/day) compared to placebo (inactive substance) in subjects with painful diabetic neuropathy.

Pregabalin is an experimental (investigational) drug that is being developed as a pain-relieving drug for patients with diabetic neuropathy. An investigational drug is one which has not been approved by the U.S. Food and Drug Administration (FDA).

You will be one of approximately 140 subjects participating in this study. Sixteen (16) of those subjects will come from this site.

This section describes, in simple terms, the purpose of the study, the total planned number of research subjects who will be enrolled in the study, and the planned number of subjects from the participants specific research location.

Duration of Study

Participation in this study will involve taking study medicine for an eight-week period. During this time you will be required to complete regular office visits so that your medical condition may be monitored. There will be three phases to the study: the baseline phase (lasting one week before taking study medicine), the eight-week double-blind phase (during which you are taking study medicine), and the one-week follow-up phase (lasting one week after you stop taking study medication). If necessary, however, the study may be stopped or you may be withdrawn at any time.

This paragraph tells you how long each phase of the study will last. It also states that the study may be stopped or that you may be withdrawn. This would happen if the drug is found to cause unacceptable side effects.

Description of the Study

A. Baseline Phase

In order to qualify for this study, you must be at least 18 years old and you must have had a history of pain associated with diabetic neuropathy for one to five years. You cannot be pregnant or nursing a baby. If you meet these qualifications, you will be scheduled for a screening visit.

During the screening visit you will undergo a medical history, a physical examination, have your vital signs taken (pulse rate, respiration rate, and blood pressure), have blood drawn, and provide urine samples, both for laboratory testing. You will also have an electrocardiogram (ECG—a tracing of the electrical activity of your heart), a visual function test (a test to check your eyes), and a neurological exam (a test of your nervous system function). For females of childbearing potential, a serum pregnancy test will be performed (and must be negative) during

> your screening visit. You will also have a chest x-ray taken unless you have had one done in the past two years. You will be asked to complete a pain questionnaire.
>
> If you are found to qualify and want to participate in the study, you will begin the seven-day baseline phase.
>
> During the baseline phase you will be given a pain and sleep diary. You will be given instructions on how to complete the diary. This diary must be completed daily in order to receive study medicine.
>
> During the baseline phase you will be required to stop most of the pain-relieving medicines and possibly other medicines that you may currently be taking. The study doctor will carefully go over with you the medicines you can and cannot take.

This section describes the basic criteria you must meet in order to qualify for the study. Remember, wanting to participate in a study is no guarantee that you will. The study is a scientific experiment. The tests performed at the screening visit are used to collect "baseline" information—that is, information about your physical condition before you start taking the study drug or placebo. For example, your blood pressure will be taken before you start taking the drug so that researchers can determine if your blood pressure increases or decreases while you are taking the study drug. Some of these tests are used to determine eligibility, as well. For example, a pregnancy test is performed. If a woman is found to be pregnant, she would be excluded from the study because the study drug's effects on the fetus are unknown and could be harmful.

The last two paragraphs in this section let you know what will be required of you if you meet the inclusion/exclusion criteria and decide to participate in the study. In this case, you would be required to maintain a diary to record any pain and sleep disturbance. It also informs you of what medications you need to stop taking. In this case, you will probably have to stop taking other pain-relieving medications (and possibly other medications, too) during the study.

> *B. 8-Week Double-Blind Phase*
>
> After you have completed the seven-day baseline phase and if it has been determined that you meet all of the entry require-

ments, you will return to the office (for Visit #2) in order to begin study medicine. At this time your pain and sleep diary will be reviewed and you will be asked to rate your pain and sleeplessness as well as answer some questionnaires and surveys. The study doctor will also examine your current symptoms of painful diabetic neuropathy. You will then be randomly assigned (like the flip of a coin) to one of two treatment groups: Group #1 pregabalin 300 mg/day; or Group #2 placebo.

You have an equal chance of being assigned to either treatment group.

You will remain in the same treatment group throughout the remainder of the study. Neither you nor the study doctor or study nurse will know the treatment group to which you were assigned; however, this information is available to the study doctor if needed in an emergency. All study medication will be in the form of pills and you will need to take it three times a day. You will begin taking the study medication the day after Visit #2. As long as you remain in the study you will continue to fill out your pain and sleep diary every day.

Throughout the eight-week double-blind phase, you will be required to attend four more office visits according to the following schedule:

Visit #3 one week after Visit #2;
Visit #4 three weeks after Visit #2;
Visit #5 five weeks after Visit #2;
Visit #6 eight weeks after Visit #2.

During your third, fourth, and fifth visits your daily pain and sleep diaries will be collected, you will be given new diaries, and you will be asked to complete a questionnaire. Additionally, you will be asked about other medicines you are taking, and you will receive additional study medicine. Also, during your fourth and fifth visits your vital signs will be taken and some blood and urine samples will be taken to check how your body is responding to the study medicine. The serum pregnancy test will be repeated at Visit #4 (if you are of childbearing ability).

You may also need to attend an extra visit at some point during the eight weeks of the study. During this visit you will be asked about other medications you are taking. Blood and urine samples will be taken to check how your body is responding to the study medicine, and you will be asked about any discomfort and pain you have experienced.

In this section, the consent form describes what will happen in the second part of the study, the eight-week double-blind phase. Especially important here is that the participants in this study will be divided randomly into two groups: one will receive the study medication and the other group will receive a placebo. The consent form calls both groups "treatment groups," but remember that one group will be receiving the placebo or an inactive substance. Some patients will improve on placebo due to what is called a "placebo" or "halo" effect. Some people respond well to any new medication, even inactive substances. For this reason, the study drug must be tested against placebo to determine if the study drug is more effective. If the study drug is not found to be more effective, then it is not considered effective. Because the study is double-blinded, neither the participants themselves nor the researchers know which participants are receiving the study medication and which participants are receiving the placebo. The consent form notes, however, that in an emergency (if you develop an allergic reaction, for example) the study doctor can find out whether you are taking the study medication or the placebo. When a blinded, placebo-controlled study has ended, the study sponsor will usually tell investigators who did and didn't receive the study drug. At that time your investigator can tell you. Keep in mind, however, that a single study protocol is used in many clinical trials over several years. If you were among the first groups testing the drug, you may have to wait years for placebo information to be "unblinded."

The double-blind phase of the study ends on your sixth visit. At this time you will no longer take study medication unless you choose to continue with the pregabalin open-label study (a study without a placebo where both you and the study doctor know which study medicine you are taking). If you choose to be in the open-label study, you will need to sign a new consent form.

This paragraph tells you that after this phase of the study, you will be able to receive the study medication by participating in another study in which no placebo is used. All participants will receive the study medication. This type of trial is called an "open-label" study, meaning that it is not blinded. Both the researchers and participants know that all of the study participants are taking the study medication.

> During your sixth visit you will have a physical exam, a neurological exam, an ECG, a visual exam, blood and urine samples will be collected, a serum pregnancy test will be given, and you will be asked about other medicines you are taking. Your daily pain and sleep diaries will be collected and you will be asked to fill out the same surveys and questionnaires you completed during Visit #2. Also, you will be asked to give your overall opinion of any change in your symptoms during the entire study.

During the sixth visit, the investigator will examine study participants. They will have tests performed and will be asked to complete questionnaires and surveys. This information is gathered to help researchers assess how the study medication has affected participants.

> At any time, if you wish to take additional non-study pain medication, you must inform the study doctor (or study nurse). At this time you will discontinue the study and begin taking the alternative medication.

Because this study is designed to test the effectiveness of a particular pain medication, the researchers don't want you to take any other pain medications during the study. If you did, researchers wouldn't be able to distinguish the effects of the study medication from the effects of the other pain medication you are taking.

> *C. Follow-up Phase*
>
> If you do not continue into the open-label study, you will be asked to complete a seventh, follow-up visit one week after your sixth visit. At this time additional blood and urine samples will be taken and you will be asked about other medicines you are taking. The study doctor or study nurse will review any medical conditions that may have begun during the study.

Risks, Inconveniences and Discomforts

The side effects seen with Pregabalin include headaches, dizziness, lightheadedness, sleepiness, euphoria (an unrealistic feeling of well-being), nausea, impaired concentration, drowsiness, blurred vision, tingling sensations, and impaired coordination. In addition, this study drug can cause tremors, clumsiness, confusion, and seizures. Mild elevations in some liver function tests have been observed. These have returned to normal levels after stopping medication. Your study doctor will discuss these with you.

This section discloses the risks and problems that can sometimes arise after taking the investigational medication Pregabalin. The first paragraph describes the side effects that other people have experienced after taking the study medication. If you were to participate in the study, you would want to ask the investigator detailed questions about known side effects and how they may affect your life—for example, your ability to work, to function, to sleep, and to eat.

A two-year study of Pregabalin in mice has shown an increased number of a type of tumor called hemangiosarcoma. This type of tumor tends to occur in mice spontaneously. It is unknown if this indicates an increased risk for cancer in humans.

This paragraph informs you of a finding from earlier animal studies of the drug: Some mice developed a type of tumor called hemangiosarcoma. You may want to ask the investigator to explain what hemangiosarcoma is. You may also want to ask how big a dose the mice received and how much time elapsed before hemangiosarcoma developed. Then ask how that compares to the dose that you will receive.

Because of potential interactions between medications, you should not start taking a new medication or change the dose of an existing medication without first discussing the new medication or medication dose change with the study doctor or a member of his study staff. Medication interactions can have serious, even fatal, consequences.

Drug interactions pose an important risk in clinical trials. If your doctor were to prescribe an already approved medication, information would exist on how that drug interacts with other commonly prescribed drugs. But because the investigational drug in a clinical trial is new and has been taken by few people, little may be known about its interactions with other drugs. If you are in a clinical trial, never begin taking another medication without first discussing it with the study doctor.

> There may be side effects which are unknown at this time. Serious allergic reactions that can be life-threatening may occur. You should exercise special caution when driving or using machinery since the study medications may cause drowsiness, lack of coordination, or slowed reaction time. Obtaining blood can cause pain, bruising, or redness where the skin is punctured. Fainting sometimes occurs and infection rarely occurs.

This paragraph tells you that the study entails risks beyond the risks of the investigational drug. Sometimes tests that are done as part of a clinical trial have risks. It's possible, for example, that you could develop an infection in your arm where blood was drawn. This is a small risk, and one that you always face when you get your blood drawn whether or not you are participating in a trial, but the researchers are acting ethically by informing you about it.

> Your pain may not improve or may worsen while participating in the study. The study drug must be taken only by the person for whom it has been prescribed, and it must be kept out of the reach of children and persons of limited capacity to read or understand.
>
> If you are a woman of childbearing potential: If you are or become pregnant, the treatment involved in this study may involve unknown risks to you or the fetus. Therefore, you must be using an effective method of birth control before, during, and immediately after the study. Acceptable methods of birth control include being post-menopausal or surgically sterile; using oral contraceptive implants or injections; ITUD; diaphragm or cervical cap with spermicide; abstinence; condoms with contraceptive foam/gel/cream; or male sterilization. If you suspect that you have become pregnant you must notify the study doctor immediately.

Because the study drug is new, the risks to a fetus are unknown. The researchers will want to be sure that women enrolled in the study are not pregnant and will not become pregnant during the study.

> You will be notified of significant new findings that may affect your willingness to continue in this study.

During the course of the study, if the investigational drug is found to cause side effects that had not been anticipated, this new information must be conveyed to you. In light of this new information, you may want to reconsider your decision to participate in the study.

> **Safeguards**
>
> For your own safety, you must tell the study doctor all your past and present diseases, allergies you are aware of, and all drugs and medications you are presently using.
>
> **Benefits**
>
> Your participation in this study may decrease the pain you feel from diabetic peripheral neuropathy. However, you may not receive direct benefit from your participation in this study and no direct medical benefits are guaranteed. Your participation in this study may provide knowledge that may be of benefit to you or to others.
>
> **Costs**
>
> There will be no cost to you for the study doctor's time, procedures, and supplies related to this study. The study medication will be provided to you without charge.

This paragraph describes the benefits that you may gain by participating in the study. It is careful to point out that you may not benefit at all. Typically you should not have to pay for any costs associated with your participation in a clinical trial.

Alternative Treatments

You do not have to participate in this study to receive pain medication. Instead, you may choose to receive standard treatment as prescribed by your doctor.

If you are considering participating in a clinical trial because the medication you are taking for your condition isn't helping you, there may be other drugs available that have been tested and approved by the Food and Drug Administration. Participating in a clinical trial usually isn't the only option available to you. Researchers should be able to tell you more information about these alternative treatments.

Confidentiality

Information from this study will be gathered and submitted to Parke-Davis Pharmaceuticals (sponsor) and to the U.S. Food and Drug Administration (FDA). It may be submitted to governmental agencies in other countries where the study drug may be considered for approval. Medical records which identify you and the consent form signed by you, will be inspected and/or copied by the sponsor and an agent for the sponsor, and may be inspected and/or copied by the FDA, the Department of Health and Human Services (DHHS) agencies, governmental agencies in other countries, the University of Rochester, and the Western Institutional Review Boards (WIRB).

Because of the need to release information to these parties, absolute confidentiality cannot be guaranteed. The results of this research study may be presented at meetings or in publications; however, you will not be identified by name in any publication or presentation.

This section informs study participants about who will have access to the information collected as part of the clinical trial. Absolute confidentiality cannot be guaranteed. The sweeping federal privacy regulations that went into effect on April 14, 2003 do not apply to research records that exist separate and apart from your medical record. But research information, as a rule, is still very tightly secured. Results of investigational treatments will go into your medical record and they will be as well protected as any other part of your medical history. Clinical trials are generally designed to protect study participants from loss of privacy and breach of confidentiality. This includes the removal of names and other identifying information about illnesses and behaviors, limiting access to the data, and hiding the personal identities of study participants when research results are presented at meetings and in medical publications. Investigators can get a Certificate of Confidentiality that provides protection even against a court subpoena for data from any FDA-regulated research. The provision was initially designed to shield the identities of study participants who use illegal drugs or commit crimes. Today, it is considered equally important in preventing the leakage of genetic information about study participants that could threaten their employment, health insurance, or social standing.

The new privacy regulations contained in the Health Insurance Portability and Accountability Act (HIPAA) may substantially limit access to archived medical records, which researchers need for the design of safe and sensible clinical trials. Protected health information may also be "de-identified" by removing key information like your name and social security number. Waivers for access are to be granted only if a strict set of criteria is met, including that the disclosure of information involves no more than "minimal risk" to you and the research would be impractical to conduct without access to that information. Clinical investigators will need to obtain not only your consent to participate in a trial (as was the case previously), but also your permission to use and disclose personal health information in your past and future medical records.

Questions

If you have any questions concerning your participation in this study, or if at any time you feel you have experienced a research-related injury or a reaction to the study medication, contact:

Dr. James Smith at (800) 555-1234 (24-hour number).

If you have questions about your rights as a research subject, you may contact:

Western Institutional Review Board (WIRB)
Telephone: (800) 562-4789.

Do not sign this consent form unless you have had a chance to ask questions and have received satisfactory answers to all of your questions. Do not sign this consent form if you do not wish to participate in this study.

There should always be two people for you to contact in order to discuss your questions and concerns. The first contact is the principal investigator. The second contact is a representative from the institutional review board (IRB) or a patient advocate that is responsible for ensuring the safety and ethical treatment of volunteers in the study. This section also reminds you again not to sign the consent form until you have had your questions answered.

Consent

I have read and I understand the information in this consent form. All my questions regarding the study and my participation in it have been answered to my satisfaction. I have been informed of the risks involved and my rights as a research subject.

I voluntarily agree to participate in this study. I understand that I will receive a signed and dated copy of this consent form. I authorize the release of my medical records to Parke-Davis, Kendle, the FDA, DHHS agencies, governmental agencies in other countries, the University of Rochester, and WIRB.

By signing this consent form, I have not waived any of the legal rights which I otherwise would have as a subject in a research study.

Subject's Name (Printed):

Subject's Signature:

Date:

The above-named subject has been fully informed of the study.

Signature of Person Conducting:

Date Informed Consent Discussion:

Investigator's Signature:
(if different from above)

Date:

At the conclusion of the consent form, you provide your consent in writing. And the study staff involved in this process also sign. This completes the contract that you have now entered into with the investigator and the research center.

Exceptions to the Rules

If the study participant is a child or an individual under the care of another person, a parent, caregiver, or legal guardian will usually sign the consent form. This would be the case with most Alzheimer's disease patients.

"My mom participated in the decision as much as she was able to. But the Alzheimer's made her pessimistic," Karen said. "She worried about everything. What if she flunked the [screening] test? What if we got lost on the way there? Are you sure you have time to do this? If left to decide on her own, she would have said no. She hates doctors. I just told her we were going to do this; we were going to go get this new medicine. The only drug [then] on the market...was effective for fewer than half the people who took it. So I thought, 'Why not try something new?' It took me maybe 10 minutes to decide, although the doctor made me take home the consent papers to read through them before I signed."

In special circumstances, FDA regulations allow doctors to provide "emergency" research before informed consent is obtained from a volunteer or caregiver. A trauma patient who shows up in a hospital emergency room in shock, for example, might be immediately placed on a resuscitation study. This would happen only because the patient is physically unable to give consent at the time the investigational treatment must be given to potentially save his or her life. The patient, or a family member, generally signs consent papers a short time later.

Take Your Time

Unlike study volunteers, investigators have usually gone through the informed consent process countless times before. Research staff may zip through explanations and give you too little time to think of questions that you might want to ask. They may also explain things in a way you don't understand. There is absolutely nothing wrong with asking a researcher to slow down and repeat something. It is also not out of line to ask them to explain something in another way, using everyday words. If English is not your first language, you need to speak up. Research centers can, and should, produce documents in your first language upon request.

It is the principal investigator's responsibility to make sure that you completely understand everything that you've read in the consent form. It is also the investigator's responsibility to give you enough time to think of any questions that you may still have. This may not necessarily happen in a single visit. When given time to think over your decision, you may raise important concerns that no one else ever thought to bring up.

Questions to Ask Before Giving Your Consent to Participate

Following is a comprehensive list of questions for you to consider asking. More than anything else, this checklist of questions may assist you in beginning your conversation with research center staff. You may want to invite along a friend or relative for support—and to help you recall answers to your questions. You may even want to record answers to these questions so you can replay them at a later date.

About the Clinical Trial

- What is the main purpose of the study?
- Why is this study important to me?
- What are the chances that this drug will work?
- Is the drug already being used in other countries?
- How long will the clinical trial last?
- What kinds of risks are involved?
- What are the eligibility requirements?
- What kinds of medical problems would prevent me from participating in the study?
- What kind of screening do I have to go through to qualify as a study subject?
- Where is the study being conducted?
- Who else is participating in the study?
- How much of my time will this take?
- Does the study involve a placebo or a treatment already on the market?
- What are my chances of getting a placebo?
- Have other studies already been done on this drug?
- What has been learned about this drug so far and where have those results been published?

- How many adverse events have been associated with this drug to date?
- What kind of side effects have other people (or animals) experienced?
- (If pregnant) What kinds of effects might this drug have on my unborn child?
- Who will be watching out for my safety?
- What other kinds of treatments are available to treat my condition?
- What can you tell me about the drug company sponsoring this study?
- Who has reviewed and approved this study? How can I contact them?
- Will I be able to find out the results of the study?

About Your Care

- How will the treatment be given to me?
- What kind of tests will be done? Will they hurt? If so, for how long?
- How will the tests in the study compare to tests I would have outside the study?
- Will I be able to see my own doctor?
- Will the research staff work with my doctor while I am in the clinical trial?
- Will I be able to take my regular medications during the study?
- Will I require support from family and friends for daily activities or daily needs (such as assistance shopping or childcare) while in the trial?
- If the study drug doesn't work, will I be able to take anything else for my symptoms?
- Will everything be done on an outpatient basis, or will I have to be hospitalized?
- What happens if I miss a dose of the study drug?
- If I have side effects, can they be treated during the study?
- Is it possible my condition will worsen during, or after, the study?
- Will I receive any follow-up care after the study ends?
- Who will provide it?
- Whom can I call with questions and concerns during the study?
- Who on the research staff will be with me in the event of an emergency?
- If the treatment works for me, can I keep using it after the study ends? For free?

- Who will provide my medical care after the study ends?

About Your Personal Matters

- Can anyone find out if I'm participating in the clinical trial?
- How might this study affect my daily life?
- Who will review my information collected during the trial?
- Can I talk to other volunteers in the trial?
- What support is available in the community for me and my family?
- What happens if I decide to quit the study?
- Can I be withdrawn from the study for any reason?
- Who can I contact with questions about the trial and my rights as a participant?

About Your Compensation and Costs

- Do I have to pay for any part of the study? If so, will insurance cover these costs?
- Do I have to talk to my health insurance company before enrolling in the study?
- How much will I be paid for my participation?
- Will I be reimbursed for gas, or will transportation be provided?

About the Research Staff

- Why did the investigator decide to get involved in clinical research?
- What is the investigator's background and training?
- What sort of research training and certification have the investigator and coordinator had?
- How many studies has the investigator done before?
- Was the investigator involved in the design of the study?
- Has the investigator or study coordinator ever participated in a clinical trial?
- Does this facility have any special credentials or experience in research?
- Do the investigator and study coordinator have any formal training in research safety and ethics?
- Does the investigator have a financial interest in the drug being studied?
- Is the investigator or study coordinator paid a bonus for recruiting me into the trial?

If a study involves a great deal of risk and close patient monitoring, for instance, it will probably be very important to the study volunteer (or their legal guardian) to know how much research training and experience the principal investigator has had. Two-thirds of our country's 30,000 investigators have limited experience conducting clinical trials. Being a researcher is a tough job, even for otherwise well-schooled medical doctors.

The U.S. Department of Health and Human Services requires that investigators involved in any of the studies it funds (through the NIH, for example) be instructed on how to conduct research responsibly. Although the FDA intends to become more specific about its educational requirements, the onus is currently on pharmaceutical companies to ensure that clinical investigators are sufficiently qualified with experience and training. Investigators have a medical or professional degree, but it is not always enough because many investigators have not received formal training in clinical research. A pathologist accustomed to working all day in a lab, for instance, wouldn't be well suited for clinical trials with pediatric populations.

Although there are no certification exams for physicians as proof of their competency in conducting clinical trials, there is plenty of accredited coursework being offered by universities, trade associations, and training companies. A number of medical schools also offer research training during doctors' internship and residency years. At least 10 medical colleges and universities now offer doctors a two-year program leading to a Master's degree of Science in Clinical Research. Some research institutions require that all investigators undergo a fairly rigorous educational program covering the basics of clinical research. The NIH and several universities (Case Western Reserve University and the University of Rochester among them) make investigators take an online test that demonstrates their knowledge of human research protections before they can seek IRB approval of a protocol.

Study coordinators and other support staff have a wide variety of accredited courses to choose from. Study coordinators can be certified. This distinction adds the letters "CCRC"—Certified Clinical Research Coordinator—to their titles. Coordinators tend to be the ones who handle informed consent discussions. In fact, at some universities, informed consent discussions exclude investigators who are also healthcare providers. This is done to lower the chance that potential study volunteers will be influenced to participate in research simply because it's being done by people they know and respect as healers.

Beginning a Dialogue

When people either blindly or half-heartedly commit to participate in a clinical trial, neither science nor an individual's health may gain anything. One reason why a high number of volunteers drop out of a study is because many don't fully understand what they're consenting to from the outset. That's why you need to find out all that you can before you give your consent. Informed consent papers and new drug brochures will answer many—but not all—of your important questions.

When it comes to study risks, in particular, you may have to dig for the full story. Families have told stories of needlessly losing a loved one in a clinical trial where earlier deaths and serious adverse events went unreported on informed consent documents because the study's sponsor didn't identify the study drug as the culprit. FDA guidelines say that study volunteers should understand the risks they're taking, but they don't require a drug's complete track record be shared. If you want to know details, such as the number of deaths and serious side effects observed in earlier clinical trials even if the study drug was not implicated, you have to make a point to request that information.

Not everyone has the time, interest, or even capability of understanding everything that is uncovered. You may want to bring some of this information to a trusted, impartial family physician or health professional for their medical opinion. Another good option is to consult with the IRB. They decide whether or not a clinical trial gets done. The IRB is also your chief advocate and troubleshooter throughout the course of the trial.

You need to always remember that you are the one volunteering for a clinical trial. The study drug may make you feel better. And your study visits may seem just like any other visit to the doctor's office, but the main purpose of research is to collect data, not to treat your illness. You should therefore participate in a clinical trial only if you feel that it is in your best interest—not in the interest of your doctor, employer, researchers, college professor, or anyone else.

From the perspective of patients, the business of becoming "informed" about a trial can be daunting and confusing:

> *"The informed consent form was really difficult for me," said Paula, a participant in several Crohn's disease clinical trials. "It was a bureaucratic, legal document done to protect the study site and pharmaceutical company—not so much to inform the patient. I was given the form to read and sign, and asked if I had any questions by the*

study nurse. Each visit or so I was given an 'updated' form. I of course would ask what had changed, as it was not marked in the document, and the nurse would explain as best she could."

"To read informed consent documents is hilarious," added Frederick, who has volunteered for a series of trials for his gastrointestinal cancer. "They say 'the doctor is going to give you this drug because he believes it may be able to help. We [the sponsoring drug company] make no such promise.' All of which leaves me to wonder, 'What am I doing here?' But I have no choice, so I laugh and sign."

During and After a Trial

Informed consent doesn't stop the moment a form is signed and witnessed. It's something you are entitled to during—and even after—the clinical trial has ended. Experienced investigators and study coordinators will repeat, remind, and reassure you frequently about what is happening to you. If they don't (and even if they do), it's okay to ask questions and expect answers from researchers. It's their job.

Any time you feel that your questions and concerns have not been sufficiently addressed, you have the option to seek help from the IRB. The pharmaceutical company sponsoring the clinical trial may also have a consumer hotline that participants can call with any unanswered concerns or general questions specifically about the drug. A list of sponsor companies and their contact information is provided in the appendix.

If a clinical trial gets suspended for reasons unrelated to the study drug, volunteers who have a medical need to continue taking the drug may be allowed to do so. If a trial is suspended due to serious adverse events related to the study drug, or production problems on the part of the pharmaceutical company, then you would be required to stop taking the drug and to seek care from your regular doctor. But the principal investigator and study staff would continue to keep an eye on you, at least until the study drug is out of your system.

Your consent means that you can withdraw from a clinical trial at any time. This is your fundamental right as a study participant. If your withdrawal may prove harmful to you, the investigator and study coordinator must tell you so. Investigators and study coordinators should not coerce you to continue to participate in a clinical trial if your decision to withdraw is final. Informed consent regulations forbid investigators who are practicing doctors from denying future care to their patients who have withdrawn from a clinical trial. If you drop out of a clinical trial, you should still be told anything that is later learned about the investigational drug that could affect your health.

Compassionate Use of Experimental Treatments

For most people, access to a study drug ends when the clinical trial does. But there are some notable exceptions. Study volunteers with serious or life-threatening illnesses who have completed a phase III study are sometimes rolled into an "open-label" study, allowing them to take an effective investigational drug, for free, until the FDA approves it or for a fixed time period such as six months or a year.

Such compassionate use, as it is often called, is only occasionally extended to patients with debilitating but not necessarily life-shortening medical conditions. And even then, this only happens if the pharmaceutical company hasn't abandoned plans to take the drug to market for one reason or another.

Even if a pharmaceutical company is willing to provide compassionate use of a helpful drug, the process doesn't necessarily happen quickly. The research investigator would need to send in a special FDA form to the company, whose attorneys might mull it over for weeks or even years.

In the meantime, patients can check with the FDA or pharmaceutical companies to learn about where investigational drugs are in the development process. If approval of the desired drug isn't far off, the best course of action may be to wait it out. There may even be another drug with a similar composition and action under study. Patients can always ask the pharmaceutical company about other promising trials it is conducting, or start a wider search on their own.

Consent and Your Obligations

By signing the consent form and agreeing to participate, you also assume certain responsibilities. Consent is a covenant of trust between researchers and research subjects. It is your responsibility to tell the truth and to comply with the rules of the clinical trial.

If you fail to meet these obligations, the data collected during the clinical trial have no integrity.

You should never lie to qualify for a clinical trial.

No matter how badly you want to qualify to participate in a clinical trial, you must tell the truth. Some people might neglect to mention things, like a prior medical condition or daily treatment of pain symptoms, which would automatically exclude them from some studies. Others might knowingly participate in two drug studies at the same time—a standard exclusion criterion. Dishonesty invalidates the study results and it is dangerous. Taking two drugs at the same time, for instance, exposes a person to unknown and difficult-to-detect interactions that can cause serious health problems—even death. One drug also may be mistakenly credited for the action of the other, or mask its harmful side effects. Faulty data lead to faulty conclusions about a drug's safety and, in the end, may endanger public health.

You should never disregard the study protocol.

Protocols are very carefully designed. Failure to comply with the protocol can endanger you and can harm the results of the trial. Study volunteers who are instructed not to drink any alcoholic beverages but do so anyway may skew important lab results. Volunteers who fail to take the study medication as instructed or ignore their promise to use birth control and become pregnant (not to mention the unknown harm done to the fetus) may invalidate the clinical trial results and put themselves at risk. Researchers need to understand how a study medication is working, whether doses need to be adjusted and what side effects you are experiencing.

Maintaining a diary is important if it is required in the protocol. If you aren't willing to devote time to keeping a diary, you shouldn't volunteer to participate. Hastily made diary entries won't benefit the research effort. To help you comply with this requirement, investigators and study coordinators often have to call to remind you to record your experiences in your diary.

Your informed consent is a fundamental right as a participant in a clinical trial. It is a major responsibility that you and your support network must assume when you decide to volunteer to participate in a clinical trial.

The Clinical Trial Participant's Bill of Rights

Any volunteer who gives his or her consent to participate in a clinical trial or who is asked to give his or her consent on behalf of another has the following rights:

1. To be told the purpose of the clinical trial.
2. To be told about the risks, side effects, or discomforts that might be reasonably expected.
3. To be told of any benefits that can be reasonably expected.
4. To be told what will happen in the study and whether any procedures, drugs, or devices are different than those that are used as standard medical treatment.
5. To be told about options available and how they may be better or worse than being in a clinical trial.
6. To be allowed to ask any questions about the trial before giving consent and at any time during the course of the study.
7. To be allowed ample time, without pressure, to decide whether to consent or not to consent to participate.
8. To refuse to participate, for any reason, before and after the trial has started.
9. To receive a signed and dated copy of the informed consent form.
10. To be told of any medical treatments available if complications occur during the trial.

CHAPTER EIGHT

Clinical-Trial Care and Compensation

The medical care that you'll receive for your treatment condition will most likely be excellent during a clinical trial. Study volunteers typically report that the principal investigator and study staff monitors them more closely than a physician and nurse would during visits for routine care. Study volunteers also report that study staff tends to be more responsive to their medical needs during a clinical trial. All of this extra attention is due, in large part, to the fact that study protocols require very detailed procedures and frequent patient assessments. Study volunteers can also expect to have valuable interactions with principal investigators who are often some of the most knowledgeable physicians about a disease or condition under investigation.

Medical care during a study also tends to be excellent because research sponsors—government agencies and pharmaceutical and biotechnology companies—place high standards on their clinical trials. They want to make sure that the research centers are conducting clinical trials to the best of their abilities. And sponsors want to make certain that their research centers are fully compliant with federal guidelines, especially as they relate to the care, safety, and ethical treatment of study volunteers.

Your care in a clinical trial also depends on the support network that you build to help you through the volunteer experience. Family, trusted friends, and advisors are extremely important members of your support network. They can help you stick with the clinical trial and stay with it through completion; comply with the protocol; offer moral support; and provide assistance in managing daily activities so that you can participate relatively easily. You may need support from family and friends to do routine errands, provide transportation and babysitting, cook and clean, and care for pets.

Coordinating Your Medical Care

Before you begin participating in a clinical trial, you should contact your doctor(s) and put them in touch with the principal investigator. It is extremely important that you coordinate your medical care among all of your doctors treating you inside and outside your clinical trial. For starters, make sure to give your personal doctors and the principal investigator permission to share medical information. This will help ensure your safety during a clinical trial. Periodically touch-base with your routine doctors to remind them to stay connected to the principal investigator of your clinical trial.

Be sure to tell the principal investigator and study coordinator if you will need to receive routine care for a medical condition other than the one being treated in the clinical trial. The research center staff will speak with your regular physician at the outset of the study to coordinate your care. The IRB will also be informed of your medical needs so that they can ensure that adequate reporting and safety oversight is in place.

If you're already participating in a study and you need medical care unrelated to your clinical trial, you should contact and visit with your primary or specialty care doctor. Study volunteers do experience unrelated medical conditions. Sometimes these conditions may be caused by, or made worse by, the treatment under investigation. Even a routine treatment for an unrelated condition might interact with the study drug during a clinical trial.

There have been instances where study volunteers have been hospitalized at a different medical-care facility for unrelated conditions. In these instances, a physician from the new facility can contact the principal investigator through the volunteer's regular doctors and quickly identify which experimental drugs are being used. In relatively rare instances, principal investigators may un-blind the volunteer's treatment group in order to assist physicians at a different medical-care facility in determining the possible causes of an unrelated medical condition.

The principal investigator remains responsible for your safety during the clinical trial. Be sure to tell him or her about any visits that you have with your routine doctors or any hospitalizations. The principal investigator may also need to report any adverse events that may be associated with the experimental treatment.

Insurance Coverage

Research sponsors cover the cost of the investigational drug, medical attention, and procedures performed to fulfill the protocol requirements. There is often a cost to the volunteer for medical devices used in clinical trials.

Many health insurers pay for costs, especially in phase III studies, that are not covered by research sponsors. These are typically costs for routine care and non-experimental care given during a clinical trial. Routine costs usually include the visit with the physician, physical exams, and tests and procedures that are required to complete a diagnosis. Non-experimental care might include additional office visits and tests.

All expected out-of-pocket costs as well as costs that will be billed to the study volunteer must be outlined in the informed-consent form. Plan to contact your health insurer to discuss your coverage once you have a good sense for the costs that you're expected to pay. Health insurers don't typically have standard procedures for handling bills for clinical trial activities. Health insurers also don't have standard policies for handling complications or side effects caused by participation in a clinical trial. Instead, they usually consider inquiries and requests on a case-by-case basis. When you call, be sure to have copies of the protocol and the informed-consent form accessible. In some states, laws have been passed requiring health insurers to cover various costs associated with care received during clinical trials. The America's Health Insurance Plans (AHIP) monitors state laws and occasionally publishes information on its web site (www.ahip.org).

There are tangible and intangible costs to consider as well. Tangible costs might include transportation, lodging, and time away from work while participating in a clinical trial. Volunteers may receive payment for some of these costs in the form of compensation. Intangible costs include the effects of participation on one's quality of life.

Medicare is mandated to cover certain patient costs of care in clinical trials. Most of the routine costs of participation in federally-funded and -approved clinical trials are covered by Medicare. If your trial is not federally funded or federally approved, you'll need to contact the Medicare office to determine whether the costs will be covered. The study investigator and study coordinator will also likely have information about Medicare coverage of costs for patient care in specific clinical trials.

Compensation for Participation

Along with complimentary medical care, and reimbursement for transportation costs, sometimes you will receive compensation for your participation. The FDA and the National Institutes of Health (NIH) carefully regulate compensation conditions in order to ensure that payments are reasonable and not coercive.

Payment for participation is considered compensation for your time and commitment to comply with the protocol. Healthy volunteers in phase I studies of a new treatment or device are usually paid for their participation. Study volunteers in phase IV studies of drugs already on the market often receive compensation. And payments in clinical trials are often given to study volunteers when the health benefits of an experimental treatment or new device are not known or are remote.

The compensation amount varies widely and depends on many factors including the length of the clinical trial, the number of visits that you'll need to make during the study, and the number and types of procedures that will be performed. Compensation can range from a hundred dollars to one or two thousand dollars. Partial payments are made over the course of participation, and are usually tied to individual visits or milestones reached during participation. The clinical-trial sponsor proposes the amount and schedule of payments to the IRB overseeing the study. The IRB will review, and in some cases revise, the proposal to ensure that it does not coerce or influence someone to agree to participate.

Patient recruitment advertisements usually list compensation amounts. The informed consent document also lists compensation amounts and payment schedules. You can also ask whether a trial is offering compensation and the amount when calling a research center to inquire about participation.

Examples of compensation levels offered

Condition	Number of visits	Compensation range
Arthritis	1-24	$100- $1,450
Breast Cancer	5-45	$150 - $1,350
Depression	1-50	$200 - $1,036
Type II Diabetes	2-28	$50 - $1,300
HIV	4-16	$50 - $1,160

Once participation begins, the research center typically writes each volunteer a check as the study progresses—usually on a per-visit basis. A small bonus may also be paid to volunteers who complete the entire study. In some cases, study doctors may dispense approved medication samples and provide additional care free of charge after the trial to show their appreciation to study volunteers.

Any financial compensation paid to study participants is considered taxable income by the Internal Revenue Service (IRS). However, research centers are obligated to report to the IRS only payments to individuals that total $600 or more for a given year. These Form 1099s for "Miscellaneous Income" are generally sent out to participants in January, the same month employers are sending out W-2 forms to their employees. If a volunteer decides to withdraw from the study before completing the trial, the research center will usually provide partial compensation.

Clinical Trial Completion

A clinical trial ends when the principal investigator has recruited enough volunteers and conducted all of the procedures and planned activities to collect the necessary study data. For each individual volunteer, the trial ends when he or she has received all of the treatment, procedures, and follow-up as described in the protocol. But it's important to remember that although the trial may have ended for you, it may still be going on for volunteers who started their participation after you did.

The trial is not officially over until the very last volunteer who entered the study has completed the requirements of their participation. Research sponsors, IRBs, the FDA and the NIH may each—or may collectively—decide to prematurely end a clinical trial for a number of reasons. When very positive results are observed during the course of the clinical trial, research sponsor may decide to unblind the study and administer the experimental treatment to all volunteers in the clinical trial. A clinical trial may be halted in order to protect volunteer safety if too many serious adverse events associated with the experimental treatment are observed. In rare instances, clinical trials are terminated early when clinical research professionals have failed to comply with federal regulations. The trial is halted to protect the safety and ethical treatment of study volunteers.

Clinical-trial volunteers are immediately notified if a clinical trial is stopped. Study staff is morally and ethically bound to protect your safety and it is their duty to advise you on what to do if the clinical trial ends prematurely. The principal investigator will consult with your primary or specialty doctor or any other doctor to whom your care is referred.

In some instances, after the clinical trial has ended, patients can continue to receive experimental treatments if they're deemed safe and effective. Pharmaceutical companies and the FDA can sometimes offer these treatments to patients who will likely benefit under "continued access" while the drug or device is awaiting FDA approval. Study staff will continue to monitor these patients and collect data during this period. As this period of the study has no control group and everyone in the original trial who might benefit will receive the experimental treatment, it is called an "open-label" phase. Continued access and open-label studies ensure continuity for volunteers who are responding well to new treatments before they are marketed commercially.

CHAPTER NINE

A Closer Look at IRBs

The Institutional Review Board (IRB), also called an Ethical Committee in other parts of the world, approves clinical trials and is the primary body protecting your safe and ethical treatment. The IRB is your advocate and you can contact them to discuss any questions that you have about your safety and protection. At the present time, there are 4,600 IRBs and ethical committees operating around the world to protect patient safety and ethical treatment. More than half of that number—2,600—are operating in the US alone.

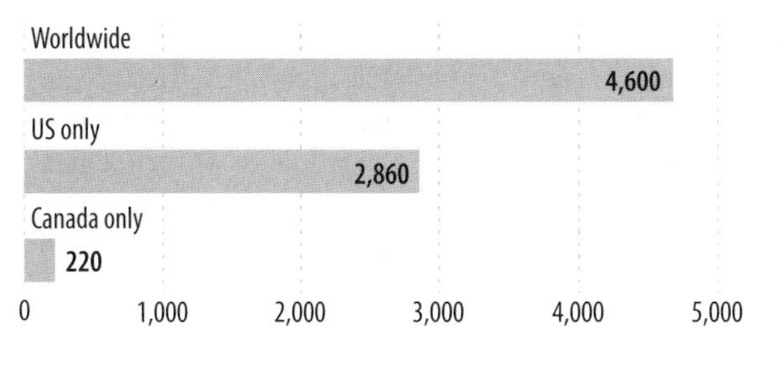

Number of institutional review boards/ethical committees operating in the US, Canada, and worldwide in 2013

FDA regulations first began requiring IRB approval of research studies in 1971. IRBs may be created and run by a hospital or university (which generally oversee all studies conducted by its network of faculty and affiliated investigators). Some IRBs are independent for-profit enterprises that oversee clinical trials conducted by independent research centers. By law, an IRB must include five or more people that are representative of the community demographics. It also must have at least one member whose primary interest is scientific, one member whose primary interest is non-scientific (a lawyer, clergyman, or ethicist, for example), and one "public member" who isn't connected with the institution, hospital, or business sponsoring the IRB.

Before any clinical trial can begin, the IRB must do a "risk/benefit assessment" to be certain that the trial does not pose a level of risk that outweighs potential benefits. The majority of IRB members must agree that it is ethical—meaning the study protocol follows the highest scientific and medical standards for conducting experiments with humans. This includes the appropriateness of using a placebo, or whether a study should be done at all. The IRB would probably reject a study designed to test a drug on very young children before the drug was tested on adults and older children.

The majority of IRB members also must be convinced that the rights of children and other "vulnerable" populations (e.g., prisoners, pregnant women, mentally disabled persons, and economically or educationally disadvantaged persons) are given special attention. Finally, the IRB must be convinced that it makes sense to conduct a clinical trial within a particular community.

A well-run IRB spends a great deal of time reviewing the informed-consent form. It is the IRB's responsibility to ensure that the consent form truthfully covers all important points about the clinical trial using words that are easy to understand. How well IRBs do their job has become a matter of considerable debate during the past several years. The IRB is also responsible for approving any advertisement that research centers use to recruit study volunteers. The IRB checks these advertisements to make sure that they are accurate and not coercive. One IRB's decision to approve a protocol or advertisement may be countered by another IRB's decision to reject them. What happens is that a large trial will be conducted at many research centers. Each center may have its own IRB reviewing its protocols and advertisements. The committee members on each IRB may have different opinions about a protocol or an advertisement. For instance, some years ago an IRB for the University of Rochester in Upstate New York pulled a national ad for a breast cancer trial because it was asking women to be study volunteers for their "daughters' sake." To the ears of those IRB members, that sounded coercive. But IRBs in other cities had no problem with the ad and let it run.

IRBs must also make a judgment call on whether the payment offered to study volunteers is reasonable or, conversely, whether it represents "undue influence" on volunteers to participate. The concern is that monetary compensation that is too attractive may blind potential subjects to the risks of participating or tempt them to lie or hide information about themselves that would disqualify them from enrolling in the study. There are no federal rules governing the matter. The idea is to arrive at some "reasonable" arrangement with study volunteers to compensate them for their time.

Of particular concern are people who may be induced to enter a trial even for a $25 payment. Just the prospect of free healthcare can entice people with major medical problems who are having a tough time making ends meet. IRB members must therefore decide, based on the number of "economically vulnerable" people who agree to volunteer, whether the opportunity to get free care is too large an incentive as to be ethically questionable.

Study volunteers who are unable to give informed consent—including some people who have had a stroke or abused drugs, have Alzheimer's disease and certain psychiatric illnesses, or are in a coma—are usually given special attention by IRBs. As long as these individuals are selected fairly and the study is not abnormally risky, many IRBs will allow consent documents to be signed by a legally-authorized representative.

Study volunteers should make it a point to get to know their IRB representatives. The oversight responsibilities of the IRB last for the duration of the study. IRB members receive regular updates on the study's progress, approve any needed changes to the study protocol and are among the first to know if any serious, adverse events happen. The IRB also decides which patients are allowed to have open-label or "compassionate use" of study drugs awaiting approval by the FDA. And IRBs typically appoint a "patient liaison" or "study participant liaison" to answer volunteer questions and to advocate on behalf of the volunteer throughout the duration of the clinical trial.

The FDA has the right to inspect IRBs and review their records in order to determine if they are following their own written procedures, as well as FDA regulations.

How an IRB Works

Before a researcher can begin a clinical trial, the principal investigator must submit the study protocol to the IRB for approval. The protocol describes the clinical trial in detail, including the purpose and objectives of the study and how the study is to be carried out. In a typical clinical trial, the protocol includes:

- The number of volunteers who will participate in the trial;
- The eligibility criteria the volunteers must meet in order to be enrolled;
- The potential risks and benefits of the trial and how they will be communicated to volunteers;

- The informed-consent form that volunteers will be asked to read and sign;
- The design of the study and whether some volunteers will receive placebo or a standard treatment;
- The study drug dosage levels, how often and for how long;
- A description of how the effects of the drug will be measured;
- A description of all study activities.

When the researcher submits the protocol to the IRB for review, the protocol is usually assigned to one member of the IRB. This member is asked to review the protocol and the consent form, and then make a presentation about them at a future IRB meeting. This individual will review the protocol and consent form carefully, usually over a period of several days or more. If any information in the protocol or consent form is unclear, the reviewer may contact the investigator for clarification.

Protocols are not presented to the IRB by the principal investigator because their presence could make it uncomfortable for IRB members to rigorously question and scrutinize the protocols put before them. IRB meetings are conducted privately. No outside observers are allowed to attend IRB meetings. Research investigators may attend IRB meetings to provide information, but they must leave the meeting during the discussion and approval or rejection of their study protocols.

At an IRB meeting, each member gives a presentation to the board members about the protocol(s) that they have been asked to review. The members of the board then have an opportunity to ask the reviewer questions about protocol and the consent form. These questions usually lead to a discussion among members of the group about issues that may affect the safety and ethical treatment of volunteers in the research study.

After IRB members have reviewed the protocol and consent form, and the group has had an opportunity to discuss any concerns, the members vote on whether to approve the protocol. Approval by a majority of the IRB members present at the meeting is necessary in order for the IRB to approve a protocol.

It is unusual for an IRB to withhold their approval of a protocol. It is more typical for the IRB to require modifications to a protocol so that the study can be conducted safely, ethically, and according to federal regulations. In these situations, the investigator is responsible for making changes that have been requested by the IRB before the protocol can be resubmitted for board approval. Typically, an IRB at a research institution, such as a university or hospital, meets every other week. Some IRBs meet more frequently. The meetings typically last two to three hours.

Once a protocol is approved by the IRB, the IRB sends the investigator a written notification of the approval. The research project is then permitted to proceed and to begin enrolling volunteers.

CHAPTER TEN

Historical Events that Have Shaped Study Participant Protection

During my first studies, I wasn't told very much. I didn't know what kind of medication I was on, where it came from, or anything. Now, doctors tell me how they're going to do the study, who and what they're doing it for, and the effects it might have on me—positive and negative. If I see something I don't like, I tell them I don't want to go any further.

Lillian, 20-year veteran of clinical trials

This chapter offers a brief overview of the evolution of human subject protections and highlights some important recent events. These protections have evolved in response to abuses and atrocities that were carried out against vulnerable members of our population, including children, prisoners, the mentally ill, and the poor.

For hundreds of years, children were typically recruited for scientific studies. They were easy to recruit precisely because they were vulnerable. This practice reached its most appalling point in Europe in the late 1930s, when children diagnosed with various defects were sometimes left to die because they were deemed too costly for the government to care for.

At the beginning of World War II, Germany was the most scientifically and technologically advanced country in the world and even had a proposed code of research ethics. In the field of medicine, the Nazi government supported midwifery, homeopathy, and nutrition programs as well as research into ecology, public health, human genetics, cancer, radiation, and asbestos. They were the first to ban smoking in public buildings. Women were denied tobacco ration coupons because of concern about the effect of nicotine on the fetus. German physicians stressed the importance of preventive medicine rather than curative medicine.

The Nazi party, however, exploited people's trust in the medical community and public health by performing unethical experiments and atrocities on populations they discriminated against. The German Air Force, for example, was concerned about the survival of pilots at extremely high altitudes. One question they wanted the answer to was: What was the maximum safe altitude for bailing out of a damaged aircraft? To answer this question, researchers designed a series of experiments involving internees at the Dachau concentration camp. In one series of experiments, researchers placed the victims in vacuum chambers that could duplicate the low air pressure and anoxia (lack of oxygen) at altitudes as high as 65,000 feet (about two to three times the maximum altitude that aircraft were flying). Approximately 200 internees at Dachau were used in these experiments, and about 40% died as a result. Some deaths were caused by extended anoxia; others were attributable to lungs rupturing from the low pressures in the chamber.

The German Air Force was also concerned with survival time after parachuting into the cold water of the North Atlantic. Some victims of this research were immersed for hours in tubs of ice water; others were fed nothing but salt water for days. Still others were penned outside, unclothed and unsheltered in sub-freezing temperatures for 12 to 14 hours. Some of these "freezing victims" were sprayed with cold water. No attempts were made to relieve the tremendous pain and suffering caused by these experiments. Approximately 33% or 100 out of 300 Dachau internees in these studies died.

Experiments involving battlefield medicine included treatment of gunshot wounds, burns, traumatic amputations and chemical and biological agent exposures. In these experiments, the wound was first inflicted upon the victim (by gunshot, stabbing, amputation, or other traumatic method) and then treated using various techniques. For example, in a study of sulfanilamide at the Ravensbrueck camp, Polish women were shot and slashed on the legs. The resulting wounds were stuffed with glass, dirt, and various bacteria cultures, and sewn shut. The infected wounds were then treated with experimental anti-infective agents.

Nazi experiments on treating exposure to chemical-warfare agents were ongoing throughout the war years. Concentration-camp internees were forced to drink poisoned water and to breathe noxious gases. Some were shot with cyanide-tipped bullets or given cyanide capsules. It was not uncommon for one out of every four internees in these studies to die as a result of their involvement in the experiments.

Representatives of the British, French, Soviet, and United States governments established the International Military Tribunal in Nuremberg, Germany, in 1945. After the initial Nuremberg Trial of Nazi leaders, a series of supplemental trials was held. The trial, officially known as United States v. Karl Brandt et al., and commonly referred to as "The Nazi Doctors Trial," was held from December 9, 1946, to July 19, 1947. As the title indicates, the judges and prosecutors in this court trial were all from the United States. The 23 defendants (including 20 physicians)—all members of the Nazi Party—were charged with murder, torture, and other atrocities committed in the name of medical science.

When the final judgment in the Nazi Doctors Trial was delivered on July 19, 1947, 15 of the 23 defendants were found guilty. Seven were sentenced to death. Four American judges presiding issued a ten-point code that described basic principles of ethical behavior in the conduct of human experimentation. This ten-point code is known as the Nuremberg Code. The Code is an "ethical standard" and reflects the modern thinking that:

1. Informed consent should be obtained without coercion.
2. The experiment should be useful and necessary.
3. Human experiments should be based on previous experiments with animals.
4. Physical and mental suffering should be avoided.
5. Death and disability should not be expected outcomes of an experiment.
6. The degree of risk to be taken should not exceed the humanitarian importance of solving the problem.
7. Human subjects should be protected against even remote possibilities of harm.
8. Only qualified scientists should conduct medical research.
9. Human subjects should be free to end an experiment at any time.

10. The scientist in charge must be prepared to end an experiment at any stage.

In 1953, the World Medical Association began drafting a document that became known as the Declaration of Helsinki. This statement of ethical principles, first issued in 1964, defined rules for "therapeutic" and "non-therapeutic" research. It repeated the Nuremberg Code requirement for consent for non-therapeutic research, but it did allow for enrolling certain patients in therapeutic research without consent. The Declaration of Helsinki also allowed legal guardians to grant permission to enroll subjects in research (both therapeutic and non-therapeutic) and recommended written consent—an issue not addressed in the Nuremberg Code. In addition, the Declaration of Helsinki required review and prior approval of a protocol by an IRB. The Declaration of Helsinki is included in the appendix for you to read.

In 1966, following the publication of the Declaration of Helsinki, Henry K. Beecher, M.D., reported in the New England Journal of Medicine (NEJM) on 22 studies that had serious ethical problems. Beecher cited various problems related to study design and to informed consent. Probably even more than the Nuremberg Trial and Code, this article (and his other earlier publications) helped to spur debate on research ethics throughout the United States.

As late as the 1960s, few research institutions had heeded requests by the NIH to set up a system for protecting research subjects. Numerous safeguards have since been added, many as a result of what is known as the "thalidomide tragedy." Thalidomide, approved as a sedative in Europe in the late 1950s, disfigured over 10,000 babies worldwide whose mothers took the drug during their first trimester of pregnancy. Congressional hearings in the United States revealed that women were not told the FDA hadn't approved the drug and that they weren't asked to give their consent. In 1962, the NDA for thalidomide was withdrawn by its U.S. manufacturer. The Kefauver-Harris Amendment was signed into law in 1962 and made the following demands on clinical trials:

- Proof of efficacy as well as safety
- Mandated reporting of adverse events
- Disclosure of risks in advertisements
- Required reproduction studies in two species of animal using two dose levels of drug

Long after the Nuremberg Code was announced and informed-consent laws were being issued and rewritten, human research subject protection was far from guaranteed. The Centers for Disease

Control and Prevention (a Department of Health and Human Services agency), for example, was actively overseeing an ongoing study that involved withholding treatment to more than 400 black sharecroppers diagnosed with syphilis. The experiment, then known as the Tuskegee Study of Untreated Syphilis in the Negro Male, began in 1932 and didn't end until 1972. In the beginning, the disease was untreatable and the prevailing belief was that it behaved differently in black than white men. The men involved were not told they had the disease, the purpose of the study, or the fact that the research would not benefit them. Even when penicillin was accepted as a treatment for syphilis, it was purposefully withheld from the study subjects. Not long after the story came to light in the *New York Times* and the *Washington Star*, the study stopped and the men—together with the wives and children who contracted the disease—were given free antibiotic treatment and lifetime medical care. But the damage to their health, as well as their trust in the medical research community, was beyond repair. In a formal White House ceremony in 1997, President Clinton apologized to subjects and their families who had participated in the Tuskegee Study, and called for renewed emphasis on research ethics.

Sadly, the list of historical abuses is long. Prisoners were routinely coerced into phase I safety testing of drugs until their use as study subjects began to be regulated in the late 1970s. In the 1940s and 1950s, the Atomic Energy Commission secretly fed people breakfast cereal containing radioactive tracers and intentionally released radioactive substances, while researchers at several major universities injected plutonium into unknowing patients to study the effects of the atomic bomb. Institutionalized patients in the 1960s became the victims of CIA brainwashing experiments with LSD. The U.S. Army carried out further experiments with the drug on soldiers as recently as 1970.

In 1974, Congress passed the National Research Act. The Act required regulations for the protection of human subjects that included requirements for informed consent and review of research by Institutional Review Boards (IRBs). IRBs were given the charge to conduct peer review of research involving human subjects. For the first time, individual physician investigators could not make decisions about the use of human volunteers in clinical research without being granted approval by colleagues in the medical community. This Act led to the creation of the National Commission for the Protection of Human Subjects of Biomedical and Behavioral Research. This commission was composed of 11 members, the majority of whom were individuals outside the medical community. Commission members included clergy, lawyers, ethicists, and philosophers. In 1979, the National Commission issued the Belmont Report, which is the cornerstone statement of ethical principles upon which the federal regulations for the protection of subjects are based.

In 1982, the Council for the International Organization of Medical Sciences (CIOMS) published the International Ethics Guidelines for Biomedical Research Involving Human Subjects (CIOMS Guidelines). These guidelines were designed to provide direction for researchers from technologically advanced countries when conducting research in developing countries. The guidelines sought to correct perceived omissions in the Nuremberg Code and the Declaration of Helsinki, especially as they applied to cross-cultural research. The CIOMS Guidelines address cultural differences in ethical standards.

Today, there are many overlapping layers of oversight and scrutiny by the FDA, by IRBs, and by pharmaceutical and biotechnology companies. The federal agency governing clinical drug trials is the FDA's Center for Drug Evaluation and Research (CDER) and, if federal funds are involved, the Office for Human Research Protections (OHRP). Either agency can temporarily—or permanently—end a study if it believes patient welfare is at risk.

Good Clinical Practice Guidelines

Government laws, regulations, and guidelines meant to protect the safety and rights of study volunteers, while ensuring the accuracy of collected study data, are collectively known as Good Clinical Practices (GCPs). These GCPs apply to many different groups, including drug companies and their employees, the contract review organizations that manage studies for them, Institutional Review Boards (IRBs), investigators, and all those who work at research centers.

GCPs essentially follow the Declaration of Helsinki. The latest, most controversial version of the Declaration holds that placebo-controlled trials should in general be used only in the absence of an existing, proven treatment. The change reflects growing fear that, without some type of prohibition, people in developing countries will be exposed to inferior treatments as research moves onto international soil. The World Medical Association recently issued a clarification, saying a placebo-controlled trial may be acceptable, even if an effective treatment is available, so long as it meets one of two conditions: either it must be scientifically necessary; or it has to be a study for a minor condition in which patients receiving the placebo face no more risk of serious harm than anyone else in the trial.

GCPs continue to recognize that placebo-controlled trials, in certain circumstances, constitute better science. It would be hard to make a case for a placebo-controlled study if, for example, the subjects are people with a life-threatening illness or a raging, deadly bacterial infection and are already taking an effective treatment. But it would be acceptable to test an investigational drug for a chronic illness against a placebo if the standard treatment is only mildly effective. Many researchers believe it is the only way to measure the true effects of drugs used for diseases like chronic fatigue syndrome and depression that have lots of "self-reported" symptoms like low energy or moodiness.

The Belmont Report

The ethical principles upon which human subject protection regulations are based appear in a formal document written in 1979 by the National Commission for the Protection of Human Subjects of Biomedical and Behavioral Research. The report outlines three fundamental principles: (1) Respect for Persons, (2) Beneficence, and (3) Justice.

Respect for Persons

The first principle basically states that individuals should be respected regardless of their age, race, gender, and socioeconomic status. This principle also recognizes that certain individuals are incapable of making decisions without the assistance of a guardian or caregiver.

Beneficence

This second principle means that the goal of research is to maximize the benefits of a drug under investigation while minimizing the risks to study subjects. Clinical trials should be properly designed to prevent harm—a primary responsibility of the principal investigators. This principle also means that the potential for risks must be justified by the greater good to society—a primary responsibility of the IRB.

Justice

The third principle means that the benefits and risks of research are shared fairly among different types of people. Regulations make both investigators and IRBs concerned about selecting sufficient numbers of men, women, children, and minorities as research subjects. It also makes them cautious when dealing with disadvantaged people—the poor, the sick, and the institutionalized—on matters of informed consent.

On April 18, 1979, the commission issued a report of its findings and recommendations. The document, called "The Belmont Report: Ethical Principles and Guidelines for the Protection of Human Subjects of Research," serves as the backbone of the Department of Health and Human Services (HHS) as well as Food and Drug Administration (FDA) regulations governing IRBs.

In 1991, a common set of regulations sprang from these three principles. Although this so-called "Common Rule" applies only to research conducted or paid for by federal agencies, similar FDA human subject protections govern all research with drugs, biologics and medical devices. Every clinical trial, therefore, requires review by an IRB, informed consent from study volunteers, and the signed promise of researchers and research sites to comply with human subject research laws.

An up-to-date, comprehensive list of patient protection guidelines is outlined in detail in the Code of Federal Regulations, and a 1991 revision to the Code spells out federal policy for human subject protection. A summary of the Code of Federal Regulations is provided in the appendix.

The Role of the FDA

The FDA reviews study protocols and study results. It regularly sends out inspectors to research centers to make sure that investigators are following the protocol, treating study volunteers well, maintaining the required records, and following standard operating procedures for conducting research. The FDA also inspects sites that it suspects have not followed Good Clinical Practice guidelines. Some investigations are sparked by complaints filed with the FDA by drug companies, IRBs, research staff members, and patients.

If fraudulent or deceptive practices are uncovered, investigators can be "blacklisted" by the FDA, preventing them from ever conducting clinical research. Principal investigators can be criminally prosecuted—meaning they can be fined, imprisoned, and/or have their medical license revoked.

The FDA also conducts routine and "for-cause" inspections of IRBs, study sponsors, and study monitors to be sure they are fulfilling all their responsibilities. Unless it has been newly formed, an established IRB may be visited once every five years if it is found to be fully compliant.

Regulations require that all adverse events associated with an investigational drug be reported to the FDA. Serious adverse events that occur during a clinical trial must be reported within seven days. If a study drug raises safety concerns, the FDA has the power to either halt the study or require the pharmaceutical company to conduct additional studies to answer questions about side effects and dosage levels. The FDA frequently instructs pharmaceutical companies to conduct a phase IV study as a condition of marketing their drug, which the companies usually do. The Food and Drug Administration Modernization Act requires the FDA to keep lists of these requests and track how well companies adhere to them. That gives the agency the power to enforce compliance.

Whether or not a drug eventually gets the FDA's stamp of approval to be sold is heavily based on the opinion of an advisory committee of scientists who review the study data. To ensure its opinion is unbiased, committee members who have any conflict of interest associated with the clinical trials or company whose product is being reviewed are excluded from these discussions.

Monitoring Clinical Trials

Pharmaceutical companies routinely send their own study monitors out to the research centers. Companies do this to be sure that they get good, accurate information about a study drug. And companies do this to ensure that study staff is complying with Good Clinical Practice guidelines. Pharmaceutical companies are very concerned that volunteers enrolled in studies actually meet the inclusion and exclusion criteria, as spelled out in the study protocol. The inclusion criteria may include an age range, such as ages 55 to 75, and a disease state or condition, such as "must be diagnosed with a specific type and stage of cancer." The exclusion criteria, or reasons you wouldn't be able to participate, might include if you are taking a certain type of medication or have a disease in addition to the one being studied. The list of inclusion and exclusion criteria is generally fairly long. An investigator who "qualifies" every person screened for a study would immediately draw suspicion and would himself be disqualified from participating in the study if breaches in protocol were detected.

Study monitors—also called clinical research associates (CRAs)—perform a variety of monitoring activities. The CRA's primary role is to help ensure that the investigator and study staff properly conduct the trial and accurately and efficiently collect the results. Study monitors interact regularly with the study staff and they are an important way that pharmaceutical companies promote quality and good clinical practices.

Pharmaceutical companies spend enormous sums developing medicines; it is estimated that companies spend more than $800 million for each drug that they successfully develop from discovery to approval. This estimate assumes that the cost of drugs that fail must be paid for by those drugs that succeed. With so many dollars invested, pharmaceutical companies are eager to learn about their drugs in clinical trials. They want to know about the successes and shortcomings of their investigational medications. Clinical-research professionals employed by pharmaceutical companies are scientists and people who want to know all of the facts—both positive and negative.

Pharmaceutical companies are businesses and one of their primary goals is to generate profits and satisfy their shareholders. But it is in a company's best interest to develop safe and effective drugs. Companies will have already invested hundreds of millions of dollars on any given drug before they even begin clinical trials for that drug. Unsafe drugs will halt their research and delay the approval process, resulting in the loss of significant investment. It is far less costly, over the long term, to quickly end a study and pay for any unintended injuries than to continue testing a marginal drug and risk greater loss.

Concerns about side effects by the FDA have caused pharmaceutical companies to abandon multi-million dollar projects just months before a medication was to make its debut on the market. If the side effect happens very infrequently, or there is question about whether it is even caused by the drug, the risk of having that side effect will instead be recorded and, upon approval of the drug by the FDA, be listed on the drug's label. Physicians would therefore be more cautious when prescribing the drug.

The Most Responsible Party: The Principal Investigator

Physicians get involved in clinical research for many reasons. For some, it's the desire to be on the "cutting edge" of medicine. For others, it's a break from the routine of day-to-day medical practice, the opportunity to become better at treating specific diseases, or simple intellectual curiosity. For still others, it's a way to avoid the restrictions on treatment choices imposed by some insurance companies. Some physicians do clinical studies, at least in part, to make money. Select investigators can earn tens to hundreds of thousands of dollars conducting clinical trials. But being the principal investigator in a clinical trial requires a major commitment, long hours, hard work, and a great deal of patience. It is reasonable that a physician be paid for the time that is dedicated to conducting clinical trials. Physician investigators must review and modify protocols, solicit IRB approval, explain a trial in detail to patients, determine which potential volunteers meet the eligibility criteria, perform required medical evaluations, and record and evaluate the findings. After covering the cost of a research nurse and additional testing, many investigators will spend more money than they earn. University-affiliated researchers, who are salaried, don't benefit directly from research profits, all of which get funneled to the institution. However, they can earn large sums of money lecturing about a drug at medical conferences. But even researchers who do studies mostly "for the money" have a powerful incentive to do it right. Failure to follow the rules will severely damage their reputation and almost guarantees that they'll never do another clinical trial again.

The principal investigator on every study is required to complete a "1572 Statement of Investigator Form" that the pharmaceutical company files with the FDA. In this form, the investigator promises to strictly adhere to Good Clinical Practice guidelines (GCPs) and the requirements of the protocol. The 1572 Form holds the principal investigator personally accountable for every aspect of the clinical trial. For example, GCPs forbid investigators from changing the study protocol unless a patient's safety is at stake. They demand that investigators explain the clinical trial clearly and honestly to study volunteers. The investigator is required to maintain accurate, detailed records for each and every volunteer. And the investigator is required to promptly report any unexpected or "serious" adverse events—including those that are fatal or life-threatening, permanently disabling, or that result in hospitalization—to the IRB and the sponsor company.

Recent Events

Conflicts of Interest Disclosure

Of growing public concern are clinical investigators who have a financial relationship with a commercial sponsor of a study. Influenced by a financial incentive, a doctor may—even if unwittingly—downplay risks or overstate benefits during informed-consent discussions. Being paid a per-participant "recruitment bonus" or a "finder's fee" for referral of potential participants may also color a doctor's judgment or willingness to report adverse reactions and even his or her analysis of research data.

The FDA keeps an especially close watch on clinical investigators with a reported conflict of interest to ensure that conflict doesn't influence your enrollment in a clinical trial or the data collection methods. In fact, the FDA has had regulations requiring "financial disclosure" for investigators since 1998. But this information has typically only been reported to the FDA—not to study volunteers.

In the past, if an investigator had a financial interest in an investigational drug or the pharmaceutical company sponsoring the research, study participants would typically not hear about it. Under the new Sunshine Act, which went into effect in August 2013, potential conflicts of interest must be far more transparent to professionals, patients, and the public as health providers, drug manufacturers, and purchasers must report payments or gifts of $10 or more made to physicians or hospitals (with some exceptions including educational materials) as well as ownership interests. The Sunshine Act, part of the Patient Protection and Affordable Care Act (PPACA), requires manufacturers to submit to the federal government detailed listings of payments—including those associated with clinical research studies—and other "transfers of value" made to physicians once a year. The detailed listings are to be placed on a website accessible to the public. The first detailed reports were submitted on March 31, 2014.

Academic research sites are increasingly and voluntarily making financial conflict-of-interest disclosures about their investigators within informed consent documents. Some of this response is due to well-publicized cases of conflicts of interest as well as several revealing articles published in peer-review journals. In one article published in 2007, researchers at Harvard University's Institute for Health Policy found that 94% of physicians reported having a relationship with the pharmaceutical industry. 78% reported regularly receiving drug samples, and 35% reported receiving fees for consulting and lecturing.

Many academic institutions exclude IRB members from decision-making on protocols for which they have a potential or actual financial conflict of interest. Some, but not all, institutions have a policy against accepting funding from pharmaceutical companies in which their investigators have a financial interest.

The Department of Health and Human Services (HHS) released a guidance paper in May 2000 hoping to promote "openness and honesty" on the part of study sponsors, institutions, and investigators. Specifically, the guidance cites the usefulness of a Conflict of Interest Committee—alone or together with the IRB—in managing conflicts. The guidance also notes the wisdom of freeing IRBs from pressures (real or perceived) to okay research activities in which its affiliated institution has a financial stake or other interest in the outcome of the research.

If the research institution itself has a financial stake in the outcome of a trial, HHS suggests that the institution either set up "special safeguards" to protect the scientific integrity of the study and its participants or to let the trial be carried out elsewhere. A financial stake may be anything from an additional upfront payment for carrying out a protocol to part ownership in the pharmaceutical or biotechnology company sponsoring the study.

In a later "final guidance document" published in May 2004, HHS recommends that IRBs, institutions, and investigators consider whether specific financial relationships create financial interests in research studies that may adversely affect the rights and welfare of subjects. Suggested actions for mitigating the impact of conflicts include separating the responsibilities of research activities and financial interests within institutions; establishing conflict-of-interest committees; and setting criteria to determine what constitutes conflict of interest. Among other recommendations were reminding IRB members of conflict-of-interest policies and including in the informed-consent document information such as the source of funding for the research and financial arrangements of institutions or investigators.

Recent steps have been taken to improve oversight and monitoring of conflicts of interest including the National Institutes of Health's inclusion of a review during visits to institutions. Also, FDA now lists the review of financial disclosures in its guidance to reviewers of drug-marketing applications.

Some institutions and independent researchers have established policies against accepting special "payment incentives" from drug companies for recruiting volunteers or referring patients to investigators. Such payments aren't specifically prohibited by federal regulations, but they are on the list of items scrutinized by IRBs. They may also run afoul of certain state medical licensing board regulations and the strict standards of practice set by the American Medical Association against the payment of referral fees. Ethically, incentive fees aren't necessarily a problem. It all depends on why the special fees are being paid. Is the money meant to cover the time needed to fill in special paperwork, prepare a report, or to do preliminary data analysis? Or is it simply to pass on names? These are questions worth asking—especially of doctors who seem anxious to sign up patients for trials.

There is as yet no agreement about how much study investigators should be paid per enrolled subject. Ethicists worry that if the payment per study volunteer is excessive, investigators' financial interests could compromise their judgment of who should and who shouldn't be asked to participate. There are several ways to weed out potential conflicts of interest in your clinical trial: First, if an investigator suggests that you participate in a clinical trial, among the questions you should ask is how he or she is compensated for enrolling patients into the trial. Your investigator should be paid for those services by the company sponsoring the clinical trial just as your insurance company would pay for the doctor's time if he or she were giving you an annual physical exam or treating your illness.

If the payment your investigator receives for enrolling you in a clinical trial is substantially more than the payment he or she would receive for treating your illness, this may indicate a conflict. Compensation should also be limited to payment for services. If the investigator or study staff is paid a special bonus simply for enrolling volunteers into the study (in addition to payment for the services provided during the study) this may also signal a conflict.

Clinical researchers can benefit in ways other than direct compensation. For example, if the investigator developed the new therapy under investigation, then he or she may stand to benefit financially once the product reaches the market. Similarly, if the investigator holds stock or part ownership in the company developing the investigational drug or device, the researcher may benefit financially. The lure of profits from the eventual success of an experimental product can unduly influence an investigator to enroll volunteers in clinical studies so that the product can be brought to market as quickly as possible.

Before you agree to participate in a clinical trial, you will want to be confident that the principal investigator is recommending the trial for the right reasons. Discuss ahead of time how your doctor is being compensated for his or her role in the clinical trial. Try to find out if there are other incentives that could be influencing his or her recommendation. If you think your doctor may have a potential conflict of interest, run the information by a physician you trust and ask his or her opinion, or contact the IRB.

Patient Privacy and Safety

In January 2013, the department of Health and Human Services (HHS) approved a new rule to improve and strengthen patient-privacy protections initially established under HIPAA—the Health Insurance Portability and Accountability Act. The new rule went into effect in March 2013 and addresses a number of recent trends in health care and clinical research that impact patients.

One key change is that patients can now request copies of their electronic health records (EHR) and their personal health information (PHI) in digital formats. If this information is not available in a digital format, patients can request an alternative format. Under the new rule, patients can also restrict what personal health information is disclosed to health insurance providers including Medicare, retail pharmacies, and labs.

Although patients and their families give their consent for tissue and genetic samples to be used in future research, there are still cases when patients and their families are not asked for permission. Specifically, research conducted during an emergency medical treatment leaves little to no time for patients and their family to give their consent. Research conducted during emergencies can be invaluable in helping health professionals determine how to care for patients with life-threatening injuries.

In 1996, HHS and the FDA passed regulation that allowed research in emergency situations to occur without requiring patient consent. Since 2010, there has been growing pressure to change this regulation. Much can be attributed to the book *The Immortal Life of Henrietta Lacks*, published in 2010, by Rebecca Skloot. The book told the amazing story of a poor black tobacco farmer whose cancer cells were taken without her knowledge or consent in 1951. These "HeLa" cells became one of the most important aids to laboratories around the world in developing the polio vaccine, cancer treatments, gene mapping, and in-vitro fertilization. Henrietta's cells have generated billions of dollars in medical treatments and advances, yet she remains virtually unknown and her family can't afford health insurance.

Looking ahead at the near future, HHS and the FDA are expected to explore new ways to ensure that patients and their families are better informed and given opportunities to provide their permission.

New Safety Standards

There are many national programs that offer their seal of approval—or accreditation—of programs, institutions and organizations that conduct human trials. These programs offer patients and study volunteers reassurances that regulatory requirements are being met.

The Association of American Medical Colleges (AAMC), together with a variety of other academic organizations, launched the

Association for the Accreditation of Human Research Protection Programs (AAHRPP) in 2002. This voluntary, education-oriented accreditation program goes beyond current regulations to collectively examine the performance of the research organization, investigators, and the IRB. Since its founding, AAHRPP has accredited 182 institutions and organizations nationwide.

Some investigators and study coordinators seek certification on their own. The Association of Clinical Research Professionals (ACRP) certifies and renews certification for hundreds of principal investigators and study coordinators every year. Certification offers some assurance that these individuals are knowledgeable in good clinical practices and the regulations to protect research subjects. In March 2009, the FDA in collaboration with the Clinical Trials Transformation Initiative and the Critical Path Initiative launched a new intensive clinical investigator training program.

On July 19, 2012, the FDA signed the Safety and Innovation Act (FDASIA) into law. This Act touches on many areas including expediting generic drug and medical-device review times and expanding post-marketing surveillance. Most notably, FDASIA reauthorized and expanded the agency's ability to collect fees from industry to fund FDA reviews of new drugs, medical devices, generic drugs, and biosimilars (i.e., generic biologics). At the present time, the FDA receives a substantial amount of funding from industry—more than half a billion dollars annually—in funding from pharmaceutical, biotechnology, and medical-device companies.

FDASIA also streamlined the approval process for drugs targeting "serious or life-threatening" conditions. It also gave the FDA the authority to designate a new drug candidate as a "breakthrough therapy" if early clinical evidence indicated that the drug demonstrated substantial improvement over existing therapies for serious or life-threatening conditions. If and when a drug is classified as a breakthrough therapy, the FDA will work closely with the drug manufacturer to expedite development and review.

Transparency of Clinical Trial Results

Studies have shown consistently that the vast majority (90%) of all study volunteers want to receive the results of their clinical trial. Studies have also shown that principal investigators and research center staff want to provide trial results to their patients. The Declaration of Helsinki and federal regulations (FDAAA 2007) obligate pharmaceutical, biotechnology, and medical-device companies to publicly post clinical trial results online when the drug or device is approved, or within a year of study completion.

The law specifically requires pharmaceutical and biotechnology companies to disclose phase II–IV clinical trial results summaries, whether the results are conclusive or inconclusive, published or not. The mandate stipulates that failure to comply may result in a substantial civil penalty of up to $10,000 per day or the withholding of NIH grant funding if noncompliance remains uncorrected thirty days after the violation has been cited. Research sponsors are permitted to delay reporting results for up to three years for clinical trials conducted before drugs are initially approved and for studies of unapproved new clinical indications for those drugs already approved.

Most research sponsors are complying with the law and they are posting technical summaries. Nevertheless, these companies are not routinely communicating clinical trial results in understandable, lay language to study volunteers and patients.

In an effort to improve disclosure and enforce transparency of clinical trial results information, the Food and Drug Administration (FDA) adopted new regulations in March 2011, requiring informed consent forms to include a statement indicating that data from the clinical trial has been or will be entered into the ClinicalTrials.gov registry. The FDA enforces this rule for informed consent documents that are initiated on or after March 7, 2012.

Since 2011, the Center for Information and Study on Clinical Research Participation (CISCRP) has been working closely with nearly three dozen pharmaceutical and biotechnology companies to develop patient-friendly summaries of clinical-trial results for study volunteers worldwide. These non-technical, lay-language summaries are sent to investigative sites who distribute the summaries directly to study volunteers. Since its introduction, the CISCRP clinical trial results communication program has demonstrated marked improvement in study volunteer comprehension of and satisfaction participating in clinical trials.

Given regulatory mandate and growing public interest in disclosing clinical trial results to study volunteers, within the next five years it is likely that pharmaceutical and biotechnology companies will be routinely providing clinical trial results to their study volunteers around the world. During the next several years, research sponsors will primarily provide general findings. But in the future, as communication technologies improve and disclosure requirements expand, research sponsors will likely be piloting efforts to communicate patient-specific study findings and customized feedback to study volunteers.

Compassionate Use

In 2007, FDAAA 1997 was amended in part to improve patient access to investigational drugs. The draft Expanded Access to Investigational Drugs for Treatment Use guidance states that compassionate use for patients not participating or no longer participating in clinical trials and with no other alternative for treatment of a life-threatening condition or disease must be reviewed and approved by an IRB. The FDA encourages the use of central IRBs for review of expanded access cases in order to facilitate faster patient access. The draft guidance completed the comment period in July 2013 and will likely go into effect in 2015.

What You Don't Know Can Hurt You

One area of "misconduct" during clinical trials that has not been addressed is the underreporting of patient deaths and adverse events to federal regulators. It's human nature to avoid responsibility for hurting others, and easy for investigators to place the blame for a bad outcome on an underlying illness or the frailty of a study subject rather than the study drug. So adverse events, when they happen, tend to get underreported and misunderstood. That leaves doctors with a false sense of security about using certain drugs and patients with an incomplete picture about the risk of taking them. Since 2012, the Veterans' Administration and some academic institutions have made efforts to improve their adverse-event reporting policies.

Bioethicists are especially concerned about government-funded studies because of the absence of monitoring by pharmaceutical companies. These studies often take place at a relatively small number of research centers, reducing the number of clinical opinions about whether an adverse event is related to the investigational medicine. IRB members have also had trouble coping with the responsibility of monitoring adverse events that occur during hundreds, if not thousands, of trials at individual institutions each year.

Between 1990 and 2000, "thousands of deaths and tens of thousands of adverse events" during NIH-sponsored clinical trials went unreported to the OHRP, according to Adil Shamoo, editor-in-chief of the journal *Accountability in Research* at the University of Maryland School of Medicine. Part of the explanation may be that only "unexpected" bad effects are reportable. Also, some investigators only report problems that they consider serious and study-related. Perhaps more disturbing is that a significant amount of human research has limited oversight because it isn't sponsored by a drug or device manufacturer and doesn't receive federal funds. Some human studies are also done before an "investigational new drug" application is filed with the FDA.

Shamoo has been a steadfast advocate of the need for better reporting of adverse events through standardized reporting, development of a national database, tracking trends and safety profiles, and a single federal oversight and management agency. Currently, adverse-event reporting happens disjointedly between the FDA and OHRP, and informed consent discussions generally fail to communicate actual adverse event risks. For federally-funded research, reporting requirements are at best vague, he said. With the FDA, problems arise because there is a confusing patchwork of requirements related to adverse-event reporting that differ "as to whom it should be reported and the timeframe for reporting." (*DIA Today*, April 2005) The FDA, together with the National Institutes of Health, took a positive first step with the 2004 launch of a web database for the reporting and monitoring of adverse reactions in gene-transfer research.

Paul Gelsinger, vice president of Citizens for Responsible Care and Research (CIRCARE), strongly believes the current system for protecting humans in research is ineffective. Because of the failure of investigators to report unanticipated serious adverse events, IRBs are prevented from minimizing risks to human subjects. CIRCARE is calling for a handful of national reforms, including: safeguards for human subjects "at least equal to" those provided to laboratory animals; better protection of vulnerable subjects; "real-time" oversight by the OHRP with the addition of unannounced visits and random audits of research sites; a toll-free hotline number for anonymous reporting of potential violations; and an improved informed consent process that is witnessed by an independent party and videotaped. Based on a review of several hundred new drug applications sponsored by industry and approved by the FDA, CenterWatch found a high incidence of adverse events across all disease categories—an average of one adverse event reported for every volunteer. But these events include many minor complaints like headache and diarrhea, some of which investigators couldn't even connect to the study drug.

Among study volunteers, CenterWatch estimates that the chances of dying due to an investigational drug during a clinical trial are low. Approximately one out of every 10,000 volunteers dies in a clinical trial. "That's on par with the odds of a mother dying while giving birth to a single child," according to John Paling, M.D., a risk communication consultant in Gainesville, FL. The risk probably isn't a bad tradeoff—at least when measured against the possibility of significant benefit, like relief from constant and debilitating pain or an extended lifetime.

The odds of your having a serious adverse event—any reaction that may be fatal, life-threatening, permanently disabling or that results in hospitalization—are one in 30. But keep in mind that the majority of these events happen in trials for people with cancer, heart disease, and immunology/infectious diseases like AIDS. Volunteers may be willing to take drugs that are likely to have unpleasant side effects because the alternative is worse: almost certain death.

No one knows how risky trials are that never make it past the early phases of testing. But it is very likely that there will be more benefit than harm by the time a drug reaches phase III trials, said Joseph Lau, M.D., professor of medicine at Brown University. The problem remains that there is no one place to go for comprehensive adverse event and death information and no independent observer making sure the reporting is accurate.

Then there's the problem of what the numbers mean. Most people simply trust the judgment of the investigator and the study staff. Most volunteers assume that they have their best interests in mind. Theoretically, the most important decision-making information—namely, the relative risk of taking a particular drug at a certain dose and specific time and setting—should be divulged during the informed-consent process. But "investigators have a conflict of interest," said Leonard Glantz, professor of health law at Boston University School of Public Health. "They want people to be in a study." Someone other than the investigator ought to be talking to potential volunteers. Even consent forms may subtly understate the risks of participation, or may mislead readers with scientific jargon.

Clinical trials are simply getting too complex for all information to flow from a single investigator, said Myrl Weinberg, president of the National Health Council in Washington, D.C. The best way for patients to understand both the benefits and risks of participation is to get the message through multiple communication vehicles—written words, dialogue, and videos—and more than one person. In practice, this rarely happens. Until it does, many research subjects will remain uninformed about the true risk of their participation.

There are inescapable conflicts between medical practice—where the aim is to heal—and medical research—where the goal is to learn. That's a difficult, but very important, thing to remember when an investigator is also a study participant's personal physician, social worker, or teacher. The line between practice and research can get very blurry when both happen at the same time. Some diabetics, for example, might get treated as patients for blood sugar, receive foot examinations, and get treated as study participants during blood pressure readings and surveys connected with an investigational hypertension drug they're taking—all within the same visit.

Your doctors' main intent is to gather information when they are wearing their "research-investigator" hat and to enhance your well-being when they're wearing their "doctor" hat. The aim of some study protocols, after all, is to induce symptoms (often by taking patients off their current prescription) so that the effect of the investigational medication can be measured. Clinical research might best be likened to a journey down a new, unexplored, and potentially dangerous path. As pioneering medical ethicist Paul Ramsey once said, investigators need to ask study participants to be "co-adventurers" with them on that journey.

CHAPTER ELEVEN

Considerations for Special Populations

"The study coordinator told him he may experience reactions to the medicine, so he would constantly say, 'I have a stomachache.' It was like he thought we were looking for him to get a stomachache and wanted to please us. It was amazing how he'd come to me and say, 'I have a fever,' and I'd say, 'No you don't,' and he'd then say, 'Oh, I meant a stomachache.' He'd come up with some reactions we didn't even talk about. We used the cough medicine once, but I was never sure if it was a forced or real cough."

Cathy, mother of Josh, a pediatric subject in a cold remedy trial

For many years, research with children and pregnant women was virtually nonexistent. People living in prisons and institutions, who could not fully participate in the consent process, were disproportionately overrepresented. These vulnerable populations are now given special consideration and, in some cases, extra protection from the federal government.

Children

Only a small fraction of all prescription drugs marketed in the United States come with instructions on the proper dosage to give children and even some of those don't come in a liquid or chewable form. This can make administering treatment to children difficult—almost like a guessing game. If a medicine isn't labeled for children, pediatricians will usually prescribe a dose based on a child's weight. But they never know exactly how effective or safe the drug is when given in a smaller dose to a smaller person.

FDA data from studies conducted in the past has shown that, when compared to actual study data, the "expert opinion" of pediatricians is correct only two-thirds of the time. Wrong doses, bad outcomes, and unexpected toxicity and interactions are relatively commonplace. An important lesson has become increasingly clear: Medications need to be dispensed to children at far different doses than pediatricians might have assumed.

Researchers are learning that children's age can have a big effect on how they handle a drug. So can their gender, both because of differences in size and body composition and changes that accompany puberty in girls. Simply reducing the adult dose, therefore, is not a medically sound idea.

Pediatric studies of a popular drug for epilepsy, for example, found that some children react with aggressive behavior—an adverse event not seen in studies on adults. The drug had to be given at a higher-than-expected dose to be effective in kids under the age of five. A similar discovery was made about an adult anti-depression medication used to treat obsessive-compulsive disorder in kids. When prescribed on a per-weight basis, adolescents were being given a dose that was too low. Conversely, girls ages eight to 11 were routinely being given a dose that was too high. It has also been found that some children need higher or more frequent doses (and sometimes both) of several important antibiotics, including penicillin.

Antidepressant drugs, as a whole, were recently found to increase the risk of suicidal thinking and behavior in children and adolescents with psychiatric disorders, prompting the FDA to require the drugs' manufacturers to make labeling changes with expanded warning statements to alert healthcare providers. These warnings include a statement regarding whether the drug is FDA-approved specifically for pediatric illnesses and, if so, which ones. Patient information sheets are also now provided directly to patients and their families and caregivers by pharmacists.

During the past decade, the Food and Drug Administration has added and expanded its regulation of medical therapies to help ensure that doctors get the information they need to appropriately and safely prescribe new medications to kids. Pharmaceutical companies paid little attention to testing their drugs in children because doctors were already prescribing them—off-label—to youngsters. Almost all pediatric studies were funded by the U.S. government, and children in those trials were protected under regulations developed during the 1970s and 1980s.

Since the late 1990s, the FDA has had multiple "pediatric rules," including one that required pediatric clinical trials be conducted for all new medications that will—or could potentially—be used to treat conditions or diseases in children. A judge struck down that rule stating that the FDA lacked the "authority" to demand pediatric studies. That decision prompted passage of the Pediatric Research Equity Act in December, 2003, giving the FDA the authority to require pediatric studies, defer them, or say they are not necessary. It also requires that such studies do not delay adult drug development. The legislation also established an FDA Office of Pediatric Therapeutics and a Pediatric Advisory Committee to monitor and oversee the growing number of pediatric studies.

The Pediatric Exclusivity portion of the FDA Modernization Act of 1997 (FDAMA) prompted pharmaceutical companies to voluntarily put about 165 medicines and vaccines in clinical trials involving pediatric volunteers. The law allowed pharmaceutical companies to extend patent protection on existing drugs by doing safety and dosing studies with children. Extending patent protection gives companies the opportunity to generate more sales without competition. Dozens of clinical research studies have already been completed on critical drugs used to treat a variety of conditions like gastroesophageal reflux disease, diabetes, pain, asthma, and hypertension.

FDAMA was allowed to sunset, but pediatric exclusivity was reestablished in January 2002 with passage of the Best Pharmaceuticals for Children Act (BPCA). The law was designed to ensure that many more drugs already on the market will continue to be carefully studied in children. It not only gives pharmaceutical companies longer patent protection in exchange for conducting pediatric studies; it requires them to share what they learn as a result of those studies, good or bad. For some older drugs whose patent has expired—meaning that generic versions of the drug are allowed to be produced—the FDA "requests" that the manufacturer conduct pediatric studies.

Because of the BPCA, information available on ClinicalTrials.gov now includes a description of whether, and through what procedure, the sponsor of the research will respond to requests for access to therapy outside of the clinical trial setting, particularly in children. This type of treatment information is especially important for young patients with serious or life-threatening diseases.

In 2007, Section IV of the Food and Drug Administration Amendments Act (FDAAA) reauthorized the Pediatric Research Equity Act and added new requirements including the creation of the Pediatric Review Committee (PeRC). This oversight body initially conducted reviews of pediatric assessments performed between 2003 and 2007. On July 9, 2012, the FDA Safety and Innovation Act (FDASIA) was signed into law and for the first time, the PREA began requiring sponsors to submit a pediatric study plan (PSP) early in the investigation new drug (IND) application phase to the FDA.

Today, the FDA will not even approve products for use in adults until pharmaceutical companies have shared their plans for studying the same drugs in children. The exceptions are for drugs that treat adult diseases, such as prostate cancer, and drugs that are used to treat conditions that manifest differently in adults than in children.

The push is now on to get pediatric cancer drugs to market more quickly. In 2005, for the first time, the FDA gave fast-track approval for a cancer drug for children to begin selling even before testing in adults is finished—a trend that Philip Walson, M.D., a pediatric clinical pharmacologist at Cincinnati Children's Hospital expects will continue. "Essentially all children with tumors are in trials, compared to only 3% to 5% of adults," he said. "That is why pediatric tumor survival improvement so far outshines adult advances." But it will take more novel approaches to help the hardest-to-treat children.

The pediatric market has represented a new growth area for pharmaceutical and biotechnology companies during the past ten years. According to the Pharmaceutical Research and Manufacturers of America association, in 2012 there were more than 300 drugs in clinical trials specifically for children—30% more than the total number of drugs in 2006.

Total number of drugs in clinical trials for children

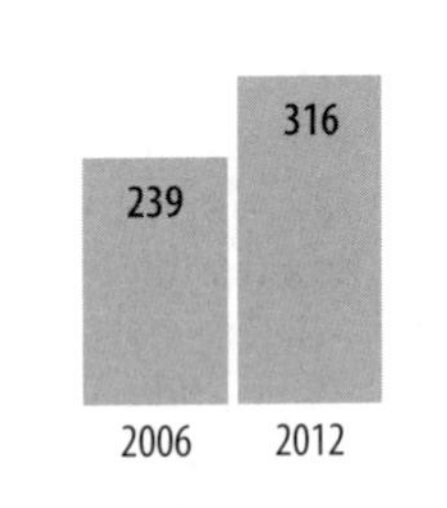

Source: Pharmaceutical Research & Manufacturers of America

Increasing numbers of children are needed to participate in clinical trials. Their involvement, however, creates a whole new set of concerns and issues. Because of their size, as well as their legal inability to consent to what happens to them, they are the most vulnerable of all vulnerable populations. Is it safe to expose children to potentially harmful procedures and unknown side effects? Are children more easily coerced to participate in clinical trials with the promise of cash, toys, and attention? The answers to these issues aren't as clear as parents and researchers would like. It's one thing for parents to enroll their children in studies that could save their life, especially if there are no other options. It's quite another to enroll them for treatment of a cold and flu, or routine ear infections for which there are already available medications.

Children's safety in clinical trials of all types has been exceedingly well protected by federal rules laid out over the past two decades. Until recently, federal protections were so strict that pharmaceutical companies were prohibited from labeling products with known information unless at least two adequate, scientific studies were done. With the exception of clinical trials specifically designed to modify a package insert, pediatric research findings have never translated into prescribing recommendations on medication labels, said Walson. A child's every encounter with a doctor, therefore, became "an uncontrolled experiment" since so few objective, scientific data were readily available to make decisions.

Although the general principles of respect, justice, and beneficence apply to clinical trials enrolling children, at least three significant differences from adult studies exist that are not widely enough known or appreciated, said Steve Hirschfeld, M.D., Ph.D., a medical officer with the FDA. For starters, "the metabolism of children changes with age and developmental stage. A premature infant is different from a 12-month-old, who is in turn different from a 3-year-old, a 6-year-old, or a 12-year-old child." Thus, to completely understand the pediatric use of a new therapy may require enrolling enough children of different ages in a clinical study and doing appropriate measurements of the effect in each age group.

Secondly, interest in conducting pediatric research exceeds the number of research centers with sufficiently trained personnel to get credible results. Most clinical trials, for example, involve blood sampling to watch the effects of an investigational drug on the body. But a child's small body size limits the amount of blood that can be taken to no more than about one-third of a teaspoon—six times less than normally would be taken from an adult. Processing smaller volumes of blood requires special machinery and specially trained staff, which many research sites do not have. Even some hospital emergency rooms lack such expertise, Hirschfeld noted.

Research sites also need to create an environment where a child feels comfortable. Those that specialize in pediatric research have people in their playrooms trained to show children how different procedures are done and get them used to the idea of undergoing the procedures themselves. It's called "medical play" and is credited with helping to make the clinical trial experience for children fun and interesting, said Hirschfeld. It also helps children better understand that the research process is partially, if not solely, about helping other children.

Thirdly, pediatric research, unlike research with adults, never fits the "ideal" situation for the protection of the study subject, continued Hirschfeld. Ideally, "the same person who takes on the risk accrues the benefit and gives consent. In reality, the child always takes the risk, may not accrue a benefit, and never is able to consent to participate in a study."

To ensure a child is protected, the principal investigator should not be an investor in or principal of a company sponsoring the research, hold the patent on the product, or have any other real or perceived conflict of interest. "If the investigator is the same physician who takes care of a child's other health needs, another doctor should be given the job of monitoring the study to maintain separation of roles and avoid any conflict of interest," Hirschfeld said.

For federally funded research, the Department of Health and Human Services (HHS) has set forth standards by which institutional review boards (IRBs) can determine if proposed pediatric clinical trials can be safely and ethically conducted. For research involving FDA-related products not covered by the HHS regulations, the FDA has adopted similar regulations. One of the key points is that kids that are capable (usually considered to be 6 years or older) should assent to participate in a clinical trial—basically, to say they agree to do it—and their parents or guardians should give fully informed permission for them to do so. "Technically, consent can only be provided by the person agreeing to participate in a study and that person must be of majority age in the jurisdiction where the study takes place," said Hirschfeld. "If a patient has a parent or guardian and the patient is unable to legally provide consent, then the parent or guardian gives permission to participate in a study."

Recruitment of study participants using "coercive inducements"—financial or otherwise—is deemed inappropriate. "However," Hirschfeld added, "if compensation for time, travel expenses, and a modest token of appreciation for participation in a study are offered, that can be considered acceptable." But not all studies provide compensation.

NIH-funded AIDS treatment trials over the past two decades have generated fresh debate about who provides consent for participants who are children in foster care. Laws on the matter vary greatly from state to state. In a few states, foster children are allowed to participate in studies with oversight by an independent advocate to help prevent even the appearance of unethical behavior. Since 1983, the federal government has also provided special protections for child wards, including independent advocates for any foster child enrolled in a narrow class of studies that involve greater-than-minimal risk and lack the promise of direct benefit.

The Office of Human Research Protections (OHRP) recently investigated the practice of using foster children in four AIDS experiments at New York Presbyterian Hospital/Columbia University Medical Center (NYPH/CUMC). In a May 2005 letter, OHRP stated that Columbia's IRB failed to obtain sufficient information to properly approve the research and ensure the children's rights and welfare were safeguarded. It required NYPH/CUMC to submit detailed corrective actions, which had already begun, but did not reprimand the facilities for failing to appoint advocates. To date, it is the only such OHRP case. Properly assessing risk in pediatric trials may never be a perfect science because there are so many variables to consider. But both the FDA and OHRP have been publishing extensive guidance to help IRBs do the best possible job of protecting children involved in clinical trials.

Federal regulations essentially place most pediatric research in one of three risk categories. If the risk is no different than what a healthy child would encounter in daily life, the research is considered to be of minimal risk. But some medical experts believe this standard can create a false sense of security: the daily risk the average child faces is fairly high due to factors including participation in sports and automobile accidents.

Currently, additional safeguards are required only for studies involving greater-than-everyday risk. In the eyes of the FDA, a child is not a "research subject" but a "patient," said Hirschfeld. That's because of the overriding belief that normal and healthy children should not be in research studies. "They're for children who have a disease, are likely to get a disease, or have just recovered from it." A good example would be an epileptic child on an anti-convulsive medication who wants to try a new drug.

Studies posing more-than-minimal risk beg the question: Will there be any benefit to the child? "If benefits are likely to occur to the patient participating in the study, then additional safety monitoring based on the perceived risk should be instituted, an IRB must approve the study, the parents or guardians must be fully informed and give permission, and the patient, if capable, should provide assent," said Hirschfeld. If benefits are considered unlikely, the parents or guardians need to understand that the child would need to go into a trial with the idea that he won't necessarily feel better but other children with the same condition, one day, might. "Just as in the circumstance when direct benefit can be expected, an IRB must determine that all appropriate safety monitoring is in place, the parents or guardians are fully informed, and that the child, if capable, has assented to participate." The child's medical condition may benefit in any type of study from the careful observation that occurs during a study and result in improved understanding of the disease for the patient and the parents or guardians.

IRBs are expected to consider a host of other factors before allowing a pediatric study to proceed, including the need for the study. If the investigational medicine will be treating a serious condition without good alternative therapies, for example, the study would probably be viewed as somewhat urgent. The IRB would look at any pediatric safety concerns about the drug, often based on the experience of adult patients. The formulation—liquid, suspensions, chewable tablets—would also have to make sense for the age of the children for whom it is intended.

Specific Questions Every Parent Should Ask About Pediatric Clinical Trials

- Does the study need to be done? If the necessary information can be gleaned from studies with adults or on animals, is there a need to put children at risk?
- What are the obligations and expectations for child volunteers?
- Are overnight stays in a hospital required?
- Is a diary required?
- How many visits to the research center are required? How often are the visits?
- What adverse event or other type of discomfort has to happen for my child to be removed from the study? If that happens, will some alternative therapy be offered?
- Are there "study-stopping rules" regarding what might prematurely end the entire study? What safety-related events, or frequency of adverse events, would close the study?
- Will study results be reviewed periodically by an independent third party?
- Are there any alternative clinical trials under way?

As a practical matter, research sites and IRBs try to seek out study protocols that have therapeutic value and may actually help a child get better. They try to avoid protocols that are "invasive," such as requiring tubes to be run from the nose to the stomach or an unnecessarily high number of blood draws. They also attempt to minimize the overall number of study participants needed. Any number of strategies may be employed to make the whole experience less distressing to children. These include conducting studies in health settings where they normally receive their care, providing age-appropriate furniture and play equipment in study areas, and using research staff who are accustomed to performing pediatric procedures.

Whether or not placebo-controlled trials are appropriate for children is a matter of some debate. But the FDA's pediatric advisors, as well as a group of medical ethicists and international experts, agreed that they're acceptable if there are no approved or adequately studied treatments for children with the condition under study. A placebo study does not mean a child receiving the placebo gets no treatment, but rather that the experimental therapy is not given to every patient. Several strategies can be used, such as:

- Patients can be provided standard care with or without the new drug (an "add-on study");
- Patients may receive the new drug and then have it removed (a "withdrawal study"); or
- Patients may receive various combinations of drugs and only some combinations have the new drug.

For serious or life-threatening conditions, special monitoring is recommended along with "study-stopping rules" for investigational drugs that prove to be either too risky or unquestionably effective and would not need further testing. Even for minor illnesses and conditions with symptoms, studies should be designed to minimize exposure to ineffective treatment.

The ways pediatric studies are developed and designed vary by the age category of patients needed. A clinical trial involving preterm newborns, for instance, would have the input of neonatologists and neonatal pharmacologists because of the unique way their tiny bodies, with their immature organs and small volume of circulating blood, respond to drugs. A study on toddlers would have to consider the great variation in maturity level from child to child. In older children, protocols need to measure the impact of a medicinal product on growth and development. They also need to allow for needed dosage changes once they hit puberty, which can affect the way drugs are broken down by the body.

The hormonal changes associated with puberty can influence the behavior of patients and their diseases and, consequently, the findings of clinical studies. Recreational drug use and noncompliance—forgetting to take a drug as instructed or an unwillingness to show up for important tests and visits—are also factors that have to be carefully and thoughtfully planned for.

With few exceptions, such as treatments for cancer or other life-threatening illnesses, most investigational products are not studied in children until they reach later phases of clinical development, or are already being marketed for the same disease in adults. This is a consequence of both international regulatory guidance and the objectives of the pharmaceutical firm. Once clinical trials on a drug are underway, most companies won't initiate studies in children until they see if it works as intended in adults.

Top areas where drugs are in clinical trials specifically for children

	Number of drugs
Infectious diseases	55
Cancer	53
Genetic diseases	52
Neurological disorders	29
Respiratory disorders	26
Cardiovascular diseases	18
Skin disorders	15
Psychiatric illnesses	14
Diabetes	11
Arthritis	7

Source: Pharmaceutical Research & Manufacturers of America, 2012

Today, pediatric studies touch virtually every category of disease and condition. Clinical trials on new treatments for infectious diseases, attention-deficit hyperactivity disorder, asthma, and allergies are particularly common. So are vaccine trials, including new "combination" therapies that immunize children against several diseases at the same time.

The majority of pediatric trials is conducted by well-trained investigators at large academic medical centers with access to kid-friendly radiology and EKG units and labs. Office-based pediatricians, if they do research at all, tend to focus on studies of vaccines, nutritional formulas, infectious diseases, and common illnesses seen in the community. A lot of clinical trials are done in conjunction with nearby medical centers.

The Age of Assent

Children aren't expected to give their consent, but they're often asked to give their assent. This will generally be recorded on a simplified form, separate from the longer, more detailed one their parents sign. But older children, depending on their level of maturity, may sign the very same form that their parents do.

The written permission of children's parents or legal guardians is also required before they can be enrolled in any study. IRBs consider parental permission sufficient if the research is going to be done on young children who lack the intellectual and emotional ability to understand what they're agreeing to. The "right" age to start asking children for their assent is when they're developmentally able to understand cause and effect, said Walson. But a multitude of other factors come into play, including whether a particular child has been in a clinical trial before, knows what to expect, and knows how to weigh the benefits and risks of participation.

IRBs don't require assent when children have a life-threatening illness, such as leukemia or a heart abnormality, and the study is considered likely to benefit them—no matter how much they may protest the idea. But recruitment of handicapped or institutionalized children is frowned upon unless the study is for diseases or conditions found mostly, or exclusively, in those populations.

For researchers, one of the harder parts of informed consent/assent among children is avoiding medical jargon and not assuming anything is understood. They also have to put themselves in the child's place to understand their motivations, fears, and desires. "Personally, the most difficult part for me is dealing with parental fear and guilt," said Walson.

As for a situation that involves a screaming three-year-old, the thoughtful researcher would probably discourage parents from enrolling the child—unless, of course, the child is seriously ill and no other good treatment option is available. It's also the more practical parental decision. Without the hope of great medicinal benefit, it's doubtful that many parents would be able to endure the ranting of an already cranky toddler past his first or second blood draw.

Compensation in Pediatric Clinical Trials

Parents are often pleased that their child's research-related visits, tests, and medications are provided free of charge. Children couldn't care less. To reward them for their participation, researchers will often give them gifts and even hourly fees. But whether children should be paid at all remains a matter of debate. The FDA takes no official position on the matter, leaving such matters to the discretion of the IRB.

"It is not wrong to compensate children and their parents for the inconvenience of being in a trial, but it is wrong to make the amount of payment or presents so much as to become an undue influence," said Walson. "Experienced institutions are likely to have unbiased people on the committees (IRBs) that decide what is 'too much.' This is not a simple question. The risks and benefits of the trial determine it. No inducement may be necessary or proper for a life-saving treatment offered nowhere else but through a clinical trial. A study requiring nightly trips to the hospital to test a new flavor of an approved, effective medication might justify a lot of payment for travel, babysitters, and missed work."

Many research centers will provide payments for pediatric studies that they believe are proportional to the time required to participate and appeal directly to the child rather than the parent. The "honorarium" might be a savings bond, toy, movie pass, gift certificates for CDs, or cash. But a few university-affiliated research centers have policies against making payments or gifts of any size to subjects of any age.

Money won't buy a child's cooperation for the entire length of a study. Children will back out of studies simply because they're in a bad mood or don't like what happened to them during their last visit. Overly active toddlers literally have to be held down for blood draws. Sometimes children, and their parents, will also underestimate the time consumed by follow-up visits and tests.

Choosing What Is Best for Your Child

The most important thing parents can do for their children is seek out an investigator they know and trust, rather than blindly responding to an advertisement, said Diane Murphy, M.D., associate director for pediatrics in the FDA's Center for Drug Evaluation and Research. "Parents need to know who they're getting involved with." Professional, well-recognized research centers, she added, are the safest bet.

The Rights of the Mentally Ill

Federal regulations on the protection of human subjects do not yet specifically address clinical trials among people whose mental status is impaired. This vulnerable population includes people with psychiatric illnesses like schizophrenia, manic depression, neurological conditions like Alzheimer's disease, and substance abusers. In the absence of regulatory guidance, the main concerns of the IRB are that subject selection is fair, risks are reasonable relative to potential benefit and that information about the trial is understandable to those capable of consenting or refusing to participate.

As a general rule, all adults regardless of their diagnosis or condition are presumed competent to consent unless there is evidence of serious mental disability that would impair reasoning or judgment. A legally responsible adult signs the consent form for subjects who are not competent. A "subject advocate" may participate in the consent process if there is question about the competency of an adult. Even subjects who are declared legally incompetent generally maintain their right to refuse participation in trials that involve no potentially beneficial diagnostic or therapeutic procedures.

As a result of greater IRB attention to the vulnerability of the mentally ill, volunteers in this population are less likely than in the past to be used as research subjects for drug and vaccine trials unrelated to their disorders or institutionalization.

Prisoners

Prisoners in federally-funded trials were given their own set of regulatory protections in 1978. The chief concern was that they might, given limited choice as a prisoner, be at greater risk of being coerced into participating in a clinical trial. To guard against this, federal regulators have instructed IRBs to more carefully review all clinical trials using prisoners as research subjects. IRB duties include ensuring:

- That compensation isn't coercive. Better amenities and the opportunity to make money in prison may unduly impair a prisoner's ability to weigh the benefits and risks of a clinical trial;
- The risks of participating would be acceptable to non-prisoner volunteers;
- The selection of subjects within the prison system is fair and does not affect decisions regarding parole;
- That adequate follow-up care is provided, if needed.

The Department of Health and Human Services published an amendment to the Code of Federal Regulations in December, 2001. These regulations provide the following additional protections for prisoners:

- A majority of the IRB (excluding prison members) cannot have an association with the prison involved, apart from membership on the IRB;
- At least one member of the IRB must be a prisoner or a prisoner representative.

For the bulk of drug studies that are sponsored by pharmaceutical companies, prisoners have no specific regulatory protections due largely to the objection of prison advocacy groups. Still, the FDA recognizes prisoners as a "vulnerable population" in need of special IRB oversight. The types of clinical trials for which prisoners volunteer depend largely on the policy and available facilities of the particular prison where they reside.

The Elderly

A growing number of clinical trials are being conducted on treatments for illnesses that affect senior Americans. Older generations of Americans have typically held a more trusting view of health professionals. As a result, this population may be more vulnerable to being influenced to participate in clinical trials. Support networks are an extremely important part of the informed consent process for senior Americans interested in volunteering for clinical trials.

In 2012, there were 467 drugs in clinical trials targeting diseases that specifically affect the elderly. That is a 50% increase over the number of drugs targeting this group in 2005. These drugs in development include treatments for diabetes, rheumatoid arthritis, Alzheimer's disease, and heart disease.

Total number of drugs in clinical trials for adults 65+

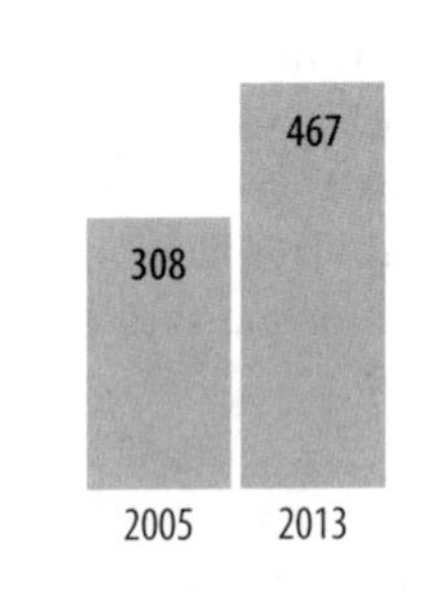

Source: Pharmaceutical Research & Manufacturers of America

Top areas where drugs are in clinical trials specifically for adults 65+

	Number of drugs
Diabetes	142
Rheumatoid arthritis	92
Alzheimer's sisease	82
Heart disease	48
Chronic obstructive pulmonary disease	40
Depression	34
Chronic kidney disease	20

Source: Pharmaceutical Research & Manufacturers of America, 2012

Special Considerations for Pregnant Women

The Department of Health and Human Services (HHS) also published an amendment to the Code of Federal Regulations in 2001 to provide additional protections for pregnant women and their fetuses involved in clinical research. The amendment builds upon special protections for pregnant women and fetuses that have existed since

1975 and clarifies the role of the father's consent when research is conducted involving unborn children.

Although it is still relatively rare to find pregnant women in studies, this group—and more specifically, their unborn children—was the first to be given special protection by HHS in 1975. The protections, however, apply only to federally-funded research, since HHS oversees government-sponsored clinical trials. The protections limit the involvement of pregnant women to trials that pose no more than a minimal risk to the fetus or intend to meet the mother's health needs and put the fetus at risk only to the minimum extent necessary. A new regulatory change, put into effect at the end of 2001, says the father's informed consent is needed only if the research is solely to benefit the fetus. Previously, the father's consent was also needed if the research was likely to also benefit the mother or simply to provide important medical knowledge.

The FDA—at least for now—has no specific regulation on the matter. If the study drug is not designed specifically for pregnant women, the FDA expects pharmaceutical companies to first test the product in non-pregnant subjects. Researchers are advised not to play a role in decisions about the termination of a pregnancy or to offer inducements to end a pregnancy for purposes of a clinical trial. Study subjects who are pregnant are also expected to be given all information about the potential risk of fetal toxicity as gathered from animal studies or experience with similar types of drugs. If the effects of a study drug on a fetus are unknown, the mother must be told. It is also the reason the FDA is silent on the issue of paternal consent.

CHAPTER TWELVE

What to Do When Things Go Wrong

Although there are cases where things have gone wrong during clinical trials, the majority of them are conducted safely and ethically. There are many professionals and procedures in place to ensure that your rights are protected and that the risk of participation is minimized. However, some violations still occur. The responsibilities of research-center personnel, the institutional review board (IRB), and the study sponsor are mandated by federal guidelines. A review of these responsibilities shows a number of checks and balances designed to protect study volunteers.

Study Coordinator responsibilities include, among other things:

- Managing daily study tasks
- Educating research center personnel about study requirements
- Submitting documents to the IRB
- Screening and enrolling study volunteers
- Collecting data and recording information on the study report forms
- Coordinating volunteer visits
- Following up and periodically touching base with study volunteers
- Storing, maintaining, and dispensing investigational drugs
- Collecting and processing lab samples
- Maintaining volunteer and data confidentiality
- Communicating with the investigator, sponsor, and study monitor

Investigator responsibilities include, among other things:

- Instructing and supervising staff compliance with the study protocol

- Submitting protocol, amendments, consent forms, and advertising material to the IRB
- Obtaining IRB approval
- Ensuring that volunteers meet eligibility criteria
- Adhering to study randomization and blinding requirements
- Maintaining patient case records and ensuring their completion
- Ensuring that data are complete and accurate
- Responding to data queries
- Documenting, conducting, and delegating study tasks
- Notifying the IRB of serious adverse events (SAEs)
- Providing periodic progress reports to the IRB

IRB responsibilities include, among other things:

- Ensuring that study risks to volunteers are minimized and reasonable in relation to the anticipated benefits
- Reviewing and approving or rejecting research studies and related activities
- Requiring modification of research activities
- Ensuring and documenting that volunteers have provided their informed consent
- Providing investigators and research center personnel with written documentation of approval, disapproval, and modifications of research activities
- Ensuring that IRB committee membership complies with regulations
- Maintaining complete records of IRB activities (e.g., meeting minutes, correspondences with research center personnel, and statements of significant new study findings communicated to volunteers during the study)

Sponsor responsibilities include, among other things:

- Selecting qualified investigators and research centers
- Providing investigators and study staff with information to conduct the protocol
- Ensuring proper and effective study monitoring
- Ensuring that the study follows the protocol and plans in the Investigational New Drug (IND) application
- Providing prompt information about serious adverse events to the FDA and participating investigators
- Disclosing to the FDA the financial interests of participating investigators

Most offenses are minor and they result in a warning letter from the FDA's Division of Scientific Investigations, which instructs them to take certain corrective actions. The FDA then monitors the situation to make sure the proper corrective steps were implemented. Each year, the FDA receives about 250 to 300 complaints. The vast majority of these complaints are for careless—though potentially dangerous—mistakes. Examples of mistakes include: Not all of the investigational drug could be accounted for; a 72-year-old is enrolled in a study when the cutoff age is 69; the investigator and the study coordinator conducted a step in the protocol out of order; a patient visited the research center several weeks later than the protocol allowed. And the opposite is also true—some FDA investigations for complaints will not turn up even a single minor violation.

Overall, fewer than 3% of unsolicited FDA audits uncover serious violations. However, in cases where inspections were solicited due to complaints filed against research centers, more than a quarter of them received serious violations of good clinical practices (GCPs). These violations included falsification of records or the failure to report adverse events. When serious violations are cited, the FDA must suspend and even consider disqualifying the investigator from conducting future research. One or two investigators are actually disqualified each year and a few others "voluntarily" remove themselves from conducting clinical research. Sometimes, investigators instead consent to having restrictions placed on how they conduct future studies—to perform no more than two studies simultaneously, for example, or to participate in trials only as a sub-investigator.

Nearly 30,000 clinical investigators are individually conducting at least one clinical trial each year. Since 1964, the FDA has disqualified approximately 130 investigators for failing to comply with Good Clinical Practice guidelines. Another 45 have had restrictions placed on them by consent. At least 20 have been prosecuted criminally. As a result of more "for-cause"—or solicited—inspections conducted annually by the FDA, the agency is actively uncovering more serious problems now than in the past. Given the increasing number of investigators and trials being conducted today, there are proportionately fewer violations than in the past.

The Office for Human Research Protections (OHRP) also receives about 100 complaints each year alleging misconduct by government-funded, university-affiliated institutions. Of these, about half move forward to a formal compliance oversight investigation.

The number of serious violations uncovered is small compared to the number of clinical trials conducted at these institutions. As many as 3,000 protocols are conducted annually at each of our nation's top 130 academic medical centers. Permanent suspension of studies or federal grant funding because of wrongdoing is rare, although oversight investigations have resulted in several research institutions being constrained from carrying out certain kinds of research or certain research projects. No research institution has had restrictions placed on its funding because of noncompliance with human subject protections regulations since 2000. But when it does happen, it is quite serious.

In recent years, two universities have had restrictions placed on their Multiple Project Assurances—the permit needed to conduct federally-funded research that holds institutions responsible for all trials involving human participants—for noncompliance with federal regulations. In 2002, the OHRP found numerous occasions in which the IRB at Oregon Health & Science University failed to conduct continuing review of research at least once per year. The IRB was additionally cited for inappropriately applying "expedited review" to research that involved greater-than-minimal risk, including a pediatric trial involving bone-marrow aspiration, and a waiver of child assent. In another pediatric trial, investigators failed to properly protect the identities of study subjects. In other cases, informed consent was not obtained until subjects underwent screening or other research-related procedures. Informed-consent documents for numerous studies also failed to adequately address the purpose of the research and completely describe the procedures to be followed. For several studies, the informed-consent document included complex language that would not be understandable to all subjects.

The Joan and Sanford I. Weill College of Medicine of Cornell University was also determined by OHRP in 2004 to have a similarly long list of regulatory breaches associated with five research protocols. Among the findings: IRB failure to adequately review the risks and potential benefits when children are involved as research subjects; enrollment of subjects prior to IRB approval of a protocol; failure to obtain informed consent from one subject; failure of the IRB to keep appropriate research-related records and minutes of meetings; and failure to report suspension of several research studies.

What You Can Do

In situations where you feel that your safety and ethical treatment are in jeopardy, your best guide is the informed-consent form. It states your rights as a volunteer. If you feel, for example, that you have been subjected to unreasonable risk, that your concerns and wishes are not being respected, or that you have witnessed unethical behavior, you need to contact the IRB immediately. A contact number for the IRB or patient advocate is usually provided with your informed-consent form. The study staff can also provide this information for you at any time.

If you are not satisfied after talking with your IRB or patient advocate, or if it appears that the IRB and the study staff are unable to help, then you need to file a complaint directly with the FDA or OHRP.

To lodge a complaint with the FDA

For studies of biologics, including gene therapy and vaccine studies, you should contact the Division of Communication and Consumer Affairs in the Center for Biologics Evaluation and Research.

CBER: Division of Communication and Consumer Affairs, Office of Communication, Outreach and Development
Phone: 301-827-2000
Fax: 301-827-3843
Email: ocod@fda.hhs.gov
Address: Division of Communication and Consumer Affairs
Office of Communication, Outreach and Development
Food and Drug Administration
1401 Rockville Pike
Suite 200N/HFM-47
Rockville, MD 20852-1448

For drug studies, the FDA contact is the Division of Scientific Investigations in the Office of Medical Policy at the Center for Drug Evaluation and Research.

CDER: Division of Scientific Investigations, Office of Compliance
Phone: 301-796-3100
Fax: 301-847-8747
Email: DSI@fda.hhs.gov
Address: Office of Compliance
10903 New Hampshire Avenue
Bldg. 51, Rm 5271
Silver Spring, MD 20993-0002

For medical device studies, the contact is the Division of Bioresearch Monitoring in the Office of Compliance at the Center for Devices and Radiological Health.

CDRH: Office of Compliance, Division of Bioresearch Monitoring
Phone: 301-796-5490

Fax: 301-847-8149
Email: bimo@cdrh.fda.gov
Address: Food & Drug Administration
Center for Devices and Radiological Health
Office of Compliance
10903 New Hampshire Avenue
WO66-3521
Silver Spring, MD 20993-0002

To lodge a complaint with the Office for Human Research Protections at the Department of Health and Human Services

DHHS: Office of Human Research Protections
Phone: (240) 453-6900
Toll free: (866) 447-4777
Fax: (240) 453-6909
Email: OHRP@hhs.gov
Address: Office for Human Research Protections
1101 Wootton Parkway, Suite 200
Rockville, MD 20852

And the Office of Inspector General at the Department of Health and Human Services

DHHS: Office of Inspector General
Phone: 1-800-HHS-TIPS (1-800-447-8477)
Fax: 1-800-223-8164
TTY: 1-800-377-4950
Email: HHSTips@ oig.hhs.gov
Online Hotline Form:
http://oig.hhs.gov/report-fraud
(may submit information anonymously)
Address: US Department of Health and Human Services
Office of Inspector General
ATTN: OIG HOTLINE OPERATIONS
PO Box 23489
Washington, DC 20026

It usually does not make sense to file a complaint with the pharmaceutical company sponsoring the research, although you can try. Most pharmaceutical companies have limited resources established to handle direct contact with study volunteers. This is changing, however. A growing number of companies—particularly the largest ones—do offer toll-free hotlines that you can call to report an emergency. Contact information for pharmaceutical and biotechnology companies is provided in the appendix.

Self-help and various advocacy groups—health and medical associations—may be of some assistance in handling your reports and complaints. Associations that set national and local health policies may also be good contacts. These groups may be better equipped to help you locate and choose clinical trials than to help you deal with misconduct issues. Still, they can help you better understand your rights as a volunteer, and they may help you contact other more helpful organizations and institutions. A list of some of these associations and groups are also included in the appendix.

It's impossible to test the safety of a drug in people with every conceivable combination of disease, drug interaction, age, and genetic predisposition. Therefore, some general and all long-term side effects aren't discovered until after a drug has been on the market and used by millions.

Physicians, pharmacists, and even patients themselves routinely report adverse events to the FDA through an ongoing drug safety program known as MedWatch. A drug causing an adverse event in sufficient frequency, relative to how often it's prescribed, will usually have its label changed so that doctors are informed about the new information and about what, if anything, they can do to minimize the risk. Many safety-related labeling changes are made every year. Specific side effects are dangerous enough to take two or three prescription drugs off the market each year. There are a number of web sites that post MedWatch information online for you to refer to.

Although this may not address immediate concerns about safety and ethical treatment, you can play a more active role in the future by joining or participating in an IRB. This experience will help you increase your network of support. Motivated parents—especially those who have had a child in a clinical trial—make ideal IRB members.

Being involved on an IRB is no small task. Although each IRB is different, members often have to do a lot of reading and attend numerous meetings. Some have a fixed number of members who look over, and comment on, every protocol. Others have a pool of members from which they draw, based on their area of interest and expertise.

The Tufts Center for the Study of Drug Development estimates that there are approximately 3,000 IRBs operating within the United States overseeing government- and industry-funded clinical trials. Boards are established, trained, and licensed differently from place to place. The OHRP offers general IRB training that focuses on research ethics (http://www.hhs.gov/ohrp).

Steve Hirschfeld, M.D., Ph.D., medical officer with the FDA, said his hope is that people will start demanding quality in clinical trials as they do in nearly everything else,from their automobiles and food to their regular medical care. Joining an IRB is a good starting point. Even people who are completely untrained in science and statistics can make substantial contributions to discussions about studies after only a few hours of training, he said.

A History of Specific Misconduct Examples

The incidence of misconduct and noncompliance is rare. When these acts are uncovered, the government and industry typically respond by modifying practices and adding new policies and procedures.

There are a lot of pressures placed on researchers today to enroll patients quickly, to conduct clinical trials faster, to review and approve study protocols in less time, and to compete against other research centers for new studies from industry and government study sponsors. Some research professionals are tempted, for example, by the potential to increase their salaries by doing more and larger clinical trials. Despite these pressures and temptations, history has shown that only a very small number of investigators, coordinators, and IRB personnel have been led astray. What follows are a few examples of their misconduct that have helped to shape new policies and legislation.

In 1999, California physician Robert Fiddes was disqualified as a clinical investigator and sent to prison for 15 months after he and two of his study coordinators conspired to falsify drug trial results by "inventing" patients and their medical data. He also lost his medical license. The whistleblower was one of Dr. Fiddes's employees.

Similarly, a disgruntled employee tipped off the Medical College of Georgia in Augusta that Drs. Richard Borison and Bruce Diamond—a prominent psychiatrist and pharmacologist, respectively—were secretly conducting schizophrenia drug trials for eight years using university resources and pocketing the proceeds. They "coaxed" psychotic patients into trials with money and cigarettes, but gave scant attention to their care. Untrained staff took blood draws and adjusted doses of study drugs. The two were finally incarcerated in 1997, fined $125,000 each, and ordered to pay millions of dollars back to the college.

Jesse Gelsinger's Story

One of the largest concerns today relates to conflicts of interest. Investigators and universities that have an economic interest in the drug they're investigating tend to be less vigilant—consciously or unconsciously—about patient safety and ethical treatment. This is considered one of the many factors associated with the death of 18-year-old Jesse Gelsinger in a 1999 gene-therapy experiment at the University of Pennsylvania. Jesse had a massive and fatal immune system reaction to a common-cold virus used to deliver a particular gene to his liver.

Jesse had an inherited metabolic disorder that had landed him in a coma several times. But he was doing relatively well on medications before entering the trial. The university and principal investigator wanted to test a treatment for newborn babies, but they first needed adults to participate in a clinical trial focusing on how suitable the common-cold virus was for gene-transport delivery. They also stood to profit if the drug worked. But the Gelsinger family was not informed about this conflict of interest—or all of the drug's dangers. Questions were raised later about whether Jesse fit the inclusion criteria and even whether federal regulators were notified of adverse events during earlier studies of the experimental intervention.

A subsequent investigation by the FDA revealed that established safety rules were not followed and that the study should have ended months earlier than it did. It ordered a halt to nine clinical research projects at the university's Institute of Human Gene Therapy. The family ultimately sued and won an out-of-court settlement. The university wrote a letter of apology to Jesse's family and was determined thereafter to make itself a model for human subject protection.

"Jesse just wanted to help," said his father, Paul, now vice president of Citizens for Responsible Care and Research (CIRCARE). "There was nothing in it for him—no money and no treatment that was even applicable to him. His heart was totally in this, and it really impressed me. It was his chance to make a difference. When he died, I tried to adopt some of the heart he had and befriended the doctors. They were not bad men. They had simply become blind to the real purpose of what they were doing."

It was only when he became aware of lapses in the protocol that he sued. "Litigation was the only way to get their attention. The clinical trial should never have taken place," said Paul Gelsinger. "It was too dangerous and of no benefit to those who participated." Perhaps most disturbing, he added, is that Jesse would probably still be alive today if a gene-therapy information network had been set up. The FDA and National Institutes of Health (NIH) were discussing the idea back in 1995 but later dropped it. The reason, an FDA official confided in him, was because his supervisors "answered to industry." And industry fears that sharing information—including adverse events and deaths associated with certain types of trials—will cost them their competitive edge.

After examining close to 100 other gene-therapy protocols, the FDA determined that gene-therapy trials are no better or worse than standard drug trials in complying with federal research rules. "What happened in the Gelsinger case, and other serious cases we've had, is that the system was compromised in more than one area," commented David Lepay, the FDA's senior advisor for clinical science. Of greatest concern are uninformed IRBs, inadequate adverse event reporting, and clinical investigators who double as study sponsors and thus conduct trials shy of a critical "control point." Education, and a special monitoring unit, may present at least a partial solution. Integrity in the doctor-patient relationship—something regulators can't control—also has to be there.

Another Case of Conflict of Interest

Allegations similar to those in the Gelsinger case have been reported at other universities and research centers since Jesse's death. These include an alleged breach of trust by the Fred Hutchinson Cancer Research Center, a top bone-marrow transplant center in Seattle. The center's principal investigators—including a Nobel Prize winner—received consulting fees from the firm producing the drug for leukemia trials conducted there in the 1980s and 1990s. The center was given shares of stock in the company and rights to study drugs owned by the company for 20 years. Nearly all of the study's 85 participants have since died. A quarter of them would still be alive, family members believe, had they received an alternative therapy. But the doctors never fully informed them about the dangers of the experimental drug or other available treatments, they say. So they filed a lawsuit against the center. A jury found in favor of the cancer research center in 2004, saying patients were sufficiently informed. But it did fine the center one million dollars for negligence in the death of one patient whose donor bone marrow was lost in a laboratory mishap.

The "whistleblower" in the case was a member of the research center's IRB. An independent review of patient-protection practices, coordinated by the Hutchinson Center, suggested a host of changes be made. One major recommendation was that all individuals involved in human-subject trials be prohibited from having a financial interest in for-profit corporations that may benefit from the result of such trials.

There is now growing concern among regulators, professionals, and the public that financial conflict of interest—including stock ownership in the sponsoring drug company—are biasing the way studies are designed and conducted. There is also growing concern that conflicts of interest are biasing the way study findings are written up in prestigious medical journals. These kinds of influences are potentially harmful both to human research subjects and those who use the drugs once they're approved for sale. The U.S. General Accounting Office, in its November 2001 report on financial conflicts of interest in research, found that editors of major medical journals were concerned about the "competitive economic environment" in which some clinical research is conceived and conducted. In response, the International Committee of Medical Journal Editors has "revised and strengthened" its position on publication ethics. Many medical journals refer to this position as the basis for their own editorial policies. As part of the revised reporting requirements, authors need to disclose details of their own and the sponsor's role in the study.

Other Cases Involving Misconduct

Participants in a clinical trial for a melanoma vaccine sued the IRB at the University of Oklahoma Health Sciences Center for failure to adequately protect them. The lawsuit alleged that the IRB was negligent in its duties, including stopping the center from conducting the trial. The IRB was faulted for not reviewing the conduct of the trial, the informed consent documents that understated risks to subjects, and the recruitment advertisements that falsely represented the vaccine as a "cure for cancer." When the trial closed prematurely in the spring of 2000, the IRB permitted researchers to tell participants that the reason was a shortage of the vaccine rather than safety violations discovered by the FDA. The university dismissed everyone involved in the alleged wrongdoing, and the suspension was lifted. While a federal judge dismissed the case in 2002, the lawsuit was re-filed in state court and "settled quite favorably for the plaintiffs," according to Alan Milstein, the attorney who represented them.

In a report issued in 1998, the inspector general of the U.S. Department of Health and Human Services concluded that many IRBs were operating over capacity. Following that report, OHRP has suspended research programs at a number of institutions. In 1999, it briefly shut down all 2,000 medical experiments at Duke University because of safety concerns, including inadequate informed consent procedures. In recent years, research has also been temporarily suspended at a number of university-affiliated sites because of human-subject safety concerns. Violations have been made across several areas including informed-consent noncompliance, poor record keeping, and poor reporting of serious adverse events.

One of the most recent suspensions was at Johns Hopkins University School of Medicine and its affiliated institutions following the death of Ellen Roche, a healthy 24-year-old woman, during an asthma experiment. She died of adult respiratory distress syndrome not long after being given an inhaled dosage of a non-marketed drug known as hexamethonium. The principal investigator said he could find no recent articles in the medical literature associating the drug with severe pulmonary disease, and no articles at all connecting it to pulmonary toxicity when delivered by inhalation. And researchers on the 1978 study attesting to the drug's safety failed to report that two of five volunteers in the study became sick.

An OHRP investigation found that Johns Hopkins's IRBs weren't providing adequate review of many new research programs and, when they did, the deliberations included board members with financial conflicts of interest. The OHRP briefly took away Johns Hopkins' Multiple Project Assurance. Previously enrolled subjects were allowed to continue in a trial only if it was in their best interests. After four days, with a new plan in place to correct deficiencies, all research in which there was no more than a minimal risk to volunteers was allowed to resume.

Regulatory scrutiny of Johns Hopkins has changed the clinical-trial process there in several significant ways. Informed-consent documents have been simplified and better cover key points. The number of IRBs reviewing studies has increased and IRB membership is more ethnically diverse. Studies that don't involve the FDA are more closely scrutinized. Investigators are also routinely reminded that changes in study protocols require IRB review and approval and that unanticipated problems involving risks to subjects must be promptly reported.

Reform is not always prompted by a complete suspension of research. An OHRP investigation, for example, led the University of Arkansas and Arkansas Children's Hospital to expand its IRB staff and require its investigators to be educated about their responsibilities to protect the safety of study volunteers. The move followed the death of a 3-year-old boy who had been placed in the wrong study group a kidney-cancer trial.

Other academic institutions and federal research agencies have undertaken similar reforms when OHRP has investigated alleged violations or suspended trials due to poor investigator compliance or IRB judgment. CIRCARE advocates that 51% of IRB membership come from—and be selected by someone—outside research institutions. It also proposes mandatory accreditation of IRBs by an independent agency. Gelsinger has further suggested that the NIH establish a user-fee program to fund the establishment of IRBs independent of institutional influence.

Unintended harm might sometimes occur from a drug long after it has been approved for sale on the open market. The incidence of these occurrences is extremely rare. The FDA shelved the popular cholesterol-lowering drug Baycol (cerivastatin) after linking it to 31 deaths in the United States from a rare muscle-destroying side effect. Volunteers involved in clinical trials for the popular diet pill "fen-phen" were informed years after the trials ended, and the drug had been prescribed to more than 7 million patients, that it was causing heart and lung problems in some patients who took it. By then, the drug had caused problems in 45,000 patients and approximately 300 deaths. People who took the drug and survived were compensated, but the damage to their health was permanent.

The widely prescribed arthritis drug Vioxx was pulled from the market following revelations that the drug increased patients' risk of heart attack and strokes. Competing drugs, including Celebrex and Bextra, were connected to the same side effects. In 2005, there was a wave of safety concerns about antidepressants—especially when they are used by children. The once-a-day pain management drug, Palladone, was also withdrawn from the market when it was learned that potentially fatal adverse reactions can occur when the drug is taken together with even one alcoholic drink.

In March 2006, in its very first clinical trial, a new drug, TGN1412, caused catastrophic organ failure among six volunteers. Although very small doses of the drug were administered during a phase I study, all six volunteers were hospitalized. An outside inquiry determined that the problems were the result of unforeseen biological reactions and not protocol violations. Still the incident caught the world's attention and led to the ultimate bankruptcy of the drug sponsor, a German-based venture-capital-backed company named TeGenero.

In the spring of 2009, the U.S. House Subcommittee on Oversight and Investigations asked the General Accountability Office (GAO) to test the integrity of the national system of human subject protection. The GAO sent out an application to a number of institutional review boards requesting approval to test a fake product—called Adhesiabloc—made by the fictitious company, Device Med-Systems. One IRB—Coast Independent Review Board—approved the application without evaluating its credibility and determining that the device was fraudulent in violation of federal and state law. In the aftermath of this investigation, Coast IRB had to close its doors.

Many of these cases show what can happen when things go wrong. Every accident and death is significant, but the likelihood of their occurring is rare. Recent responses by regulatory agencies, sponsor companies, and research centers suggest that measures are being taken to help prevent these accidents from happening again. In particular, many institutional and independent IRBs implemented initiatives designed to improve IRB effectiveness. These initiatives involved increasing IRB headcount, creating toll-free numbers for volunteers, providing more training and education, establishing greater disclosure of conflicts-of-interest, and improving standard operating procedures.

Some suggested steps that you can take to better protect yourself

- Ask who wrote the study protocol and what qualified that person to do so.
- Call the IRB to learn about how much time was spent reviewing the study protocol and what specific areas, if any, gave members cause for discussion or concern.
- Find out if there is or has been professional debate about the risks associated with the study drug. If so, ask for referrals to medical publications where these risks are discussed.
- Request that the study staff speak to you in plain English (or Spanish, French, sign language, etc.)—or find someone who can.
- Quiz the researcher and study coordinator about how many adverse events and deaths have been reported during trials of this study drug—whether or not they were actually attributed to the drug. If they don't know, call the IRB. If the IRB doesn't know, call the pharmaceutical company.
- Ask the researchers if they would advise you to enroll in the trial if you were a member of their family.
- Gather as much information as you can from published reports and news coverage about your study medication.
- If possible, go to another research center conducting the same clinical trial. Go through the same set of questions and see if you get the same answers. Seek explanations for inconsistencies.
- Share everything you learned with your family doctor and other friends and family within your support network before enrolling.

The danger of sharing these examples of misconduct is that they can increase your fears and anxieties about participating in clinical trials. But the danger of not sharing these examples is more serious. They illustrate the worst cases and the responses they prompted from the government, the public, academic institutions, and from industry. This chapter is intended to help you avoid these worst-case situations.

As in all things, knowledge is power. Whereas reading this chapter, or this book, is no guarantee that you will be protected from all the potential risks associated with a clinical trial, reading it does give you the knowledge and the power to recognize when your rights and your health are at risk and to take steps to protect yourself from these risks.

AFTERWORD

Nearly 4,000 experimental drug therapies are in active clinical trials today and that number will continue to grow as improvements are made in detecting disease, in understanding the root causes of acute and chronic illnesses, and in discovering medical innovations. And in the not-so-distant future, as electronic health records and clinical research converge, it will be more common for clinical trials to be discussed during routine visits with the doctor.

At this time, for the vast majority of people, the idea of clinical trials never enters their consciousness. Most people stumble upon clinical trials when faced with the sudden prospect of a serious, often life-threatening, illness for which no marketed medication is available or adequate. Information about clinical trials may first come from a physician or nurse, friends and family, or a personal search on the Internet or in the newspaper. Regardless of its source, patients and their support network must gather information quickly in order to make major decisions about whether to participate. This rush to navigate the unknown terrain of clinical trials invariably feels like an overwhelming and confusing undertaking.

Having interacted with many patients who've been through this harrowing experience, in 2004 I founded the Center for Information and Study on Clinical Research Participation (CISCRP). This Boston-based independent nonprofit is dedicated to helping raise public and patient awareness about clinical research. I also founded CISCRP to raise the level of public appreciation for clinical-research participants. After all, behind every medicine and intervention are thousands of patients who have volunteered to participate in clinical trials.

There is a chance that participation may bring hope to study volunteers. Yet, more often clinical trials will benefit those who will suffer from the illness in the future. And of course, our overall public health benefits from clinical trials regardless of whether an experimental treatment is safe and effective, or harmful and ineffective.

Participation is a brave act as there are numerous risks in clinical trials. Even the best-run studies are not completely free of risk despite the fact that the research process is highly regulated, managed by very experienced professionals, and has many built-in safeguards to help protect study volunteers. It is important to know all of the facts about clinical trials before choosing whether or not to participate in one. At CISCRP, our motto "Education Before Participation" guides the many programs and initiatives that we implement each year to improve public and patient literacy, to engender feelings of empowerment and control among patients and their families, and to ensure more informed decision-making.

I wrote *The Gift of Participation* to provide facts and information to help patients and their network of support make educated decisions about the importance of volunteering for clinical trials and whether or not to participate in them. I hope that you have found this book useful and that you, your family, and your friends will refer to it often for insight and guidance.

The Gift of Participation is only a road map. Choosing to be a volunteer in a clinical trial takes a great deal of courage and conviction. It also takes a lot of time and effort to gather the facts and information thoroughly and to weigh your many options thoughtfully. The decision to participate in a clinical trial is not one that you should make alone. It must be a team effort. In order to make a truly informed decision, you need to involve your family and friends, your physician and nurse, the clinical investigator and study staff.

I welcome your feedback and comments. Please send me an email at kengetz@ciscrp.org or call 617-725-2750 with your thoughts and ideas on ways to make *The Gift of Participation* better.

Ken Getz

Founder and Chairman, CISCRP

Director, Sponsored Research Programs and Associate Professor
The Center for the Study of Drug Development
Tufts University School of Medicine
Boston, MA

APPENDIX A

Glossary of Terms

Adverse Drug Reaction (ADR): An unintended reaction to a drug taken at normal doses. In clinical trials, an ADR would include any injuries due to overdosing, abuse/dependence, and unintended interactions with other medical treatments.

Adverse Event (AE): A negative experience encountered by a volunteer during the course of a clinical trial, that is associated with the drug. An AE can include previously undetected symptoms, or the exacerbation of a preexisting condition. When an AE has been determined to be related to the investigational drug, it is considered an Adverse Drug Reaction.

Biologic: A virus, therapeutic serum, toxin, antitoxin, vaccine, blood, blood component or derivative, allergenic product, or analogous product applicable to the prevention, treatment, or cure of human diseases or injuries.

Biotechnology: Any technique that uses living organisms, or substances from organisms, biological systems, or processes to make or modify a product or process, to change plants or animals, or to develop microorganisms for specific uses.

Blinding: The process through which one or more parties involved in a clinical trial are unaware of the treatment assignments. In a single-blinded study, usually the volunteers are unaware of the treatment assignments. In a double-blinded study, both volunteers and the investigator are unaware of the treatment assignments. Also, in a double-blinded study, the monitors and sometimes the data analysts are unaware. "Blinded" studies are conducted to prevent the unintentional biases that can affect subject data when treatment assignments are known.

Case Report Form (CRF): A record of pertinent information collected on each volunteer during a clinical trial, as outlined in the study protocol.

Clinical Investigation: A systematic study designed to evaluate a product (drug, device, or biologic) using human subjects, in the treatment, prevention, or diagnosis of a disease or condition, as determined by the product's benefits relative to its risks. Clinical investigations can only be conducted with the approval of the Food and Drug Administration (FDA).

Clinical Trial: Any investigation in human subjects intended to determine the clinical pharmacological, pharmacokinetic, and/or other pharmacodynamic effects of an investigational agent, and/or to identify any adverse reactions to an investigational agent to assess the agent's safety and efficacy.

Control Group: The comparison group of subjects who are not treated with the investigational agent. The volunteers in this groupmay receive no therapy, a different therapy, or a placebo.

Data Management: The process of handling the data gathered during a clinical trial. May also refer to the department responsible for managing data entry and database generation and/or maintenance.

Declaration of Helsinki: A series of guidelines adopted by the 18th World Medical Assembly in Helsinki, Finland in 1964. Addresses ethical issues for physicians conducting biomedical research involving human subjects. Recommendations include the procedures required to ensure subject safety in clinical trials, including informed consent and Ethics Committee reviews.

Demographic Data: Refers to the characteristics of study participants, including sex, age, family medical history, and other characteristics relevant to the study in which they are enrolled.

Device: An instrument, apparatus, implement, machine, contrivance, implant, in vitro reagent, or other similar or related article, including any component, part or accessory, which is intended for use in the diagnosis, cure, treatment or prevention of disease. A device does not achieve its intended purpose through chemical action in the body and is not dependent upon being metabolized to achieve its purpose.

Double-Blind: The design of a study in which neither the investigator nor the volunteer knows which medication (or placebo) the volunteer is receiving.

Drug: As defined by the Food, Drug, and Cosmetic Act, drugs are "articles (other than food) intended for the use in the diagnosis, cure, mitigation, treatment, or prevention of disease in man or other animals, or to affect the structure or any function of the body of man or other animals."

Drug Product: A final dosage form (e.g. tablet, capsule, or solution) that contains the active drug ingredient usually combined with inactive ingredients.

Effective Dose: The dose of an investigational agent that produces the outcome considered "effective," as defined in the study protocol. This could mean a cure of the disease in question or simply the mitigation of symptoms.

Efficacy: A product's ability to produce beneficial effects on the duration or course of a disease. Efficacy is measured by evaluating the clinical and statistical results of clinical tests.

Ethical Review Board: An independent group of both medical and non-medical professionals who are responsible for verifying the integrity of a study and ensuring the safety, integrity, and human rights of the study participants.

Exclusion Criteria: Refers to the characteristics that would prevent a subject from participating in a clinical trial, as outlined in the study protocol.

Food and Drug Administration (FDA): A US government agency responsible for ensuring compliance with the Food, Drug, and Cosmetic Act of 1938. All drugs sold in the U.S. must receive marketing approval from the FDA.

Formulation: The mixture of chemicals and/or biological substances and excipients used to prepare dosage forms. An excipient is a substance that is basically inert. It is used in a prescription to help give a drug its proper form.

Generic Drug: A medicinal product with the same active ingredient, but not necessarily the same inactive ingredients as a brand-name drug. A generic drug may only be marketed after the original drug's patent has expired.

Good Clinical Practice (GCP): The FDA has established regulations and guidelines that specify the responsibilities of sponsors, investigators, monitors, and IRBs involved in clinical drug testing. These regulations are meant to protect the safety, rights, and welfare of the patients in addition to ensuring the accuracy of the collected study data.

Human Subject: A human subject is an individual who voluntarily is or becomes a participant in research, either as a recipient of the test article or as a control. A subject may be either a healthy human or a patient.

Inclusion Criteria: A list of criteria that must be met in order to participate in a clinical trial.

In Vitro Testing: Non-clinical testing conducted in an artificial environment such as a test tube or culture medium.

In Vivo Testing: Testing conducted in living animal and human systems.

Informed Consent: The voluntary verification of a patient's willingness to participate in a clinical trial, along with documentation. This verification is requested only after complete, objective information has been provided about the trial, including an explanation of the study's objectives, potential benefits, risks, and inconveniences; alternative therapies available; and the volunteer's rights and responsibilities in accordance with the current revision of the Declaration of Helsinki.

Institutional Review Board (IRB): An independent group of professionals designated to review and approve the clinical protocol, informed consent forms, study advertisements, and patient brochures, to ensure that the study is safe and effective for human participation. It is also the IRB's responsibility to ensure that the study adheres to the FDA's regulations.

Investigational New Drug Application (IND): The petition through which a drug sponsor requests the FDA to allow human testing of its drug product.

Investigator: A medical professional, usually a physician but may also be a nurse, pharmacist, or other health care professional, under whose direction an investigational drug is administered or dispensed. A principal investigator is responsible for the overall conduct of the clinical trial at his or her site.

Longitudinal Study: A study conducted over a long period of time.

MedWatch Program: An FDA program designed to monitor adverse events (AE) from drugs marketed in the U.S. Through the MedWatch program, health professionals may report AEs voluntarily to the FDA. Drug manufacturers are required to report all AEs brought to their attention.

New Drug Application (NDA): The compilation of all nonclinical, clinical, pharmacological, pharmacokinetic, and stability information required about a drug by the FDA in order to approve the drug for marketing in the U.S.

Nuremberg Code: As a result of the medical experimentation conducted by Nazis during World War II, the U.S. Military Tribunal in Nuremberg in 1947 set forth a code of medical ethics for researchers conducting clinical trials. The code is designed to protect the safety and integrity of study participants.

Off Label: The unauthorized use of a drug for a purpose other than that approved of by the FDA.

Open-Label Study: A study in which all parties, (patient, physician, and study coordinator) are informed of the drug and dose being administered. In an open-label study, none of the participants are given placebos. These are usually conducted with Phase I and II studies.

Orphan Drug: A designation of the FDA to indicate a therapy developed to treat a rare disease (one which afflicts a U.S. population of less than 200,000 people). Because there are few financial incentives for drug companies to develop therapies for diseases that afflict so few people, the U.S. government offers additional incentives to drug companies (i.e. tax advantages and extended marketing exclusivity) that develop these drugs.

Over-the-Counter (OTC): Drugs available for purchase without a physician's prescription.

Pharmacoeconomics: The study of cost-benefit ratios of drugs with other therapies or with similar drugs. Pharmacoeconomic studies compare various treatment options in terms of their cost, both financial and quality-of-life. Also referred to as "outcomes research."

Phase I Study: The first of four phases of clinical trials, phase I studies are designed to establish the effects of a new drug in humans. These studies are usually conducted on small populations of healthy people to specifically determine a drug's toxicity, absorption, distribution, and metabolism.

Phase II Study: After the successful completion of phase I trials, a drug is then tested for safety and efficacy in a slightly larger population of individuals who are afflicted with the disease or condition for which the drug was developed.

Phase III Study: The third and last pre-approval round of testing of a drug is conducted on large populations of afflicted patients. Phase III studies usually test the new drug in comparison with the standard therapy currently being used for the disease in question. The results of these trials usually provide the information that is included in the package insert and labeling.

Phase IV Study: After a drug has been approved by the FDA, phase IV studies are conducted to compare the drug to a competitor, to explore additional patient populations, or to further study any adverse events.

Pivotal Study: Usually a phase III study which presents the data that the FDA uses to decide whether or not to approve a drug. A pivotal study will generally be well-controlled, randomized, of adequate size, and whenever possible, double-blind.

Placebo: An inactive substance designed to resemble the drug being tested. It is used as a control to rule out any psychological effects testing may present. Most well-designed studies include a control group of volunteers which is unwittingly taking a placebo.

Pre-Clinical Testing: Before a drug may be tested on humans, pre-clinical studies must be conducted either in vitro but usually in vivo on animals to determine that the drug is safe.

Protocol: A detailed plan that sets forth the objectives, study design, and methodology for a clinical trial. A study protocol must be approved by an IRB before investigational drugs may be administered to humans.

Quality Assurance: Systems and procedures designed to ensure that a study is being performed in compliance with Good Clinical Practice (GCP) guidelines and that the data being generated is accurate.

Randomization: Study participants are usually assigned to groups in such a way that each participant has an equal chance of being assigned to each treatment (or control) group. Since randomization ensures that no specific criteria are used to assign any patients to a particular group, all the groups will be equally comparable.

Regulatory Affairs: In clinical trials, the department or function that is responsible for ensuring compliance with government regulations and interacts with the regulatory agencies. Each drug sponsor has a regulatory affairs department that manages the entire drug approval process.

Serious Adverse Event (SAE): Any adverse event (AE) that is fatal, life-threatening, permanently disabling, or which results in hospitalization, initial or prolonged.

Sponsor: Person or entity who initiates and takes responsibility for a clinical study. This is often a pharmaceutical company, but can also be a medical device manufacturer, government agency, academic institution, private organization, or even an individual researcher.

Standard Operating Procedure (SOP): Official, detailed, written instructions for the management of clinical trials. SOPs ensure that all the functions and activities of a clinical trial are carried out in a consistent and efficient manner.

Standard Treatment: The currently accepted treatment or intervention considered to be effective in the treatment of a specific disease or condition.

Study Coordinator: The individual who assists the principal investigator and who runs the clinical trial. This person may also be called clinical research coordinator, research nurse, or protocol nurse.

Treatment IND: Amethod through which the FDA allows seriously ill patients with no acceptable therapeutic alternative to access promising investigational drugs still in clinical development. The drug must show "sufficient evidence of safety and effectiveness." In recent decades many AIDs patients have been able to access unapproved therapies through this program.

APPENDIX B

A History of Major Regulations and Guidelines Affecting Patient Protection in Clinical Research

1938

Federal Food, Drug, and Cosmetic Act: New law requires pharmaceutical companies to submit to the U.S. Food and Drug Administration (FDA) evidence of drug safety, in the form of a new drug application (NDA), before marketing a drug. The catalyst is 107 human deaths attributed to a liquid preparation of the first sulfa drug used to treat certain infectious bacteria, including pneumonia and strep throat.

1946

AMA Code of Ethics: Responding to concerns about research abuses, the American Medical Association adopts its first code of research ethics for physicians.

1947

Nuremberg Code: In reaction to atrocities committed by German scientists during World War II, the Nuremberg Military Tribunal writes a set of ten principles for research involving human participants, including an absolute requirement for informed consent. Primary responsibility for the ethical conduct of research is placed on investigators.

1961

First investigation of an investigator: FDA starts a file of clinical investigators "who have contributed incredible reports to NDAs." The first to be investigated is a general practitioner who had undertaken clinical trials on adults, infants, and children for 25 different drug companies. It was discovered that he mostly fabricated study results from his kitchen table. In subsequent years, the FDA investigated researchers who neglected any number of their responsibilities, including seeing study subjects and reporting adverse events.

1962

Kefauver-Harris Amendments to the Food, Drug, and Cosmetic Act: Changes in federal regulations are triggered by a thalidomide trial that caused women who took the experimental drug during their first trimester of pregnancy to give birth to deformed babies. The amendment requires drug manufacturers to prove effectiveness before marketing any new product and researchers to obtain informed consent of study subjects and report adverse events. FDA placed in supervisory position. With the Act's passage, the number of new-drug approvals fell dramatically.

1963

Investigational Drug Regulations: New regulations establish the Investigational New Drug (IND) application, detailed plans that pharmaceutical companies must submit to the FDA before starting human testing of their drug products. Companies must now prove efficacy as well as safety before a drug will be approved for marketing. They also must submit to the FDA-proposed study protocols, the names and qualifications of investigators who are to conduct those studies, and the research sites to be used.

Certification of informed consent: FDA regulations enacted this year also require clinical investigators to certify to sponsors of drug research that informed consent would be obtained in accordance with the 1962 amendments.

1964

Declaration of Helsinki: World Medical Association issues 32-point statement of ethical principles defining the rules for "therapeutic" and "non-therapeutic" research. Repeats many of the requirements in the Nuremberg Code but allows certain patients to be enrolled in therapeutic research without consent. The Declaration also allows legal guardians to grant permission to enroll subjects in research.

1966

HHS policy of independent review: The U.S. Department of Health and Human Services (HHS) requires independent review of research it funds by a committee of the investigator's "institutional associates." Review is to include, among other things, appropriateness of the methods used to secure informed consent.

FDA consent requirements: FDA requires consent in all nontherapeutic drug studies and in all but exceptional cases of therapeutic application of an experimental drug.

Beecher article: Henry Beecher publishes an article outlining 22 examples of "unethical or questionably ethical studies" appearing in mainstream medical journals, including the ingestion of the hepatitis virus into retarded children at Willowbrook State School in New York.

AMA ethical guidelines: Ethical guidelines for clinical investigation are adopted by the AMA.

1967

Division of Scientific Investigations: A new division of the FDA is created to do inspections of the work of clinical investigators, using the previously established suspect list, prison-based testing operations, and requests by IND and NDA reviewers.

Changes to FDA consent regulations: FDA permits oral informed consent in certain situations and clarifies the information that needs to be given to subjects, including whether they might receive a placebo.

1971

Institutional Review Boards (IRBs): FDA regulations require studies involving experimental drugs and biologics performed on institutionalized human subjects to receive review and approval by an institutional review board (IRB).

1972

Office for Protection from Research Risks (OPRR): OPRR, housed within the National Institutes of Health (NIH), is established to protect participants in research conducted or sponsored by HHS. This is the same year details emerge about the Public Health Service's (PHS's) natural history study of syphilis in poor, black males in Alabama who were misled into believing they were receiving treatment. The FDA also reiterates that a drug study's sponsor must play a more active role in monitoring trials and in making sure that researchers are competent and understand their obligations.

1974

HHS human subjects protection regulations: Researchers are required to get voluntary informed consent from all persons taking part in studies done or federally funded by HHS.

National Research Act: The National Research Act, an amendment to the Public Health Services Act, establishes the National Commission for the Protection of Human Subjects in Biomedical and Behavioral Research (the National Commission), charged with identifying basic principles of research conduct and suggesting ways to ensure those principles are followed. IRBs were established as one subject protection method for federally-funded research. The motivation is mistakes made in the PHS syphilis study.

1975

Helsinki Accords: The United States and 34 other nations sign the Declaration of Helsinki and recommendations guiding the moral treatment of patients in biomedical research. Responsibility for trial conduct is put on the shoulders of physician investigators.

Special protections for pregnant women: Special protections pertaining to federally funded research involving fetuses, pregnant women and human in-vitro fertilization is adopted by HHS. IRBs are directed to give adequate consideration to the manner in which potential subjects are selected and informed consent is handled. Research involving pregnant women is limited to trials that intend to meet the mother's health needs and put the fetus at no more risk than necessary to meet those needs.

Acceptance of foreign studies: The FDA accepts non-U.S. clinical studies as primary evidence for U.S. marketing approval of drugs for a major health gain, uncommon disease, or a strikingly favorable ratio of benefit to risk.

1976

GAO report/Expanded bioresearch monitoring: Using data from an earlier FDA survey, the General Accounting Office (GAO) concludes that human test subjects and the public are not being adequately protected. The FDA is infused with funding to expand bioresearch monitoring and come up with regulations and compliance programs.

1977

Bioresearch Monitoring Program: FDA expands on-site reviews of IRBs to include clinical investigators, research sponsors, study monitors, and non-clinical (animal) laboratories. The intent is less about noncompliance than ensuring the quality of data submitted to the FDA and protection of human subjects of research.

Inclusion of women: FDA guidelines forbid the inclusion of women of childbearing potential in phase I and early phase II studies, excepting those with a life-threatening disease.

1978

Special protections for prisoners: HHS gives additional protections to prisoners involved in research. Federally funded studies involving inmates now require the approval of the OPRR and must have a prisoner or prison representative sit on the IRB. Research cannot provide special advantages to prisoners, subject them to risks greater than would be accepted by non-prisoner volunteers, or involve unfair selection of study subjects. While the FDA has no similar set of regulations to this day, it routinely refers researchers to these protections.

1979

Belmont Report: Ethical Principles and Guidelines for the Protection of Human Subjects of Research published in the Federal Register. Written by the National Commission, the report outlines the ethical principles of respect for persons, beneficence, and justice upon which current regulations on human-subject protection are based.

1981

Federal Policy for the Protection of Human Subjects in Research: Regulations of both the HHS and the FDA are revised to reflect principles contained in the Belmont Report. They ensure broad backgrounds, and community attitudes, are represented on IRBs. Specific elements of informed consent are also spelled out.

President's Commission: The President's Commission for the Study of Ethical Problems in Medicine and Biomedical and Behavioral Research is established. One of its reports recommends a uniform federal regulatory system.

1982

CIOMS Guidelines: The Council for International Organizations of Medical Sciences publishes the first version of its International Ethical Guidelines for Biomedical Research Involving Human Subjects, aimed at researchers conducting studies in developing countries. The guidelines allow for cultural differences in ethical standards.

Consent agreement process: The FDA develops a "consent agreement" process for some investigators who might otherwise be disqualified via legal channels from conducting research. Investigators generally agree to do no further studies of drugs within FDA jurisdiction or agree to some specific restriction on their use of investigational drugs, such as conducting no more phase III studies.

1983

Special protections for children: HHS gives additional protections for children involved as subjects in federally-funded research.

1985

NDA regulations revised: With a rewrite of NDA regulations, the FDA begins accepting foreign clinical trial data as the sole basis for drug approval—sometimes with and sometimes without the need for an on-site inspection of the research site.

1987

IND rewrite: Contract research organizations (CROs) recognized as a regulated entity and can be transferred responsibility for certain parts of a study delegated to them. Trial sponsors are also required to identify studies they have audited or reviewed when submitting an NDA.

1988

Guidelines for the monitoring of clinical investigators: FDA requires sponsors to conduct quality assurance audits of the work of clinical investigators.

1990

International Conference on Harmonization (ICH): Government agencies and pharmaceutical trade organizations from Europe, Japan, and the United States create guidelines for clinical drug trials that cross national borders.

1991

Common Rule: The common rule is agreement by 15 federal departments and agencies to adopt a common set of human subject protections. It includes required review of research by an IRB, informed consent of subjects, and assurances of compliance by research institutions receiving federal support. The Common Rule has since been adopted by three additional federal agencies.

1993

Advisory Committee on Human Radiation Experiments (ACHRE): National press coverage about Cold War-era radiation experiments leads President Clinton to establish ACHRE to investigate reports of federally funded human research involving radioactive materials conducted between 1944 and 1972. The Committee urges that federal oversight of human subject protections focus on outcomes and performance, punishment be in proportion to violation and protections broaden to include research that is not federally funded.

NIH Revitalization Act: A controversial provision in the NIH Revitalization Act requires all NIH-funded studies to include representative samples of subpopulations, including women and members of diverse racial and ethnic groups, unless their exclusion is justified.

New FDA guidelines on inclusion of women: FDA sets guidelines calling for a "reasonable" number of women to be included in all new clinical trials, reversing its 1977 policy.

1995

National Bioethics Advisory Commission: On the advice of ACHRE, President Clinton establishes a think tank group composed of physicians, theologians, ethicists, scientists, lawyers, psychologists, and members of the public. Their charge is to make recommendations to government regarding ethical issues surrounding research on humans. The Commission is funded and led by HHS.

NDA regulations amended: The FDA amended the Code of Federal Regulation, requiring NDAs to include analysis of efficacy and safety data by gender, age, and racial subgroups.

1997

Food and Drug Administration Modernization Act: This new law gives pharmaceutical companies a huge financial incentive to conduct pediatric studies of drugs already FDA-approved for use in adults. In return for testing the efficacy and safety of drugs in children, companies are granted an extra six months of patent protection on those drugs. The FDA Modernization Act also expedited the development and review of applications for approval of products that treat a serious or life-threatening condition and have the potential to address an unmet medical need.

1998

FDA Financial Disclosure Regulations: FDA requires study sponsors to reveal any financial link between themselves and clinical investigators that may bias the design, conduct, or reporting of clinical studies.

Sex-related data presentation: FDA requires that safety and efficacy data be presented separately for men and women in NDA summaries. Also requires tabulation of the number of study participants by sex in investigational new drug reports.

1999

Office for Human Research Protections (OHRP): OPRR was renamed OHRP and elevated to department status within HHS to convey the importance of the function—and to avoid the appearance of a conflict of interest (since NIH also funds studies). It assumes responsibility for protection of human research subjects at institutions receiving federal funds, as well as implementing the 18-agency Common Rule.

2000

FDA Pediatric Rule: FDA's Pediatric Rule is finalized, requiring pediatric studies on any new drug that will be, or could be, used by children.

New research-suspending authority: FDA gives itself the authority to stop proposed research for life-threatening conditions if men or women are excluded because of their reproductive potential.

Medicare coverage of clinical trials: Health Care Financing Administration (now the Centers for Medicare and Medicaid Services) adopts new policy for Medicare to cover routine costs of qualifying clinical trials, as well as reasonable and necessary items and services used to diagnose and complications arising from participation in trials. Federally-funded trials and trials under an investigational new-drug application reviewed by the FDA automatically qualify. The policy also applies to enrollees in both the traditional Medicare and Medicare+ Choice programs.

2001

Clinical Investigation of Medicinal Products in the Pediatric Population: FDA establishes new rule, mandated by the Children's Health Act of 2000, that sets the standards for determining whether proposed pediatric clinical trials can be safely and ethically conducted. It is the FDA's first specific set of protections for children. The rule seeks, among other things, to assure children's assent to participate in clinical trials (when possible) and that their parents or guardians give fully informed consent to that participation. It adopts the principles, with some modifications, of HHS protections from 1983.

Public disclosure rule: FDA establishes new rule making information on all new and ongoing clinical trials involving gene therapy or xenotransplantation publicly available. Much of the gene therapy information to be disclosed is already publicly discussed in open meetings of the Recombinant DNA Advisory Committee of the NIH.

Office of Good Clinical Practice (OGCP): OGCP is opened by the FDA in order to establish consistency in policy. This office is broadly responsible for ensuring FDA's protective role in clinical research, from trial design through trial conduct, trial analyses, trial oversight, data integrity, and data quality. One of OGCP's highest priorities will be to bring about GCP compliance globally.

2002

Best Pharmaceuticals for Children Act: Best Pharmaceuticals for Children Act is designed to ensure that many more drugs already on the market will continue to be carefully studied in children. The new law not only gives pharmaceutical companies longer patent protection in exchange for conducting pediatric studies; it requires them to share what they learn as a result of those studies, good or bad. If they refuse to do a study that is requested by the FDA, a third party can do it as permitted by a fundraising organization for the NIH. A competitive bidding process for $200 million in funding is set up through the new NIH office to encourage pediatric clinical trials of older drugs whose patent has expired, meaning that generic versions of the drug are allowed to be produced.

Principles on the Conduct of Clinical Trials and Communication of Clinical Trial Results: Published by the Pharmaceutical Research and Manufacturers Association (PhRMA). In this document major pharmaceutical and biotechnology companies commit to disclosing the results, positive or negative, of later-stage clinical trials and set disclosure guidelines.

2004

Registration of Clinical Trials Requirement for Publication in Major Medical Journals: The International Committee of Medical Journal Editors (ICMJE) published a joint editorial aimed at promoting the registration of all clinical trials. The ICMJE states that it will consider a manuscript for publication only if the data presented in the manuscript comes from clinical trials that have been registered before the enrollment of the first patient. This policy applies to trials that start recruiting on or after July 1, 2005.

PhRMA Clinical Study Results Registry: PhRMA launched an online Clinical Study Results Database (ClinicalStudyResults.org) to provide a centralized repository for clinical trial results from industry-sponsored clinical trials.

2006

WHO Announces Introduction of International Registry of Clinical Trial Listings and Results: The World Health Organization announces that it will be launching a new centralized registry on the Internet in 2007 providing comprehensive international listings of government- and industry-funded clinical trials actively recruiting volunteers and the results of completed clinical trials.

2007

Food and Drug Administration Amendments Act: Mandates the creation of the internal committee called the Pediatric Review Committee (PeRC) and also mandates an expansion of ClinicalTrials.gov and requires responsible parties to register and submit study results of clinical trials to the online registry. The act also calls for expanded access—under "compassionate use"—to investigational drugs (not yet approved) for patients not participating/no longer participating in clinical trials and with no other alternative for treatment of a life-threatening condition or disease. Originally in FDAMA 1997, it is amended in the Food and Drug Administration Amendments Act of 2007 and now requires HHS to regulate how a physician may provide the drug under a risk-evaluation and -mitigation strategy (REMS).

2010

Patient Protection and Affordable Care Act: This broadly sweeping legislation requires, among many provisions, health insurers to provide coverage of routine patient costs associated with clinical trials beginning in 2014. Insurers cannot deny individual participation in trials, limit coverage in trial, or discriminate against an individual. The act creates a new office within NIH that will speed up translation of basic scientific discoveries into treatments; establishes a nonprofit organization PCORI (Patient-Centered Outcomes Research Institute) to oversee comparative effectiveness research; expands the role of the National Center on Minority Health and Health Disparities, which will become an Institute within NIH; creates a pathway for the manufacturing of safer and higher-quality generic biologics or biosimilars, and grants manufacturers 12 years of exclusivity under this new pathway; and implements a national education program to raise awareness of the threat of breast cancer in young women.

2012

FDA Safety and Innovation Act (FDASIA): Requires that research sponsors submit a pediatric study plan (PSP) early in the investigation new drug (IND) application phase. FDASIA also establishes public meetings inviting patients to provide their input into unmet medical needs; establishes the Generic Drug User Fee Act (GDUFA) to improve the availability of generic drugs; and assists sponsors in expediting the development of drugs that offer substantial health improvements for those that may suffer from serious or life-threatening diseases under a new "Breakthrough Therapies" classification.

2013

Physician Payment Sunshine Act (part of PPACA): Health providers and drug manufacturers must report payments or gifts of $10 or more made to physicians or hospitals (with some exceptions including educational materials) as well as ownership interests beginning in August 2013. The information will then be made public through the Centers for Medicare & Medicaid Services (CMS) by September 2014. This act is intended to improve conflict of interest disclosure.

APPENDIX C

Declaration of Helsinki

WMA Declaration of Helsinki
Ethical Principles for Medical Research
Involving Human Subjects

***

Preamble

1. The World Medical Association (WMA) has developed the Declaration of Helsinki as a statement of ethical principles for medical research involving human subjects, including research on identifiable human material and data.

The Declaration is intended to be read as a whole and each of its constituent paragraphs should be applied with consideration of all other relevant paragraphs.

2. Consistent with the mandate of the WMA, the Declaration is addressed primarily to physicians. The WMA encourages others who are involved in medical research involving human subjects to adopt these principles.

General Principles

3. The Declaration of Geneva of the WMA binds the physician with the words, "The health of my patient will be my first consideration," and the International Code of Medical Ethics declares that, "A physician shall act in the patient's best interest when providing medical care."

4. It is the duty of the physician to promote and safeguard the health, well-being and rights of patients, including those who are involved

in medical research. The physician's knowledge and conscience are dedicated to the fulfilment of this duty.

5. Medical progress is based on research that ultimately must include studies involving human subjects.

6. The primary purpose of medical research involving human subjects is to understand the causes, development and effects of diseases and improve preventive, diagnostic and therapeutic interventions (methods, procedures and treatments). Even the best proven interventions must be evaluated continually through research for their safety, effectiveness, efficiency, accessibility and quality.

7. Medical research is subject to ethical standards that promote and ensure respect for all human subjects and protect their health and rights.

8. While the primary purpose of medical research is to generate new knowledge, this goal can never take precedence over the rights and interests of individual research subjects.

9. It is the duty of physicians who are involved in medical research to protect the life, health, dignity, integrity, right to self-determination, privacy, and confidentiality of personal information of research subjects. The responsibility for the protection of research subjects must always rest with the physician or other health care professionals and never with the research subjects, even though they have given consent.

10. Physicians must consider the ethical, legal and regulatory norms and standards for research involving human subjects in their own countries as well as applicable international norms and standards. No national or international ethical, legal or regulatory requirement should reduce or eliminate any of the protections for research subjects set forth in this Declaration.

11. Medical research should be conducted in a manner that minimises possible harm to the environment.

12. Medical research involving human subjects must be conducted only by individuals with the appropriate ethics and scientific education, training and qualifications. Research on patients or healthy volunteers requires the supervision of a competent and appropriately qualified physician or other health care professional.

13. Groups that are underrepresented in medical research should be provided appropriate access to participation in research.

14. Physicians who combine medical research with medical care should involve their patients in research only to the extent that this is justified by its potential preventive, diagnostic or therapeutic value and if the physician has good reason to believe that participation in the research study will not adversely affect the health of the patients who serve as research subjects.

15. Appropriate compensation and treatment for subjects who are harmed as a result of participating in research must be ensured.

Risks, Burdens and Benefits

16. In medical practice and in medical research, most interventions involve risks and burdens.

Medical research involving human subjects may only be conducted if the importance of the objective outweighs the risks and burdens to the research subjects.

17. All medical research involving human subjects must be preceded by careful assessment of predictable risks and burdens to the individuals and groups involved in the research in comparison with foreseeable benefits to them and to other individuals or groups affected by the condition under investigation.

Measures to minimise the risks must be implemented. The risks must be continuously monitored, assessed and documented by the researcher.

18. Physicians may not be involved in a research study involving human subjects unless they are confident that the risks have been adequately assessed and can be satisfactorily managed.

When the risks are found to outweigh the potential benefits or when there is conclusive proof of definitive outcomes, physicians must assess whether to continue, modify or immediately stop the study.

Vulnerable Groups and Individuals

19. Some groups and individuals are particularly vulnerable and may have an increased likelihood of being wronged or of incurring additional harm.

All vulnerable groups and individuals should receive specifically considered protection.

20. Medical research with a vulnerable group is only justified if the research is responsive to the health needs or priorities of this group and the research cannot be carried out in a non-vulnerable group. In addition, this group should stand to benefit from the knowledge, practices or interventions that result from the research.

Scientific Requirements and Research Protocols

21. Medical research involving human subjects must conform to generally accepted scientific principles, be based on a thorough knowledge of the scientific literature, other relevant sources of information, and adequate laboratory and, as appropriate, animal experimentation. The welfare of animals used for research must be respected.

22. The design and performance of each research study involving human subjects must be clearly described and justified in a research protocol.

The protocol should contain a statement of the ethical considerations involved and should indicate how the principles in this Declaration have been addressed. The protocol should include information regarding funding, sponsors, institutional affiliations, potential conflicts of interest, incentives for subjects and information regarding provisions for treating and/or compensating subjects who are harmed as a consequence of participation in the research study.

In clinical trials, the protocol must also describe appropriate arrangements for post-trial provisions.

Research Ethics Committees

23. The research protocol must be submitted for consideration, comment, guidance and approval to the concerned research ethics committee before the study begins. This committee must be transparent in its functioning, must be independent of the researcher, the sponsor and any other undue influence and must be duly qualified. It must take into consideration the laws and regulations of the country or countries in which the research is to be performed as well as applicable international norms and standards but these must not be allowed to reduce or eliminate any of the protections for research subjects set forth in this Declaration.

The committee must have the right to monitor ongoing studies. The researcher must provide monitoring information to the committee, especially information about any serious adverse events. No amendment to the protocol may be made without consideration and approval by the committee. After the end of the study, the researchers must submit a final report to the committee containing a summary of the study's findings and conclusions.

Privacy and Confidentiality

24. Every precaution must be taken to protect the privacy of research subjects and the confidentiality of their personal information.

Informed Consent

25. Participation by individuals capable of giving informed consent as subjects in medical research must be voluntary. Although it may be appropriate to consult family members or community leaders, no individual capable of giving informed consent may be enrolled in a research study unless he or she freely agrees.

26. In medical research involving human subjects capable of giving informed consent, each potential subject must be adequately informed of the aims, methods, sources of funding, any possible conflicts of interest, institutional affiliations of the researcher, the anticipated benefits and potential risks of the study and the discomfort it may entail, post-study provisions and any other relevant aspects of the study. The potential subject must be informed of the right to refuse to participate in the study or to withdraw consent to participate at any time without reprisal. Special attention should be given to the specific information needs of individual potential subjects as well as to the methods used to deliver the information.

After ensuring that the potential subject has understood the information, the physician or another appropriately qualified individual must then seek the potential subject's freely-given informed consent, preferably in writing. If the consent cannot be expressed in writing, the non-written consent must be formally documented and witnessed.

All medical research subjects should be given the option of being informed about the general outcome and results of the study.

27. When seeking informed consent for participation in a research study the physician must be particularly cautious if the potential subject is in a dependent relationship with the physician or may consent under duress. In such situations the informed consent must be sought by an appropriately qualified individual who is completely independent of this relationship.

28. For a potential research subject who is incapable of giving informed consent, the physician must seek informed consent from the legally authorised representative. These individuals must not be included in a research study that has no likelihood of benefit for them unless it is intended to promote the health of the group represented by the potential subject, the research cannot instead be performed with persons capable of providing informed consent, and the research entails only minimal risk and minimal burden.

29. When a potential research subject who is deemed incapable of giving informed consent is able to give assent to decisions about participation in research, the physician must seek that assent in addition to the consent of the legally authorised representative. The potential subject's dissent should be respected.

30. Research involving subjects who are physically or mentally incapable of giving consent, for example, unconscious patients, may be done only if the physical or mental condition that prevents giving informed consent is a necessary characteristic of the research group. In such circumstances the physician must seek informed consent from the legally authorised representative. If no such representative is available and if the research cannot be delayed, the study may proceed without informed consent provided that the specific reasons for involving subjects with a condition that renders them unable to give informed consent have been stated in the research protocol and the study has been approved by a research ethics committee. Consent to remain in the research must be obtained as soon as possible from the subject or a legally authorised representative.

31. The physician must fully inform the patient which aspects of their care are related to the research. The refusal of a patient to participate in a study or the patient's decision to withdraw from the study must never adversely affect the patient-physician relationship.

32. For medical research using identifiable human material or data, such as research on material or data contained in biobanks or similar repositories, physicians must seek informed consent for its collection, storage and/or reuse. There may be exceptional situations where consent would be impossible or impracticable to obtain for such research. In such situations the research may be done only after consideration and approval of a research ethics committee.

Use of Placebo

33. The benefits, risks, burdens and effectiveness of a new intervention must be tested against those of the best proven intervention(s), except in the following circumstances:

Where no proven intervention exists, the use of placebo, or no intervention, is acceptable; or

Where for compelling and scientifically sound methodological reasons the use of any intervention less effective than the best proven one, the use of placebo, or no intervention is necessary to determine the efficacy or safety of an intervention

and the patients who receive any intervention less effective than the best proven one, placebo, or no intervention will not be subject to additional risks of serious or irreversible harm as a result of not receiving the best proven intervention.

Extreme care must be taken to avoid abuse of this option.

Post-Trial Provisions

34. In advance of a clinical trial, sponsors, researchers and host country governments should make provisions for post-trial access for all participants who still need an intervention identified as beneficial in the trial. This information must also be disclosed to participants during the informed consent process.

Research Registration and Publication and Dissemination of Results

35. Every research study involving human subjects must be registered in a publicly accessible database before recruitment of the first subject.

36. Researchers, authors, sponsors, editors and publishers all have ethical obligations with regard to the publication and dissemination of the results of research. Researchers have a duty to make publicly available the results of their research on human subjects and are accountable for the completeness and accuracy of their reports. All parties should adhere to accepted guidelines for ethical reporting. Negative and inconclusive as well as positive results must be published or otherwise made publicly available. Sources of funding, institutional affiliations and conflicts of interest must be declared in the publication. Reports of research not in accordance with the principles of this Declaration should not be accepted for publication.

Unproven Interventions in Clinical Practice

37. In the treatment of an individual patient, where proven interventions do not exist or other known interventions have been ineffective, the physician, after seeking expert advice, with informed consent from the patient or a legally authorised representative, may use an unproven intervention if in the physician's judgement it offers hope of saving life, re-establishing health or alleviating suffering. This intervention should subsequently be made the object of research, designed to evaluate its safety and efficacy. In all cases, new information must be recorded and, where appropriate, made publicly available.

APPENDIX D

The Belmont Report

Office of the Secretary

Ethical Principles and Guidelines for the Protection of Human Subjects of Research

The National Commission for the Protection of Human Subjects of Biomedical and Behavioral Research

April 18, 1979

AGENCY: Department of Health, Education, and Welfare.

ACTION: Notice of Report for Public Comment.

SUMMARY: On July 12, 1974, the National Research Act (Pub. L. 93-348) was signed into law, there-by creating the National Commission for the Protection of Human Subjects of Biomedical and Behavioral Research. One of the charges to the Commission was to identify the basic ethical principles that should underlie the conduct of biomedical and behavioral research involving human subjects and to develop guidelines which should be followed to assure that such research is conducted in accordance with those principles. In carrying out the above, the Commission was directed to consider: (i) the boundaries between biomedical and behavioral research and the accepted and routine practice of medicine, (ii) the role of assessment of risk-benefit criteria in the determination of the appropriateness of research involving human subjects, (iii) appropriate guidelines for the selection of human subjects for participation in such research and (iv) the nature and definition of informed consent in various research settings.

The Belmont Report attempts to summarize the basic ethical principles identified by the Commission in the course of its deliberations. It is the outgrowth of an intensive four-day period of discussions that were held in February 1976 at the Smithsonian Institution's Belmont Conference Center supplemented by the monthly deliberations of the Commission that were held over a period of nearly four years. It is a statement of basic ethical principles and guidelines that should assist in resolving the ethical problems that surround the conduct of research with human subjects. By publishing the Report in the Federal Register, and providing reprints upon request, the Secretary intends that it may be made readily available to scientists, members of Institutional Review Boards, and Federal employees. The two-volume Appendix, containing the lengthy reports of experts and specialists who assisted the Commission in fulfilling this part of its charge, is available as DHEW Publication No. (OS) 78-0013 and No. (OS) 78-0014, for sale by the Superintendent of Documents, U.S. Government Printing Office, Washington, D.C. 20402.

Unlike most other reports of the Commission, the Belmont Report does not make specific recommendations for administrative action by the Secretary of Health, Education, and Welfare. Rather, the Commission recommended that the Belmont Report be adopted in its entirety, as a statement of the Department's policy. The Department requests public comment on this recommendation.

National Commission for the Protection of Human Subjects of Biomedical and Behavioral Research

Members of the Commission

Kenneth John Ryan, M.D., Chairman, Chief of Staff, Boston Hospital for Women.

Joseph V. Brady, Ph.D., Professor of Behavioral Biology, Johns Hopkins University.

Robert E. Cooke, M.D., President, Medical College of Pennsylvania.

Dorothy I. Height, President, National Council of Negro Women, Inc.

Albert R. Jonsen, Ph.D., Associate Professor of Bioethics, University of California at San Francisco.

Patricia King, J.D., Associate Professor of Law, Georgetown University Law Center.

Karen Lebacqz, Ph.D., Associate Professor of Christian Ethics, Pacific School of Religion.

**** David W. Louisell, J.D., Professor of Law, University of California at Berkeley.*

Donald W. Seldin, M.D., Professor and Chairman, Department of Internal Medicine, University of Texas at Dallas.

****Eliot Stellar, Ph.D., Provost of the University and Professor of Physiological Psychology, University of Pennsylvania.*

**** Robert H. Turtle, LL.B., Attorney, VomBaur, Coburn, Simmons & Turtle, Washington, D.C.*

****Deceased.*

Table of Contents

Ethical Principles & Guidelines for Research Involving Human Subjects

Scientific research has produced substantial social benefits. It has also posed some troubling ethical questions. Public attention was drawn to these questions by reported abuses of human subjects in biomedical experiments, especially during the Second World War. During the Nuremberg War Crime Trials, the Nuremberg code was drafted as a set of standards for judging physicians and scientists who had conducted biomedical experiments on concentration camp prisoners. This code became the prototype of many later codes(1) intended to assure that research involving human subjects would be carried out in an ethical manner.

The codes consist of rules, some general, others specific, that guide the investigators or the reviewers of research in their work. Such rules often are inadequate to cover complex situations; at times they come into conflict, and they are frequently difficult to interpret or apply. Broader ethical principles will provide a basis on which specific rules may be formulated, criticized and interpreted.

Three principles, or general prescriptive judgments, that are relevant to research involving human subjects are identified in this statement. Other principles may also be relevant. These three are comprehensive, however, and are stated at a level of generalization that should assist scientists, subjects, reviewers and interested citizens to understand the ethical issues inherent in research involving human subjects. These principles cannot always be applied so as to resolve beyond dispute particular ethical problems. The objective is to provide an analytical framework that will guide the resolution of ethical problems arising from research involving human subjects.

This statement consists of a distinction between research and practice, a discussion of the three basic ethical principles, and remarks about the application of these principles.

Part A: Boundaries Between Practice & Research

A. Boundaries Between Practice and Research

It is important to distinguish between biomedical and behavioral research, on the one hand, and the practice of accepted therapy on the other, in order to know what activities ought to undergo review for the protection of human subjects of research. The distinction between research and practice is blurred partly because both often occur together (as in research designed to evaluate a therapy) and partly because notable departures from standard practice are often called "experimental" when the terms "experimental" and "research" are not carefully defined.

For the most part, the term "practice" refers to interventions that are designed solely to enhance the well-being of an individual patient or client and that have a reasonable expectation of success. The purpose of medical or behavioral practice is to provide diagnosis, preventive treatment or therapy to particular individuals.(2) By contrast, the term "research' designates an activity designed to test an hypothesis, permit conclusions to be drawn, and thereby to develop or contribute to generalizable knowledge (expressed, for example, in theories, principles, and statements of relationships). Research is usually described in a formal protocol that sets forth an objective and a set of procedures designed to reach that objective.

When a clinician departs in a significant way from standard or accepted practice, the innovation does not, in and of itself, constitute research. The fact that a procedure is "experimental," in the sense of new, untested or different, does not automatically place it in the category of research. Radically new procedures of this description should, however, be made the object of formal research at an early stage in order to determine whether they are safe and effective. Thus, it is the responsibility of medical practice committees, for example, to insist that a major innovation be incorporated into a formal research project.(3)

Research and practice may be carried on together when research is designed to evaluate the safety and efficacy of a therapy. This need not cause any confusion regarding whether or not the activity requires review; the general rule is that if there is any element of research in an activity, that activity should undergo review for the protection of human subjects.

Part B: Basic Ethical Principles

B. Basic Ethical Principles

The expression "basic ethical principles" refers to those general judgments that serve as a basic justification for the many particular ethical prescriptions and evaluations of human actions. Three basic principles, among those generally accepted in our cultural tradition, are particularly relevant to the ethics of research involving human subjects: the principles of respect of persons, beneficence and justice.

1. Respect for Persons.—Respect for persons incorporates at least two ethical convictions: first, that individuals should be treated as autonomous agents, and second, that persons with diminished autonomy are entitled to protection. The principle of respect for persons thus divides into two separate moral requirements: the requirement to acknowledge autonomy and the requirement to protect those with diminished autonomy.

An autonomous person is an individual capable of deliberation about personal goals and of acting under the direction of such deliberation. To respect autonomy is to give weight to autonomous persons' considered opinions and choices while refraining from obstructing their actions unless they are clearly detrimental to others. To show lack of respect for an autonomous agent is to repudiate that person's considered judgments, to deny an individual the freedom to act on those considered judgments, or to withhold information necessary to make a considered judgment, when there are no compelling reasons to do so.

However, not every human being is capable of self-determination. The capacity for self-determination matures during an individual's life, and some individuals lose this capacity wholly or in part because of illness, mental disability, or circumstances that severely restrict liberty. Respect for the immature and the incapacitated may require protecting them as they mature or while they are incapacitated.

Some persons are in need of extensive protection, even to the point of excluding them from activities which may harm them; other persons require little protection beyond making sure they undertake activities freely and with awareness of possible adverse consequence. The extent of protection afforded should depend upon the risk of harm and the likelihood of benefit. The judgment that any individual lacks autonomy should be periodically reevaluated and will vary in different situations.

In most cases of research involving human subjects, respect for persons demands that subjects enter into the research voluntarily and with adequate information. In some situations, however, application of the principle is not obvious. The involvement of prisoners as subjects of research provides an instructive example. On the one hand, it would seem that the principle of respect for persons requires that prisoners not be deprived of the opportunity to volunteer for research. On the other hand, under prison conditions they may be subtly coerced or unduly influenced to engage in research activities for which they would not otherwise volunteer. Respect for persons would then dictate that prisoners be protected. Whether to allow prisoners to "volunteer" or to "protect" them presents a dilemma. Respecting persons, in most hard cases, is often a matter of balancing competing claims urged by the principle of respect itself.

2. Beneficence.—Persons are treated in an ethical manner not only by respecting their decisions and protecting them from harm, but also by making efforts to secure their well-being. Such treatment falls under the principle of beneficence. The term "beneficence" is often understood to cover acts of kindness or charity that go beyond strict obligation. In this document, beneficence is understood in a stronger sense, as an obligation. Two general rules have been formulated as complementary expressions of beneficent actions in this sense: **(1)** do not harm and **(2)** maximize possible benefits and minimize possible harms.

The Hippocratic maxim "do no harm" has long been a fundamental principle of medical ethics. Claude Bernard extended it to the realm of research, saying that one should not injure one person regardless of the benefits that might come to others. However, even avoiding harm requires learning what is harmful; and, in the process of obtaining this information, persons may be exposed to risk of harm. Further, the Hippocratic Oath requires physicians to benefit their patients "according to their best judgment." Learning what will in fact benefit may require exposing persons to risk. The problem posed by these imperatives is to decide when it is justifiable to seek certain benefits despite the risks involved, and when the benefits should be foregone because of the risks.

The obligations of beneficence affect both individual investigators and society at large, because they extend both to particular research projects and to the entire enterprise of research. In the case of particular projects, investigators and members of their institutions are obliged to give forethought to the maximization of benefits and the reduction of risk that might occur from the research investigation. In the case of scientific research in general, members of the larger society are obliged to recognize the longer term benefits and risks that may result from the improvement of knowledge and from the development of novel medical, psychotherapeutic, and social procedures.

The principle of beneficence often occupies a well-defined justifying role in many areas of research involving human subjects. An example is found in research involving children. Effective ways of treating childhood diseases and fostering healthy development are benefits that serve to justify research involving children—even when individual research subjects are not direct beneficiaries. Research also makes it possible to avoid the harm that may result from the application of previously accepted routine practices that on closer investigation turn out to be dangerous. But the role of the principle of beneficence is not always so unambiguous. A difficult ethical problem remains, for example, about research that presents more than minimal risk without immediate prospect of direct benefit to the children involved. Some have argued that such research is inadmissible, while others have pointed out that this limit would rule out much research promising great benefit to children in the future. Here again, as with all hard cases, the different claims covered by the principle of beneficence may come into conflict and force difficult choices.

3. Justice.—Who ought to receive the benefits of research and bear its burdens? This is a question of justice, in the sense of "fairness in distribution" or "what is deserved." An injustice occurs when some benefit to which a person is entitled is denied without good reason or when some burden is imposed unduly. Another way of conceiving the principle of justice is that equals ought to be treated equally. However, this statement requires explication. Who is equal and who is unequal? What considerations justify departure from equal distribution? Almost all commentators allow that distinctions based on experience, age, deprivation, competence, merit and position do sometimes constitute criteria justifying differential treatment for certain purposes. It is necessary, then, to explain in what respects people should be treated equally. There are several widely accepted formulations of just ways to distribute burdens and benefits. Each formulation mentions some relevant property on the basis of which burdens and benefits should be distributed. These formulations are **(1)** to each person an equal share, **(2)** to each person according to individual need, **(3)** to each person according to individual effort, **(4)** to each person according to societal contribution, and **(5)** to each person according to merit.

Questions of justice have long been associated with social practices such as punishment, taxation and political representation. Until recently these questions have not generally been associated with scientific research. However, they are foreshadowed even in the earliest reflections on the ethics of research involving human subjects. For example, during the 19th and early 20th centuries the burdens of serving as research subjects fell largely upon poor ward patients, while the benefits of improved medical care flowed primarily to private patients. Subsequently, the exploitation of unwilling prisoners as research subjects in Nazi concentration camps was condemned as a particularly flagrant injustice. In this country, in the 1940's, the Tuskegee syphilis study used disadvantaged, rural black men to study the untreated course of a disease that is by no means confined to that population. These subjects were deprived of demonstrably effective treatment in order not to interrupt the project, long after such treatment became generally available.

Against this historical background, it can be seen how conceptions of justice are relevant to research involving human subjects. For example, the selection of research subjects needs to be scrutinized in order to determine whether some classes (e.g., welfare patients, particular racial and ethnic minorities, or persons confined to institutions) are being systematically selected simply because of their easy availability, their compromised position, or their manipulability, rather than for reasons directly related to the problem being studied. Finally, whenever research supported by public funds leads to the development of therapeutic devices and procedures, justice demands both that these not provide advantages only to those who can afford them and that such research should not unduly involve persons from groups unlikely to be among the beneficiaries of subsequent applications of the research.

Part C: Applications

C. Applications

Applications of the general principles to the conduct of research leads to consideration of the following requirements: informed consent, risk/benefit assessment, and the selection of subjects of research.

1. Informed Consent.—Respect for persons requires that subjects, to the degree that they are capable, be given the opportunity to choose what shall or shall not happen to them. This opportunity is provided when adequate standards for informed consent are satisfied.

While the importance of informed consent is unquestioned, controversy prevails over the nature and possibility of an informed consent. Nonetheless, there is widespread agreement that the consent process can be analyzed as containing three elements: information, comprehension and voluntariness.

Information. Most codes of research establish specific items for disclosure intended to assure that subjects are given sufficient information. These items generally include: the research procedure, their purposes, risks and anticipated benefits, alternative procedures (where therapy is involved), and a statement offering the subject the opportunity to ask questions and to withdraw at any time from the research. Additional items have been proposed, including how subjects are selected, the person responsible for the research, etc.

However, a simple listing of items does not answer the question of what the standard should be for judging how much and what sort of information should be provided. One standard frequently invoked in medical practice, namely the information commonly provided by practitioners in the field or in the locale, is inadequate since research takes place precisely when a common understanding does not exist. Another standard, currently popular in malpractice law, requires the practitioner to reveal the information that reasonable persons would wish to know in order to make a decision regarding their care. This, too, seems insufficient since the research subject, being in essence a volunteer, may wish to know considerably more about risks gratuitously undertaken than do patients who deliver themselves into the hand of a clinician for needed care. It may be that a standard of "the reasonable volunteer" should be proposed: the extent and nature of information should be such that persons, knowing that the procedure is neither necessary for their care nor perhaps fully understood, can decide whether they wish to participate in the furthering of knowledge. Even when some direct benefit to them is anticipated, the subjects should understand clearly the range of risk and the voluntary nature of participation.

A special problem of consent arises where informing subjects of some pertinent aspect of the research is likely to impair the validity of the research. In many cases, it is sufficient to indicate to subjects that they are being invited to participate in research of which some features will not be revealed until the research is concluded. In all cases of research involving incomplete disclosure, such research is justified only if it is clear that **(1)** incomplete disclosure is truly necessary to accomplish the goals of the research, **(2)** there are no undisclosed risks to subjects that are more than minimal, and **(3)** there is an adequate plan for debriefing subjects, when appropriate, and for dissemination of research results to them. Information about risks should never be withheld for the purpose of eliciting the cooperation of subjects, and truthful answers should always be given to direct questions about the research. Care should be taken to distinguish cases in which disclosure would destroy or invalidate the research from cases in which disclosure would simply inconvenience the investigator.

Comprehension. The manner and context in which information is conveyed is as important as the information itself. For example, presenting information in a disorganized and rapid fashion, allowing too little time for consideration or curtailing opportunities for questioning, all may adversely affect a subject's ability to make an informed choice.

Because the subject's ability to understand is a function of intelligence, rationality, maturity and language, it is necessary to adapt the presentation of the information to the subject's capacities. Investigators are responsible for ascertaining that the subject has comprehended the information. While there is always an obligation to ascertain that the information about risk to subjects is complete and adequately comprehended, when the risks are more serious, that obligation increases. On occasion, it may be suitable to give some oral or written tests of comprehension.

Special provision may need to be made when comprehension is severely limited,—for example, by conditions of immaturity or mental disability. Each class of subjects that one might consider as incompetent (e.g., infants and young children, mentally disable patients, the terminally ill and the comatose) should be considered on its own terms. Even for these persons, however, respect requires giving them the opportunity to choose to the extent they are able, whether or not to participate in research. The objections of these subjects to involvement should be honored, unless the research entails providing them a therapy unavailable elsewhere. Respect for persons also requires seeking the permission of other parties in order to protect the subjects from harm. Such persons are thus respected both by acknowledging their own wishes and by the use of third parties to protect them from harm.

The third parties chosen should be those who are most likely to understand the incompetent subject's situation and to act in that person's best interest. The person authorized to act on behalf of the subject should be given an opportunity to observe the research as it proceeds in order to be able to withdraw the subject from the research, if such action appears in the subject's best interest.

Voluntariness. An agreement to participate in research constitutes a valid consent only if voluntarily given. This element of informed consent requires conditions free of coercion and undue influence. Coercion occurs when an overt threat of harm is intentionally presented by one person to another in order to obtain compliance. Undue influence, by contrast, occurs through an offer of an excessive, unwarranted, inappropriate or improper reward or other overture in order to obtain compliance. Also, inducements that would ordinarily be acceptable may become undue influences if the subject is especially vulnerable.

Unjustifiable pressures usually occur when persons in positions of authority or commanding influence—especially where possible sanctions are involved—urge a course of action for a subject. A continuum of such influencing factors exists, however, and it is impossible to state precisely where justifiable persuasion ends and undue influence begins. But undue influence would include actions such as manipulating a person's choice through the controlling influence of a close relative and threatening to withdraw health services to which an individual would otherwise be entitle.

2. Assessment of Risks and Benefits.—The assessment of risks and benefits requires a careful arrayal of relevant data, including, in some cases, alternative ways of obtaining the benefits sought in the research. Thus, the assessment presents both an opportunity and a responsibility to gather systematic and comprehensive information about proposed research. For the investigator, it is a means to examine whether the proposed research is properly designed. For a review committee, it is a method for determining whether the risks that will be presented to subjects are justified. For prospective subjects, the assessment will assist the determination whether or not to participate.

The Nature and Scope of Risks and Benefits. The requirement that research be justified on the basis of a favorable risk/benefit assessment bears a close relation to the principle of beneficence, just as the moral requirement that informed consent be obtained is derived primarily from the principle of respect for persons. The term "risk" refers to a possibility that harm may occur. However, when expressions such as "small risk" or "high risk" are used, they usually refer (often ambiguously) both to the chance (probability) of experiencing a harm and the severity (magnitude) of the envisioned harm.

The term "benefit" is used in the research context to refer to something of positive value related to health or welfare. Unlike, "risk," "benefit" is not a term that expresses probabilities. Risk is properly contrasted to probability of benefits, and benefits are properly contrasted with harms rather than risks of harm. Accordingly, so-called risk/benefit assessments are concerned with the probabilities and magnitudes of possible harm and anticipated benefits. Many kinds of possible harms and benefits need to be taken into account. There are, for example, risks of psychological harm, physical harm, legal harm, social harm and economic harm and the corresponding benefits. While the most likely types of harms to research subjects are those of psychological or physical pain or injury, other possible kinds should not be overlooked.

Risks and benefits of research may affect the individual subjects, the families of the individual subjects, and society at large (or special groups of subjects in society). Previous codes and Federal regulations have required that risks to subjects be outweighed by the sum of both the anticipated benefit to the subject, if any, and the anticipated benefit to society in the form of knowledge to be gained from the research. In balancing these different elements, the risks and benefits affecting the immediate research subject will normally carry special weight. On the other hand, interests other than those of the subject may on some occasions be sufficient by themselves to justify the risks involved in the research, so long as the subjects' rights have been protected. Beneficence thus requires that we protect against risk of harm to subjects and also that we be concerned about the loss of the substantial benefits that might be gained from research.

The Systematic Assessment of Risks and Benefits. It is commonly said that benefits and risks must be "balanced" and shown to be "in a favorable ratio." The metaphorical character of these terms draws attention to the difficulty of making precise judgments. Only on rare occasions will quantitative techniques be available for the scrutiny of research protocols. However, the idea of systematic, nonarbitrary analysis of risks and benefits should be emulated insofar as possible. This ideal requires those making decisions about the justifiability of research to be thorough in the accumulation and assessment of information about all aspects of the research, and to consider alternatives systematically. This procedure renders the assessment of research more rigorous and precise, while making communication between review board members and investigators less subject to misinterpretation, misinformation and conflicting judgments. Thus, there should first be a determination of the validity of the presuppositions of the research; then the nature, probability and magnitude of risk should be distinguished with as much clarity as possible. The method of ascertaining risks should be explicit, especially where there is no alternative to the use of such vague categories as small or slight risk. It should also be determined whether an investigator's estimates of the probability of harm or benefits are reasonable, as judged by known facts or other available studies.

Finally, assessment of the justifiability of research should reflect at least the following considerations: **(i)** Brutal or inhumane treatment of human subjects is never morally justified. **(ii)** Risks should be reduced to those necessary to achieve the research objective. It should be determined whether it is in fact necessary to use human subjects at all. Risk can perhaps never be entirely eliminated, but it can often be reduced by careful attention to alternative procedures. **(iii)** When research involves significant risk of serious impairment, review committees should be extraordinarily insistent on the justification of the risk (looking usually to the likelihood of benefit to the subject—or, in some rare cases, to the manifest voluntariness of the participation).

(iv) When vulnerable populations are involved in research, the appropriateness of involving them should itself be demonstrated. A number of variables go into such judgments, including the nature and degree of risk, the condition of the particular population involved, and the nature and level of the anticipated benefits. **(v)** Relevant risks and benefits must be thoroughly arrayed in documents and procedures used in the informed consent process.

3. Selection of Subjects.—Just as the principle of respect for persons finds expression in the requirements for consent, and the principle of beneficence in risk/benefit assessment, the principle of justice gives rise to moral requirements that there be fair procedures and outcomes in the selection of research subjects.

Justice is relevant to the selection of subjects of research at two levels: the social and the individual. Individual justice in the selection of subjects would require that researchers exhibit fairness: thus, they should not offer potentially beneficial research only to some patients who are in their favor or select only "undesirable" persons for risky research. Social justice requires that distinction be drawn between classes of subjects that ought, and ought not, to participate in any particular kind of research, based on the ability of members of that class to bear burdens and on the appropriateness of placing further burdens on already burdened persons. Thus, it can be considered a matter of social justice that there is an order of preference in the selection of classes of subjects (e.g., adults before children) and that some classes of potential subjects (e.g., the institutionalized mentally infirm or prisoners) may be involved as research subjects, if at all, only on certain conditions.

Injustice may appear in the selection of subjects, even if individual subjects are selected fairly by investigators and treated fairly in the course of research. Thus injustice arises from social, racial, sexual and cultural biases institutionalized in society. Thus, even if individual researchers are treating their research subjects fairly, and even if IRBs are taking care to assure that subjects are selected fairly within a particular institution, unjust social patterns may nevertheless appear in the overall distribution of the burdens and benefits of research. Although individual institutions or investigators may not be able to resolve a problem that is pervasive in their social setting, they can consider distributive justice in selecting research subjects.

Some populations, especially institutionalized ones, are already burdened in many ways by their infirmities and environments. When research is proposed that involves risks and does not include a therapeutic component, other less burdened classes of persons should be called upon first to accept these risks of research, except where the research is directly related to the specific conditions of the class involved. Also, even though public funds for research may often flow in the same directions as public funds for health care, it seems unfair that populations dependent on public health care constitute a pool of preferred research subjects if more advantaged populations are likely to be the recipients of the benefits.

One special instance of injustice results from the involvement of vulnerable subjects. Certain groups, such as racial minorities, the economically disadvantaged, the very sick, and the institutionalized may continually be sought as research subjects, owing to their ready availability in settings where research is conducted. Given their dependent status and their frequently compromised capacity for free consent, they should be protected against the danger of being involved in research solely for administrative convenience, or because they are easy to manipulate as a result of their illness or socioeconomic condition.

(**1**) Since 1945, various codes for the proper and responsible conduct of human experimentation in medical research have been adopted by different organizations. The best known of these codes are the Nuremberg Code of 1947, the Helsinki Declaration of 1964 (revised in 1975), and the 1971 Guidelines (codified into Federal Regulations in 1974) issued by the U.S. Department of Health, Education, and Welfare Codes for the conduct of social and behavioral research have also been adopted, the best known being that of the American Psychological Association, published in 1973.

(**2**) Although practice usually involves interventions designed solely to enhance the well-being of a particular individual, interventions are sometimes applied to one individual for the enhancement of the well-being of another (e.g., blood donation, skin grafts, organ transplants) or an intervention may have the dual purpose of enhancing the well-being of a particular individual, and, at the same time, providing some benefit to others (e.g., vaccination, which protects both the person who is vaccinated and society generally). The fact that some forms of practice have elements other than immediate benefit to the individual receiving an intervention, however, should not confuse the general distinction between research and practice. Even when a procedure applied in practice may benefit some other person, it remains an intervention designed to enhance the well-being of a particular individual or groups of individuals; thus, it is practice and need not be reviewed as research.

(**3**) Because the problems related to social experimentation may differ substantially from those of biomedical and behavioral research, the Commission specifically declines to make any policy determination regarding such research at this time. Rather, the Commission believes that the problem ought to be addressed by one of its successor bodies.

APPENDIX E

Code of Federal Regulations

TITLE 45
PUBLIC WELFARE

DEPARTMENT OF HEALTH AND HUMAN SERVICES

PART 46
PROTECTION OF HUMAN SUBJECTS

* * *

Subpart A Basic HHS Policy for Protection of Human Research Subjects

Sec.

46.101 To what does this policy apply?

46.102 Definitions.

46.103 Assuring compliance with this policy—research conducted or supported by any Federal Department or Agency.

46.104-46.106 [Reserved]

46.107 IRB membership.

46.108 IRB functions and operations.

46.109 IRB review of research.

46.110	Expedited review procedures for certain kinds of research involving no more than minimal risk, and for minor changes in approved research.
46.111	Criteria for IRB approval of research.
46.112	Review by institution.
46.113	Suspension or termination of IRB approval of research.
46.114	Cooperative research.
46.115	IRB records.
46.116	General requirements for informed consent.
46.117	Documentation of informed consent.
46.118	Applications and proposals lacking definite plans for involvement of human subjects.
46.119	Research undertaken without the intention of involving human subjects.
46.120	Evaluation and disposition of applications and proposals for research to be conducted or supported by a Federal Department or Agency.
46.121	[Reserved]
46.122	Use of Federal funds.
46.123	Early termination of research support: Evaluation of applications and proposals.
46.124	Conditions.

Subpart B Additional Protections for Pregnant Women, Human Fetuses and Neonates Involved in Research

Sec.

46.201	To what do these regulations apply?

46.202 Definitions.

46.203 Duties of IRBs in connection with research involving pregnant women, fetuses, and neonates.

46.204 Research involving pregnant women or fetuses.

46.205 Research involving neonates.

46.206 Research involving, after delivery, the placenta, the dead fetus or fetal material.

46.207 Research not otherwise approvable which presents an opportunity to understand, prevent, or alleviate a serious problem affecting the health or welfare of pregnant women, fetuses, or neonates.

Subpart C Additional Protections Pertaining to Biomedical and Behavioral Research Involving Prisoners as Subjects

Sec.

46.301 Applicability.

46.302 Purpose.

46.303 Definitions.

46.304 Composition of Institutional Review Boards where prisoners are involved.

46.305 Additional duties of the Institutional Review Boards where prisoners are involved.

46.306 Permitted research involving prisoners.

Subpart D Additional Protections for Children Involved as Subjects in Research

Sec.

46.401 To what do these regulations apply?

46.402	Definitions.
46.403	IRB duties.
46.404	Research not involving greater than minimal risk.
46.405	Research involving greater than minimal risk but presenting the prospect of direct benefit to the individual subjects.
46.406	Research involving greater than minimal risk and no prospect of direct benefit to individual subjects, but likely to yield generalizable knowledge about the subject's disorder or condition.
46.407	Research not otherwise approvable which presents an opportunity to understand, prevent, or alleviate a serious problem affecting the health or welfare of children.
46.408	Requirements for permission by parents or guardians and for assent by children.
46.409	Wards.

Subpart E Registration of Institutional Review Boards

Sec.

46.501	What IRBs must be registered?
46.502	What information must be provided when registering an IRB?
46.503	When must an IRB be registered?
46.504	How must an IRB be registered?
46.505	When must IRB registration information be renewed or updated?

Authority: 5 U.S.C. 301; 42 U.S.C. 289(a).

Editorial Note: The Department of Health and Human Services issued a notice of waiver regarding the requirements set forth in part 46, relating to protection of human subjects, as they pertain to demonstration projects, approved under section 1115 of the Social Security Act, which test the use of cost--sharing, such as deductibles, copayment and coinsurance, in the Medicaid program. For further information see 47 FR 9208, Mar. 4, 1982.

* * *

Subpart A Basic HHS Policy for Protection of Human Research Subjects

Authority:5 U.S.C. 301; 42 U.S.C. 289(a); 42 U.S.C. 300v-1(b).

Source:56 FR 28012, 28022, June 18, 1991, unless otherwise noted.

§46.101 To what does this policy apply?

(a) Except as provided in paragraph (b) of this section, this policy applies to all research involving human subjects conducted, supported or otherwise subject to regulation by any federal department or agency which takes appropriate administrative action to make the policy applicable to such research. This includes research conducted by federal civilian employees or military personnel, except that each department or agency head may adopt such procedural modifications as may be appropriate from an administrative standpoint. It also includes research conducted, supported, or otherwise subject to regulation by the federal government outside the United States.

(1) Research that is conducted or supported by a federal department or agency, whether or not it is regulated as defined in §46.102, must comply with all sections of this policy.

(2) Research that is neither conducted nor supported by a federal department or agency but is subject to regulation as defined in §46.102(e) must be reviewed and approved, in compliance with §46.101, §46.102, and §46.107 through §46.117 of this policy, by an institutional review board (IRB) that operates in accordance with the pertinent requirements of this policy.

(b) Unless otherwise required by department or agency heads, research activities in which the only involvement of human subjects will be in one or more of the following categories are exempt from this policy:

(1) Research conducted in established or commonly accepted educational settings, involving normal educational practices, such as (i) research on regular and special education instructional strategies, or (ii) research on the effectiveness of or the comparison among instructional techniques, curricula, or classroom management methods.

(2) Research involving the use of educational tests (cognitive, diagnostic, aptitude, achievement), survey procedures, interview procedures or observation of public behavior, unless: (i) information obtained is recorded in such a manner that human subjects can be identified, directly or through identifiers linked to the subjects; and (ii) any disclosure of the human subjects' responses outside the research could reasonably place the subjects at risk of criminal or civil liability or be damaging to the subjects' financial standing, employability, or reputation.

(3) Research involving the use of educational tests (cognitive, diagnostic, aptitude, achievement), survey procedures, interview procedures, or observation of public behavior that is not exempt under paragraph (b)(2) of this section, if: (i) the human subjects are elected or appointed public officials or candidates for public office; or (ii) federal statute(s) require(s) without exception that the confidentiality of the personally identifiable information will be maintained throughout the research and thereafter.

(4) Research involving the collection or study of existing data, documents, records, pathological specimens, or diagnostic specimens, if these sources are publicly available or if the information is recorded by the investigator in such a manner that subjects cannot be identified, directly or through identifiers linked to the subjects.

(5) Research and demonstration projects which are conducted by or subject to the approval of department or agency heads, and which are designed to study, evaluate, or otherwise examine: (i) Public benefit or service programs; (ii) procedures for obtaining benefits or services under those programs; (iii) possible changes in or alternatives to those programs or procedures; or (iv) possible changes in methods or levels of payment for benefits or services under those programs.

(6) Taste and food quality evaluation and consumer acceptance studies, (i) if wholesome foods without additives are consumed or (ii) if a food is consumed that contains a food ingredient at or below the level and for a use found to be safe, or agricultural chemical or environmental contaminant at or below the level found to be safe, by the Food and Drug Administration or approved by the Environmental Protection Agency or the Food Safety and Inspection Service of the U.S. Department of Agriculture.

(c) Department or agency heads retain final judgment as to whether a particular activity is covered by this policy.

(d) Department or agency heads may require that specific research activities or classes of research activities conducted, supported, or otherwise subject to regulation by the department or agency but not otherwise covered by this policy, comply with some or all of the requirements of this policy.

(e) Compliance with this policy requires compliance with pertinent federal laws or regulations which provide additional protections for human subjects.

(f) This policy does not affect any state or local laws or regulations which may otherwise be applicable and which provide additional protections for human subjects.

(g) This policy does not affect any foreign laws or regulations which may otherwise be applicable and which provide additional protections to human subjects of research.

(h) When research covered by this policy takes place in foreign countries, procedures normally followed in the foreign countries to protect human subjects may differ from those set forth in this policy. [An example is a foreign institution which complies with guidelines consistent with the World Medical Assembly Declaration (Declaration of Helsinki amended 1989) issued either by sovereign states or by an organization whose function for the protection of human research subjects is internationally recognized.] In these circumstances, if a department or agency head determines that the procedures prescribed by the institution afford protections that are at least equivalent to those provided in this policy, the department or agency head may approve the substitution of the foreign procedures in lieu of the procedural requirements provided in this policy. Except when otherwise required by statute, Executive Order, or the department or agency head, notices of these actions as they occur will be published in the FEDERAL REGISTER or will be otherwise published as provided in department or agency procedures.

(i) Unless otherwise required by law, department or agency heads may waive the applicability of some or all of the provisions of this policy to specific research activities or classes or research activities otherwise covered by this policy. Except when otherwise required by statute or Executive Order, the department or agency head shall forward advance notices of these actions to the Office for Human Research Protections, Department of Health and Human Services (HHS), or any successor office, and shall also publish them in the FEDERAL REGISTER or in such other manner as provided in department or agency procedures.[1]

1 Institutions with HHS-approved assurances on file will abide by provisions of Title 45 CFR part 46 subparts A-D. Some of the other departments and agencies have incorporated all provisions of Title 45 CFR part 46 into their policies and procedures as well. However, the exemptions at 45 CFR 46.101(b) do not apply to research involving prisoners, subpart C. The exemption at 45 CFR 46.101(b)(2), for research involving survey or interview procedures or observation of public behavior, does not apply to research with children, subpart D, except for research involving observations of public behavior when the investigator(s) do not participate in the activities being observed.

[56 FR 28012, 28022, June 18, 1991; 56 FR 29756, June 28, 1991, as amended at70 FR 36328, June 23, 2005]

§46.102 Definitions.

(a) *Department or agency head* means the head of any federal department or agency and any other officer or employee of any department or agency to whom authority has been delegated.

(b) *Institution* means any public or private entity or agency (including federal, state, and other agencies).

(c) *Legally authorized representative* means an individual or judicial or other body authorized under applicable law to consent on behalf of a prospective subject to the subject's participation in the procedure(s) involved in the research.

(d) *Research* means a systematic investigation, including research development, testing and evaluation, designed to develop or contribute to generalizable knowledge. Activities which meet this definition constitute research for purposes of this policy, whether or not they are conducted or supported under a program which is considered research for other purposes. For example, some demonstration and service programs may include research activities.

(e) *Research subject to regulation*, and similar terms are intended to encompass those research activities for which a federal department or agency has specific responsibility for regulating as a research activity, (for example, Investigational New Drug requirements administered by the Food and Drug Administration). It does not include research activities which are incidentally regulated by a federal department or agency solely as part of the department's or agency's broader responsibility to regulate certain types of activities whether research or non-research in nature (for example, Wage and Hour requirements administered by the Department of Labor).

(f) *Human subject* means a living individual about whom an investigator (whether professional or student) conducting research obtains

(1) Data through intervention or interaction with the individual, or

(2) Identifiable private information.

Intervention includes both physical procedures by which data are gathered (for example, venipuncture) and manipulations of the subject or the subject's environment that are performed for research purposes. Interaction includes communication or interpersonal contact between investigator and subject. *Private information* includes information about behavior that occurs in a context in which an individual can reasonably expect that no observation or recording is taking place, and information which has been provided for specific purposes by an individual and which the individual can reasonably expect will not be made public (for example, a medical record). Private information must be individually identifiable (i.e., the identity of the subject is or may readily be ascertained by the investigator or associated with the information) in order for obtaining the information to constitute research involving human subjects.

(g) *IRB* means an institutional review board established in accord with and for the purposes expressed in this policy.

(h) *IRB approval* means the determination of the IRB that the research has been reviewed and may be conducted at an institution within the constraints set forth by the IRB and by other institutional and federal requirements.

(i) *Minimal risk* means that the probability and magnitude of harm or discomfort anticipated in the research are not greater in and of themselves than those ordinarily encountered in daily life or during the performance of routine physical or psychological examinations or tests.

(j) *Certification* means the official notification by the institution to the supporting department or agency, in accordance with the requirements of this policy, that a research project or activity involving human subjects has been reviewed and approved by an IRB in accordance with an approved assurance.

§46.103 Assuring compliance with this policy—research conducted or supported by any Federal Department or Agency.

(a) Each institution engaged in research which is covered by this policy and which is conducted or supported by a federal department or agency shall provide written assurance satisfactory to the department or agency head that it will comply with the requirements set forth in this policy. In lieu of requiring submission of an assurance, individual department or agency heads shall accept the existence of a current assurance, appropriate for the research in question, on file with the Office for Human Research Protections, HHS, or any successor office, and approved for federalwide use by that office. When the existence of an HHS-approved assurance is accepted in lieu of requiring submission of an assurance, reports (except certification) required by this policy to be made to department and agency heads shall also be made to the Office for Human Research Protections, HHS, or any successor office.

(b) Departments and agencies will conduct or support research covered by this policy only if the institution has an assurance approved as provided in this section, and only if the institution has certified to the department or agency head that the research has been reviewed and approved by an IRB provided for in the assurance, and will be subject to continuing review by the IRB. Assurances applicable to federally supported or conducted research shall at a minimum include:

(1) A statement of principles governing the institution in the discharge of its responsibilities for protecting the rights and welfare of human subjects of research conducted at or sponsored by the institution, regardless of whether the research is subject to Federal regulation. This may include an appropriate existing code, declaration, or statement of ethical principles, or a statement formulated by the institution itself. This requirement does not preempt provisions of this policy applicable to department- or agency-supported or regulated research and need not be applicable to any research exempted or waived under §46.101(b) or (i).

(2) Designation of one or more IRBs established in accordance with the requirements of this policy, and for which provisions are made for meeting space and sufficient staff to support the IRB's review and recordkeeping duties.

(3) A list of IRB members identified by name; earned degrees; representative capacity; indications of experience such as board certifications, licenses, etc., sufficient to describe each member's chief anticipated contributions to IRB deliberations; and any employment or other relationship between each member and the institution; for example: full-time employee, part-time employee, member of governing panel or board, stockholder, paid or unpaid consultant. Changes in IRB membership shall be reported to the department or agency head, unless in accord with §46.103(a) of this policy, the existence of an HHS-approved assurance is accepted. In this case, change in IRB membership shall be reported to the Office for Human Research Protections, HHS, or any successor office.

(4) Written procedures which the IRB will follow (i) for conducting its initial and continuing review of research and for reporting its findings and actions to the investigator and the institution; (ii) for determining which projects require review more often than annually and which projects need verification from sources other than the investigators that no material changes have occurred since previous IRB review; and (iii) for ensuring prompt reporting to the IRB of proposed changes in a research activity, and for ensuring that such changes in approved research, during the period for which IRB approval has already been given, may not be initiated without IRB review and approval except when necessary to eliminate apparent immediate hazards to the subject.

(5) Written procedures for ensuring prompt reporting to the IRB, appropriate institutional officials, and the department or agency head

of (i) any unanticipated problems involving risks to subjects or others or any serious or continuing noncompliance with this policy or the requirements or determinations of the IRB; and (ii) any suspension or termination of IRB approval.

(c) The assurance shall be executed by an individual authorized to act for the institution and to assume on behalf of the institution the obligations imposed by this policy and shall be filed in such form and manner as the department or agency head prescribes.

(d) The department or agency head will evaluate all assurances submitted in accordance with this policy through such officers and employees of the department or agency and such experts or consultants engaged for this purpose as the department or agency head determines to be appropriate. The department or agency head's evaluation will take into consideration the adequacy of the proposed IRB in light of the anticipated scope of the institution's research activities and the types of subject populations likely to be involved, the appropriateness of the proposed initial and continuing review procedures in light of the probable risks, and the size and complexity of the institution.

(e) On the basis of this evaluation, the department or agency head may approve or disapprove the assurance, or enter into negotiations to develop an approvable one. The department or agency head may limit the period during which any particular approved assurance or class of approved assurances shall remain effective or otherwise condition or restrict approval.

(f) Certification is required when the research is supported by a federal department or agency and not otherwise exempted or waived under §46.101(b) or (i). An institution with an approved assurance shall certify that each application or proposal for research covered by the assurance and by §46.103 of this Policy has been reviewed and approved by the IRB. Such certification must be submitted with the application or proposal or by such later date as may be prescribed by the department or agency to which the application or proposal is submitted. Under no condition shall research covered by §46.103 of the Policy be supported prior to receipt of the certification that the research has been reviewed and approved by the IRB. Institutions without an approved assurance covering the research shall certify within 30 days after receipt of a request for such a certification from the department or agency, that the application or proposal has been approved by the IRB. If the certification is not submitted within these time limits, the application or proposal may be returned to the institution.

(Approved by the Office of Management and Budget under Control Number 0990-0260.)

[56 FR 28012, 28022, June 18, 1991; 56 FR 29756, June 28, 1991, as amended at 70 FR 36328, June 23, 2005]

§§46.104—46.106 [Reserved]

§46.107 IRB membership.

(a) Each IRB shall have at least five members, with varying backgrounds to promote complete and adequate review of research activities commonly conducted by the institution. The IRB shall be sufficiently qualified through the experience and expertise of its members, and the diversity of the members, including consideration of race, gender, and cultural backgrounds and sensitivity to such issues as community attitudes, to promote respect for its advice and counsel in safeguarding the rights and welfare of human subjects. In addition to possessing the professional competence necessary to review specific research activities, the IRB shall be able to ascertain the acceptability of proposed research in terms of institutional commitments and regulations, applicable law, and standards of professional conduct and practice. The IRB shall therefore include persons knowledgeable in these areas. If an IRB regularly reviews research that involves a vulnerable category of subjects, such as children, prisoners, pregnant women, or handicapped or mentally disabled persons, consideration shall be given to the inclusion of one or more individuals who are knowledgeable about and experienced in working with these subjects.

(b) Every nondiscriminatory effort will be made to ensure that no IRB consists entirely of men or entirely of women, including the institution's consideration of qualified persons of both sexes, so long as no selection is made to the IRB on the basis of gender. No IRB may consist entirely of members of one profession.

(c) Each IRB shall include at least one member whose primary concerns are in scientific areas and at least one member whose primary concerns are in nonscientific areas.

(d) Each IRB shall include at least one member who is not otherwise affiliated with the institution and who is not part of the immediate family of a person who is affiliated with the institution.

(e) No IRB may have a member participate in the IRB's initial or continuing review of any project in which the member has a conflicting interest, except to provide information requested by the IRB.

(f) An IRB may, in its discretion, invite individuals with competence in special areas to assist in the review of issues which require expertise beyond or in addition to that available on the IRB. These individuals may not vote with the IRB

§46.108 IRB functions and operations.

In order to fulfill the requirements of this policy each IRB shall:

(a) Follow written procedures in the same detail as described in §46.103(b)(4) and, to the extent required by, §46.103(b)(5).

(b) Except when an expedited review procedure is used (see §46.110), review proposed research at convened meetings at which a majority of the members of the IRB are present, including at least one member whose primary concerns are in nonscientific areas. In order for the research to be approved, it shall receive the approval of a majority of those members present at the meeting.

§46.109 IRB review of research.

(a) An IRB shall review and have authority to approve, require modifications in (to secure approval), or disapprove all research activities covered by this policy.

(b) An IRB shall require that information given to subjects as part of informed consent is in accordance with §46.116. The IRB may require that information, in addition to that specifically mentioned in §46.116, be given to the subjects when in the IRB's judgment the information would meaningfully add to the protection of the rights and welfare of subjects.

(c) An IRB shall require documentation of informed consent or may waive documentation in accordance with §46.117.

(d) An IRB shall notify investigators and the institution in writing of its decision to approve or disapprove the proposed research activity, or of modifications required to secure IRB approval of the research activity. If the IRB decides to disapprove a research activity, it shall include in its written notification a statement of the reasons for its decision and give the investigator an opportunity to respond in person or in writing.

(e) An IRB shall conduct continuing review of research covered by this policy at intervals appropriate to the degree of risk, but not less than once per year, and shall have authority to observe or have a third party observe the consent process and the research.

(Approved by the Office of Management and Budget under Control Number 0990-0260.)

[56 FR 28012, 28022, June 18, 1991, as amended at 70 FR 36328, June 23, 2005]

§46.110 Expedited review procedures for certain kinds of research involving no more than minimal risk, and for minor changes in approved research.

(a) The Secretary, HHS, has established, and published as a Notice in the FEDERAL REGISTER, a list of categories of research that may be reviewed by the IRB through an expedited review procedure. The list will be amended, as appropriate, after consultation with other departments and agencies, through periodic republication by the Secretary, HHS, in the FEDERAL REGISTER. A copy of the list is available from the Office for Human Research Protections, HHS, or any successor office.

(b) An IRB may use the expedited review procedure to review either or both of the following:

(1) some or all of the research appearing on the list and found by the reviewer(s) to involve no more than minimal risk,

(2) minor changes in previously approved research during the period (of one year or less) for which approval is authorized.

Under an expedited review procedure, the review may be carried out by the IRB chairperson or by one or more experienced reviewers designated by the chairperson from among members of the

IRB. In reviewing the research, the reviewers may exercise all of the authorities of the IRB except that the reviewers may not disapprove the research. A research activity may be disapproved only after review in accordance with the non-expedited procedure set forth in §46.108(b).

(c) Each IRB which uses an expedited review procedure shall adopt a method for keeping all members advised of research proposals which have been approved under the procedure.

(d) The department or agency head may restrict, suspend, terminate, or choose not to authorize an institution's or IRB's use of the expedited review procedure.

[56 FR 28012, 28022, June 18, 1991, as amended at 70 FR 36328, June 23, 2005]

§46.111 Criteria for IRB approval of research.

(a) In order to approve research covered by this policy the IRB shall determine that all of the following requirements are satisfied:

(1) Risks to subjects are minimized: (i) By using procedures which are consistent with sound research design and which do not unnecessarily expose subjects to risk, and (ii) whenever appropriate, by using procedures already being performed on the subjects for diagnostic or treatment purposes.

(2) Risks to subjects are reasonable in relation to anticipated benefits, if any, to subjects, and the importance of the knowledge that may reasonably be expected to result. In evaluating risks and benefits, the IRB should consider only those risks and benefits that may result from the research (as distinguished from risks and benefits of therapies subjects would receive even if not participating in the research). The IRB should not consider possible long-range effects of applying knowledge gained in the research (for example, the possible effects of the research on public policy) as among those research risks that fall within the purview of its responsibility.

(3) Selection of subjects is equitable. In making this assessment the IRB should take into account the purposes of the research and the setting in which the research will be conducted and should be particularly cognizant of the special problems of research involving vulnerable populations, such as children, prisoners, pregnant

women, mentally disabled persons, or economically or educationally disadvantaged persons.

(4) Informed consent will be sought from each prospective subject or the subject's legally authorized representative, in accordance with, and to the extent required by §46.116.

(5) Informed consent will be appropriately documented, in accordance with, and to the extent required by §46.117.

(6) When appropriate, the research plan makes adequate provision for monitoring the data collected to ensure the safety of subjects.

(7) When appropriate, there are adequate provisions to protect the privacy of subjects and to maintain the confidentiality of data.

(b) When some or all of the subjects are likely to be vulnerable to coercion or undue influence, such as children, prisoners, pregnant women, mentally disabled persons, or economically or educationally disadvantaged persons, additional safeguards have been included in the study to protect the rights and welfare of these subjects.

§46.112 Review by institution.

Research covered by this policy that has been approved by an IRB may be subject to further appropriate review and approval or disapproval by officials of the institution. However, those officials may not approve the research if it has not been approved by an IRB.

§46.113 Suspension or termination of IRB approval of research.

An IRB shall have authority to suspend or terminate approval of research that is not being conducted in accordance with the IRB's requirements or that has been associated with unexpected serious harm to subjects. Any suspension or termination of approval shall include a statement of the reasons for the IRB's action and shall be reported promptly to the investigator, appropriate institutional officials, and the department or agency head.

(Approved by the Office of Management and Budget under Control Number 0990-0260.)

[56 FR 28012, 28022, June 18, 1991, as amended at 70 FR 36328, June 23, 2005]

§46.114 Cooperative research.

Cooperative research projects are those projects covered by this policy which involve more than one institution. In the conduct of cooperative research projects, each institution is responsible for safeguarding the rights and welfare of human subjects and for complying with this policy. With the approval of the department or agency head, an institution participating in a cooperative project may enter into a joint review arrangement, rely upon the review of another qualified IRB, or make similar arrangements for avoiding duplication of effort.

§46.115 IRB records.

(a) An institution, or when appropriate an IRB, shall prepare and maintain adequate documentation of IRB activities, including the following:

(1) Copies of all research proposals reviewed, scientific evaluations, if any, that accompany the proposals, approved sample consent documents, progress reports submitted by investigators, and reports of injuries to subjects.

(2) Minutes of IRB meetings which shall be in sufficient detail to show attendance at the meetings; actions taken by the IRB; the vote on these actions including the number of members voting for, against, and abstaining; the basis for requiring changes in or disapproving research; and a written summary of the discussion of controverted issues and their resolution.

(3) Records of continuing review activities.

(4) Copies of all correspondence between the IRB and the investigators.

(5) A list of IRB members in the same detail as described in §46.103(b)(3).

(6) Written procedures for the IRB in the same detail as described in §46.103(b)(4) and §46.103(b)(5).

(7) Statements of significant new findings provided to subjects, as required by §46.116(b)(5).

(b) The records required by this policy shall be retained for at least 3 years, and records relating to research which is conducted shall be retained for at least 3 years after completion of the research. All records shall be accessible for inspection and copying by authorized representatives of the department or agency at reasonable times and in a reasonable manner.

(Approved by the Office of Management and Budget under Control Number 0990-0260.)

[56 FR 28012, 28022, June 18, 1991, as amended at 70 FR 36328, June 23, 2005]

§46.116 General requirements for informed consent.

Except as provided elsewhere in this policy, no investigator may involve a human being as a subject in research covered by this policy unless the investigator has obtained the legally effective informed consent of the subject or the subject's legally authorized representative. An investigator shall seek such consent only under circumstances that provide the prospective subject or the representative sufficient opportunity to consider whether or not to participate and that minimize the possibility of coercion or undue influence. The information that is given to the subject or the representative shall be in language understandable to the subject or the representative. No informed consent, whether oral or written, may include any exculpatory language through which the subject or the representative is made to waive or appear to waive any of the subject's legal rights, or releases or appears to release the investigator, the sponsor, the institution or its agents from liability for negligence.

(a) Basic elements of informed consent. Except as provided in paragraph (c) or (d) of this section, in seeking informed consent the following information shall be provided to each subject:

(1) A statement that the study involves research, an explanation of the purposes of the research and the expected duration of the subject's participation, a description of the procedures to be followed, and identification of any procedures which are experimental;

(2) A description of any reasonably foreseeable risks or discomforts to the subject;

(3) A description of any benefits to the subject or to others which may reasonably be expected from the research;

(4) A disclosure of appropriate alternative procedures or courses of treatment, if any, that might be advantageous to the subject;

(5) A statement describing the extent, if any, to which confidentiality of records identifying the subject will be maintained;

(6) For research involving more than minimal risk, an explanation as to whether any compensation and an explanation as to whether any medical treatments are available if injury occurs and, if so, what they consist of, or where further information may be obtained;

(7) An explanation of whom to contact for answers to pertinent questions about the research and research subjects' rights, and whom to contact in the event of a research-related injury to the subject; and

(8) A statement that participation is voluntary, refusal to participate will involve no penalty or loss of benefits to which the subject is otherwise entitled, and the subject may discontinue participation at any time without penalty or loss of benefits to which the subject is otherwise entitled.

(b) Additional elements of informed consent. When appropriate, one or more of the following elements of information shall also be provided to each subject:

(1) A statement that the particular treatment or procedure may involve risks to the subject (or to the embryo or fetus, if the subject is or may become pregnant) which are currently unforeseeable;

(2) Anticipated circumstances under which the subject's participation may be terminated by the investigator without regard to the subject's consent;

(3) Any additional costs to the subject that may result from participation in the research;

(4) The consequences of a subject's decision to withdraw from the research and procedures for orderly termination of participation by the subject;

(5) A statement that significant new findings developed during the course of the research which may relate to the subject's willingness to continue participation will be provided to the subject; and

(6) The approximate number of subjects involved in the study.

(c) An IRB may approve a consent procedure which does not include, or which alters, some or all of the elements of informed consent set forth above, or waive the requirement to obtain informed consent provided the IRB finds and documents that:

(1) The research or demonstration project is to be conducted by or subject to the approval of state or local government officials and is designed to study, evaluate, or otherwise examine: (i) public benefit or service programs; (ii) procedures for obtaining benefits or services under those programs; (iii) possible changes in or alternatives to those programs or procedures; or (iv) possible changes in methods or levels of payment for benefits or services under those programs; and

(2) The research could not practicably be carried out without the waiver or alteration.

(d) An IRB may approve a consent procedure which does not include, or which alters, some or all of the elements of informed consent set forth in this section, or waive the requirements to obtain informed consent provided the IRB finds and documents that:

(1) The research involves no more than minimal risk to the subjects;

(2) The waiver or alteration will not adversely affect the rights and welfare of the subjects;

(3) The research could not practicably be carried out without the waiver or alteration; and

(4) Whenever appropriate, the subjects will be provided with additional pertinent information after participation.

(e) The informed consent requirements in this policy are not intended to preempt any applicable federal, state, or local laws which require additional information to be disclosed in order for informed consent to be legally effective.

(f) Nothing in this policy is intended to limit the authority of a physician to provide emergency medical care, to the extent the physician is permitted to do so under applicable federal, state, or local law.

(Approved by the Office of Management and Budget under Control Number 0990-0260.)

[56 FR 28012, 28022, June 18, 1991, as amended at 70 FR 36328, June 23, 2005]

§46.117 Documentation of informed consent.

(a) Except as provided in paragraph (c) of this section, informed consent shall be documented by the use of a written consent form approved by the IRB and signed by the subject or the subject's legally authorized representative. A copy shall be given to the person signing the form.

(b) Except as provided in paragraph (c) of this section, the consent form may be either of the following:

(1) A written consent document that embodies the elements of informed consent required by §46.116. This form may be read to the subject or the subject's legally authorized representative, but in any event, the investigator shall give either the subject or the representative adequate opportunity to read it before it is signed; or

(2) A short form written consent document stating that the elements of informed consent required by §46.116 have been presented orally to the subject or the subject's legally authorized representative. When this method is used, there shall be a witness to the oral presentation. Also, the IRB shall approve a written summary of what is to be said to the subject or the representative. Only the short form itself is to be signed by the subject or the representative. However, the witness shall sign both the short form and a copy of the summary, and the person actually obtaining consent shall sign a copy of the summary. A copy of the summary shall be given to the subject or the representative, in addition to a copy of the short form.

(c) An IRB may waive the requirement for the investigator to obtain a signed consent form for some or all subjects if it finds either:

(1) That the only record linking the subject and the research would be the consent document and the principal risk would be potential

harm resulting from a breach of confidentiality. Each subject will be asked whether the subject wants documentation linking the subject with the research, and the subject's wishes will govern; or

(2) That the research presents no more than minimal risk of harm to subjects and involves no procedures for which written consent is normally required outside of the research context.

In cases in which the documentation requirement is waived, the IRB may require the investigator to provide subjects with a written statement regarding the research.

(Approved by the Office of Management and Budget under Control Number 0990-0260.)

[56 FR 28012, 28022, June 18, 1991, as amended at 70 FR 36328, June 23, 2005]

§46.118 Applications and proposals lacking definite plans for involvement of human subjects.

Certain types of applications for grants, cooperative agreements, or contracts are submitted to departments or agencies with the knowledge that subjects may be involved within the period of support, but definite plans would not normally be set forth in the application or proposal. These include activities such as institutional type grants when selection of specific projects is the institution's responsibility; research training grants in which the activities involving subjects remain to be selected; and projects in which human subjects' involvement will depend upon completion of instruments, prior animal studies, or purification of compounds. These applications need not be reviewed by an IRB before an award may be made. However, except for research exempted or waived under §46.101(b) or (i), no human subjects may be involved in any project supported by these awards until the project has been reviewed and approved by the IRB, as provided in this policy, and certification submitted, by the institution, to the department or agency.

§46.119 Research undertaken without the intention of involving human subjects.

In the event research is undertaken without the intention of involving human subjects, but it is later proposed to involve human subjects in the research, the research shall first be reviewed and approved by an IRB, as provided in this policy, a certification submitted, by the institution, to the department or agency, and final approval given to the proposed change by the department or agency.

§46.120 Evaluation and disposition of applications and proposals for research to be conducted or supported by a Federal Department or Agency.

(a) The department or agency head will evaluate all applications and proposals involving human subjects submitted to the department or agency through such officers and employees of the department or agency and such experts and consultants as the department or agency head determines to be appropriate. This evaluation will take into consideration the risks to the subjects, the adequacy of protection against these risks, the potential benefits of the research to the subjects and others, and the importance of the knowledge gained or to be gained.

(b) On the basis of this evaluation, the department or agency head may approve or disapprove the application or proposal, or enter into negotiations to develop an approvable one.

§46.121 [Reserved]

§46.122 Use of Federal funds.

Federal funds administered by a department or agency may not be expended for research involving human subjects unless the requirements of this policy have been satisfied.

§46.123 Early termination of research support: Evaluation of applications and proposals.

(a) The department or agency head may require that department or agency support for any project be terminated or suspended in the manner prescribed in applicable program requirements, when the department or agency head finds an institution has materially failed to comply with the terms of this policy.

(b) In making decisions about supporting or approving applications or proposals covered by this policy the department or agency head may take into account, in addition to all other eligibility requirements and program criteria, factors such as whether the applicant has been subject to a termination or suspension under paragraph (a) of this section and whether the applicant or the person or persons who would direct or has/have directed the scientific and technical aspects of an activity has/have, in the judgment of the department or agency head, materially failed to discharge responsibility for the protection of the rights and welfare of human subjects (whether or not the research was subject to federal regulation).

§46.124 Conditions.

With respect to any research project or any class of research projects the department or agency head may impose additional conditions prior to or at the time of approval when in the judgment of the department or agency head additional conditions are necessary for the protection of human subjects.

Subpart B Additional Protections for Pregnant Women, Human Fetuses and Neonates Involved in Research

Source:66 FR 56778, Nov. 13, 2001, unless otherwise noted.

§46.201 To what do these regulations apply?

(a) Except as provided in paragraph (b) of this section, this subpart applies to all research involving pregnant women, human fetuses, neonates of uncertain viability, or nonviable neonates conducted or supported by the Department of Health and Human Services (DHHS). This includes all research conducted in DHHS facilities by any person and all research conducted in any facility by DHHS employees.

(b) The exemptions at §46.101(b)(1) through (6) are applicable to this subpart.

(c) The provisions of §46.101(c) through (i) are applicable to this subpart. Reference to State or local laws in this subpart and in §46.101(f) is intended to include the laws of federally recognized American Indian and Alaska Native Tribal Governments.

(d) The requirements of this subpart are in addition to those imposed under the other subparts of this part.

§46.202 Definitions.

The definitions in §46.102 shall be applicable to this subpart as well. In addition, as used in this subpart:

(a) *Dead fetus* means a fetus that exhibits neither heartbeat, spontaneous respiratory activity, spontaneous movement of voluntary muscles, nor pulsation of the umbilical cord.

(b) *Delivery* means complete separation of the fetus from the woman by expulsion or extraction or any other means.

(c) *Fetus* means the product of conception from implantation until delivery.

(d) *Neonate* means a newborn.

(e) *Nonviable neonate* means a neonate after delivery that, although living, is not viable.

(f) *Pregnancy* encompasses the period of time from implantation until delivery. A woman shall be assumed to be pregnant if she exhibits any of the pertinent presumptive signs of pregnancy, such as missed menses, until the results of a pregnancy test are negative or until delivery.

(g) *Secretary* means the Secretary of Health and Human Services and any other officer or employee of the Department of Health and Human Services to whom authority has been delegated.

(h) *Viable*, as it pertains to the neonate, means being able, after delivery, to survive (given the benefit of available medical therapy) to the point of independently maintaining heartbeat and respiration. The Secretary may from time to time, taking into account medical advances, publish in the FEDERAL REGISTER guidelines to assist in determining whether a neonate is viable for purposes of this subpart. If a neonate is viable then it may be included in research only to the extent permitted and in accordance with the requirements of subparts A and D of this part.

§46.203 Duties of IRBs in connection with research involving pregnant women, fetuses, and neonates.

In addition to other responsibilities assigned to IRBs under this part, each IRB shall review research covered by this subpart and approve only research which satisfies the conditions of all applicable sections of this subpart and the other subparts of this part.

§46.204 Research involving pregnant women or fetuses.

Pregnant women or fetuses may be involved in research if all of the following conditions are met:

(a) Where scientifically appropriate, preclinical studies, including studies on pregnant animals, and clinical studies, including studies on nonpregnant women, have been conducted and provide data for assessing potential risks to pregnant women and fetuses;

(b) The risk to the fetus is caused solely by interventions or procedures that hold out the prospect of direct benefit for the woman or the fetus; or, if there is no such prospect of benefit, the risk to the fetus is not greater than minimal and the purpose of the research is the development of important biomedical knowledge which cannot be obtained by any other means;

(c) Any risk is the least possible for achieving the objectives of the research;

(d) If the research holds out the prospect of direct benefit to the pregnant woman, the prospect of a direct benefit both to the pregnant woman and the fetus, or no prospect of benefit for the woman nor the fetus when risk to the fetus is not greater than minimal and the purpose of the research is the development of important biomedical knowledge that cannot be obtained by any other means, her consent is obtained in accord with the informed consent provisions of subpart A of this part;

(e) If the research holds out the prospect of direct benefit solely to the fetus then the consent of the pregnant woman and the father is obtained in accord with the informed consent provisions of subpart A of this part, except that the father's consent need not be obtained if he is unable to consent because of unavailability, incompetence, or temporary incapacity or the pregnancy resulted from rape or incest.

(f) Each individual providing consent under paragraph (d) or (e) of this section is fully informed regarding the reasonably foreseeable impact of the research on the fetus or neonate;

(g) For children as defined in §46.402(a) who are pregnant, assent and permission are obtained in accord with the provisions of subpart D of this part;

(h) No inducements, monetary or otherwise, will be offered to terminate a pregnancy;

(i) Individuals engaged in the research will have no part in any decisions as to the timing, method, or procedures used to terminate a pregnancy; and

(j) Individuals engaged in the research will have no part in determining the viability of a neonate.

§46.205 Research involving neonates.

(a) Neonates of uncertain viability and nonviable neonates may be involved in research if all of the following conditions are met:

(1) Where scientifically appropriate, preclinical and clinical studies have been conducted and provide data for assessing potential risks to neonates.

(2) Each individual providing consent under paragraph (b)(2) or (c)(5) of this section is fully informed regarding the reasonably foreseeable impact of the research on the neonate.

(3) Individuals engaged in the research will have no part in determining the viability of a neonate.

(4) The requirements of paragraph (b) or (c) of this section have been met as applicable.

(b) Neonates of uncertain viability. Until it has been ascertained whether or not a neonate is viable, a neonate may not be involved in research covered by this subpart unless the following additional conditions have been met:

(1) The IRB determines that:

(i) The research holds out the prospect of enhancing the probability of survival of the neonate to the point of viability, and any risk is the least possible for achieving that objective, or

(ii) The purpose of the research is the development of important biomedical knowledge which cannot be obtained by other means and there will be no added risk to the neonate resulting from the research; and

(2) The legally effective informed consent of either parent of the neonate or, if neither parent is able to consent because of unavailability, incompetence, or temporary incapacity, the legally effective informed consent of either parent's legally authorized representative is obtained in accord with subpart A of this part, except that the consent of the father or his legally authorized representative need not be obtained if the pregnancy resulted from rape or incest.

(c) Nonviable neonates. After delivery nonviable neonate may not be involved in research covered by this subpart unless all of the following additional conditions are met:

(1) Vital functions of the neonate will not be artificially maintained;

(2) The research will not terminate the heartbeat or respiration of the neonate;

(3) There will be no added risk to the neonate resulting from the research;

(4) The purpose of the research is the development of important biomedical knowledge that cannot be obtained by other means; and

(5) The legally effective informed consent of both parents of the neonate is obtained in accord with subpart A of this part, except that the waiver and alteration provisions of §46.116(c) and (d) do not apply. However, if either parent is unable to consent because of unavailability, incompetence, or temporary incapacity, the informed consent of one parent of a nonviable neonate will suffice to meet the requirements of this paragraph (c)(5), except that the consent of the father need not be obtained if the pregnancy resulted from rape or incest. The consent of a legally authorized representative of either or both of the parents of a nonviable neonate will not suffice to meet the requirements of this paragraph (c)(5).

(d) Viable neonates. A neonate, after delivery, that has been determined to be viable may be included in research only to the extent permitted by and in accord with the requirements of subparts A and D of this part.

§46.206 Research involving, after delivery, the placenta, the dead fetus or fetal material.

(a) Research involving, after delivery, the placenta; the dead fetus; macerated fetal material; or cells, tissue, or organs excised from a dead fetus, shall be conducted only in accord with any applicable federal, state, or local laws and regulations regarding such activities.

(b) If information associated with material described in paragraph (a) of this section is recorded for research purposes in a manner that living individuals can be identified, directly or through identifiers linked to those individuals, those individuals are research subjects and all pertinent subparts of this part are applicable.

§46.207 Research not otherwise approvable which presents an opportunity to understand, prevent, or alleviate a serious problem affecting the health or welfare of pregnant women, fetuses, or neonates.

The Secretary will conduct or fund research that the IRB does not believe meets the requirements of §46.204 or §46.205 only if:

(a) The IRB finds that the research presents a reasonable opportunity to further the understanding, prevention, or alleviation of a serious problem affecting the health or welfare of pregnant women, fetuses or neonates; and

(b) The Secretary, after consultation with a panel of experts in pertinent disciplines (for example: science, medicine, ethics, law) and following opportunity for public review and comment, including a public meeting announced in the FEDERAL REGISTER, has determined either:

(1) That the research in fact satisfies the conditions of §46.204, as applicable; or

(2) The following:

(i) The research presents a reasonable opportunity to further the understanding, prevention, or alleviation of a serious problem affecting the health or welfare of pregnant women, fetuses or neonates;

(ii) The research will be conducted in accord with sound ethical principles; and

(iii) Informed consent will be obtained in accord with the informed consent provisions of subpart A and other applicable subparts of this part.

Subpart C Additional Protections Pertaining to Biomedical and Behavioral Research Involving Prisoners as Subjects

Source:43 FR 53655, Nov. 16, 1978, unless otherwise noted.

§46.301 Applicability.

(a) The regulations in this subpart are applicable to all biomedical and behavioral research conducted or supported by the Department of Health and Human Services involving prisoners as subjects.

(b) Nothing in this subpart shall be construed as indicating that compliance with the procedures set forth herein will authorize research involving prisoners as subjects, to the extent such research is limited or barred by applicable State or local law.

(c) The requirements of this subpart are in addition to those imposed under the other subparts of this part.

§46.302 Purpose.

Inasmuch as prisoners may be under constraints because of their incarceration which could affect their ability to make a truly voluntary and uncoerced decision whether or not to participate as subjects in research, it is the purpose of this subpart to provide additional safeguards for the protection of prisoners involved in activities to which this subpart is applicable.

§46.303 Definitions.

As used in this subpart:

(a) *Secretary* means the Secretary of Health and Human Services and any other officer or employee of the Department of Health and Human Services to whom authority has been delegated.

(b) *DHHS* means the Department of Health and Human Services.

(c) *Prisoner* means any individual involuntarily confined or detained in a penal institution. The term is intended to encompass individuals sentenced to such an institution under a criminal or civil statute, individuals detained in other facilities by virtue of statutes or commitment procedures which provide alternatives to criminal prosecution or incarceration in a penal institution, and individuals detained pending arraignment, trial, or sentencing.

(d) *Minimal risk* is the probability and magnitude of physical or psychological harm that is normally encountered in the daily lives, or in the routine medical, dental, or psychological examination of healthy persons.

§46.304 Composition of Institutional Review Boards where prisoners are involved.

In addition to satisfying the requirements in §46.107 of this part, an Institutional Review Board, carrying out responsibilities under this part with respect to research covered by this subpart, shall also meet the following specific requirements:

(a) A majority of the Board (exclusive of prisoner members) shall have no association with the prison(s) involved, apart from their membership on the Board.

(b) At least one member of the Board shall be a prisoner, or a prisoner representative with appropriate background and experience to serve in that capacity, except that where a particular research project is reviewed by more than one Board only one Board need satisfy this requirement.

[43 FR 53655, Nov. 16, 1978, as amended at 46 FR 8366, Jan. 26, 1981]

§46.305 Additional duties of the Institutional Review Boards where prisoners are involved.

(a) In addition to all other responsibilities prescribed for Institutional Review Boards under this part, the Board shall review research covered by this subpart and approve such research only if it finds that:

(1) The research under review represents one of the categories of research permissible under §46.306(a)(2);

(2) Any possible advantages accruing to the prisoner through his or her participation in the research, when compared to the general living conditions, medical care, quality of food, amenities and opportunity for earnings in the prison, are not of such a magnitude that his or her ability to weigh the risks of the research against the value of such advantages in the limited choice environment of the prison is impaired;

(3) The risks involved in the research are commensurate with risks that would be accepted by nonprisoner volunteers;

(4) Procedures for the selection of subjects within the prison are fair to all prisoners and immune from arbitrary intervention by prison authorities or prisoners. Unless the principal investigator provides to the Board justification in writing for following some other procedures, control subjects must be selected randomly from the group of available prisoners who meet the characteristics needed for that particular research project;

(5) The information is presented in language which is understandable to the subject population;

(6) Adequate assurance exists that parole boards will not take into account a prisoner's participation in the research in making decisions regarding parole, and each prisoner is clearly informed in advance that participation in the research will have no effect on his or her parole; and

(7) Where the Board finds there may be a need for follow-up examination or care of participants after the end of their participation, adequate provision has been made for such examination or care, taking into account the varying lengths of individual prisoners' sentences, and for informing participants of this fact.

(b) The Board shall carry out such other duties as may be assigned by the Secretary.

(c) The institution shall certify to the Secretary, in such form and manner as the Secretary may require, that the duties of the Board under this section have been fulfilled.

§46.306 Permitted research involving prisoners.

(a) Biomedical or behavioral research conducted or supported by DHHS may involve prisoners as subjects only if:

(1) The institution responsible for the conduct of the research has certified to the Secretary that the Institutional Review Board has approved the research under §46.305 of this subpart; and

(2) In the judgment of the Secretary the proposed research involves solely the following:

(i) Study of the possible causes, effects, and processes of incarceration, and of criminal behavior, provided that the study presents no more than minimal risk and no more than inconvenience to the subjects;

(ii) Study of prisons as institutional structures or of prisoners asincarcerated persons, provided that the study presents no more than minimal risk and no more than inconvenience to the subjects;

(iii) Research on conditions particularly affecting prisoners as a class (for example, vaccine trials and other research on hepatitis which is much more prevalent in prisons than elsewhere; and research on social and psychological problems such as alcoholism, drug addiction, and sexual assaults) provided that the study may proceed only after the Secretary has consulted with appropriate experts including experts in penology, medicine, and ethics, and published notice, in the FEDERAL REGISTER, of his intent to approve such research; or

(iv) Research on practices, both innovative and accepted, which have the intent and reasonable probability of improving the health or well-being of the subject. In cases in which those studies require the assignment of prisoners in a manner consistent with protocols approved by the IRB to control groups which may not benefit from the research, the study may proceed only after the Secretary has consulted with appropriate experts, including experts in penology, medicine, and ethics, and published notice, in the FEDERAL REGISTER, of the intent to approve such research.

(b) Except as provided in paragraph (a) of this section, biomedical or behavioral research conducted or supported by DHHS shall not involve prisoners as subjects.

Subpart D Additional Protections for Children Involved as Subjects in Research

Source:48 FR 9818, March 8, 1983, unless otherwise noted.

§46.401 To what do these regulations apply?

(a) This subpart applies to all research involving children as subjects, conducted or supported by the Department of Health and Human Services.

(1) This includes research conducted by Department employees, except that each head of an Operating Division of the Department may adopt such nonsubstantive, procedural modifications as may be appropriate from an administrative standpoint.

(2) It also includes research conducted or supported by the Department of Health and Human Services outside the United States, but in appropriate circumstances, the Secretary may, under paragraph (e) of §46.101 of subpart A, waive the applicability of some or all of the requirements of these regulations for research of this type.

(b) Exemptions at §46.101(b)(1) and (b)(3) through (b)(6) are applicable to this subpart. The exemption at §46.101(b)(2) regarding educational tests is also applicable to this subpart. However, the exemption at §46.101(b)(2) for research involving survey or interview procedures or observations of public behavior does not apply to research covered by this subpart, except for research involving observation of public behavior when the investigator(s) do not participate in the activities being observed.

(c) The exceptions, additions, and provisions for waiver as they appear in paragraphs (c) through (i) of §46.101 of subpart A are applicable to this subpart.

[48 FR 9818, Mar.8, 1983; 56 FR 28032, June 18, 1991; 56 FR 29757, June 28, 1991.]

§46.402 Definitions.

The definitions in §46.102 of subpart A shall be applicable to this subpart as well. In addition, as used in this subpart:

(a) *Children* are persons who have not attained the legal age for consent to treatments or procedures involved in the research, under the applicable law of the jurisdiction in which the research will be conducted.

(b) *Assent* means a child's affirmative agreement to participate in research. Mere failure to object should not, absent affirmative agreement, be construed as assent.

(c) *Permission* means the agreement of parent(s) or guardian to the participation of their child or ward in research.

(d) *Parent* means a child's biological or adoptive parent.

(e) *Guardian* means an individual who is authorized under applicable State or local law to consent on behalf of a child to general medical care.

§46.403 IRB duties.

In addition to other responsibilities assigned to IRBs under this part, each IRB shall review research covered by this subpart and approve only research which satisfies the conditions of all applicable sections of this subpart.

§46.404 Research not involving greater than minimal risk.

HHS will conduct or fund research in which the IRB finds that no greater than minimal risk to children is presented, only if the IRB finds that adequate provisions are made for soliciting the assent of the children and the permission of their parents or guardians, as set forth in §46.408.

§46.405 Research involving greater than minimal risk but presenting the prospect of direct benefit to the individual subjects.

HHS will conduct or fund research in which the IRB finds that more than minimal risk to children is presented by an intervention or procedure that holds out the prospect of direct benefit for the individual subject, or by a monitoring procedure that is likely to contribute to the subject's well-being, only if the IRB finds that:

(a) The risk is justified by the anticipated benefit to the subjects;

(b) The relation of the anticipated benefit to the risk is at least as favorable to the subjects as that presented by available alternative approaches; and

(c) Adequate provisions are made for soliciting the assent of the children and permission of their parents or guardians, as set forth in §46.408.

§46.406 Research involving greater than minimal risk and no prospect of direct benefit to individual subjects, but likely to yield generalizable knowledge about the subject's disorder or condition.

HHS will conduct or fund research in which the IRB finds that more than minimal risk to children is presented by an intervention or procedure that does not hold out the prospect of direct benefit for the individual subject, or by a monitoring procedure which is not likely to contribute to the well-being of the subject, only if the IRB finds that:

(a) The risk represents a minor increase over minimal risk;

(b) The intervention or procedure presents experiences to subjects that are reasonably commensurate with those inherent in their actual or expected medical, dental, psychological, social, or educational situations;

(c) The intervention or procedure is likely to yield generalizable knowledge about the subjects' disorder or condition which is of vital importance for the understanding or amelioration of the subjects' disorder or condition; and

(d) Adequate provisions are made for soliciting assent of the children and permission of their parents or guardians, as set forth in §46.408.

§46.407 Research not otherwise approvable which presents an opportunity to understand, prevent, or alleviate a serious problem affecting the health or welfare of children.

HHS will conduct or fund research that the IRB does not believe meets the requirements of §46.404, §46.405, or §46.406 only if:

(a) the IRB finds that the research presents a reasonable opportunity to further the understanding, prevention, or alleviation of a serious problem affecting the health or welfare of children; and

(b) the Secretary, after consultation with a panel of experts in pertinent disciplines (for example: science, medicine, education, ethics, law) and following opportunity for public review and comment, has determined either:

(1) that the research in fact satisfies the conditions of §46.404, §46.405, or §46.406, as applicable, or (2) the following:

(i) the research presents a reasonable opportunity to further the understanding, prevention, or alleviation of a serious problem affecting the health or welfare of children;

(ii) the research will be conducted in accordance with sound ethical principles;

(iii) adequate provisions are made for soliciting the assent of children and the permission of their parents or guardians, as set forth in §46.408.

§46.408 Requirements for permission by parents or guardians and for assent by children.

(a) In addition to the determinations required under other applicable sections of this subpart, the IRB shall determine that adequate provisions are made for soliciting the assent of the children, when in the judgment of the IRB the children are capable of providing assent. In determining whether children are capable of assenting, the IRB shall take into account the ages, maturity, and psychological state of the children involved. This judgment may be made for all children to be involved in research under a particular protocol, or for each child, as the IRB deems appropriate. If the IRB determines that the capability of some or all of the children is so limited that they cannot reasonably be consulted or that the intervention or procedure involved in the research holds out a prospect of direct benefit that is important to the health or well-being of the children and is available only in the context of the research, the assent of the children is not a necessary condition for proceeding with the research. Even where the IRB determines that the subjects are capable of assenting, the IRB may still waive the assent requirement under circumstances in which consent may be waived in accord with §46.116 of Subpart A.

(b) In addition to the determinations required under other applicable sections of this subpart, the IRB shall determine, in accordance with and to the extent that consent is required by §46.116 of Subpart A, that adequate provisions are made for soliciting the permission of each child's parents or guardian. Where parental permission is to be obtained, the IRB may find that the permission of one parent is sufficient for research to be conducted under §46.404 or §46.405. Where research is covered by §§46.406 and 46.407 and permission is to be obtained from parents, both parents must give their permission unless one parent is deceased, unknown, incompetent, or not reasonably available, or when only one parent has legal responsibility for the care and custody of the child.

(c) In addition to the provisions for waiver contained in §46.116 of subpart A, if the IRB determines that a research protocol is designed for conditions or for a subject population for which parental or guardian permission is not a reasonable requirement to protect the subjects (for example, neglected or abused children), it may waive the consent requirements in Subpart A of this part and paragraph (b) of this section, provided an appropriate mechanism for protecting the children who will participate as subjects in the research is substituted, and provided further that the waiver is not inconsistent with federal, state, or local law. The choice of an appropriate mechanism would depend upon the nature and purpose of the activities described in the protocol, the risk and anticipated benefit to the research subjects, and their age, maturity, status, and condition.

(d) Permission by parents or guardians shall be documented in accordance with and to the extent required by §46.117 of subpart A.

(e) When the IRB determines that assent is required, it shall also determine whether and how assent must be documented.

§46.409 Wards.

(a) Children who are wards of the state or any other agency, institution, or entity can be included in research approved under §46.406 or §46.407 only if such research is:

(1) Related to their status as wards; or

(2) Conducted in schools, camps, hospitals, institutions, or similar settings in which the majority of children involved as subjects are not wards.

(b) If the research is approved under paragraph (a) of this section, the IRB shall require appointment of an advocate for each child who is a ward, in addition to any other individual acting on behalf of the child as guardian or in loco parentis. One individual may serve as advocate for more than one child. The advocate shall be an individual who has the background and experience to act in, and agrees to act in, the best interests of the child for the duration of the child's participation in the research and who is not associated in any way (except in the role as advocate or member of the IRB) with the research, the investigator(s), or the guardian organization.

Subpart E Registration of Institutional Review Boards

Source:74 FR 2399, January 15, 2009, unless otherwise noted.

§46.501 What IRBs must be registered?

Each IRB that is designated by an institution under an assurance of compliance approved for federalwide use by the Office for Human Research Protections (OHRP) under §46.103(a) and that reviews research involving human subjects conducted or supported by the Department of Health and Human Services (HHS) must be registered with HHS. An individual authorized to act on behalf of the institution or organization operating the IRB must submit the registration information.

§46.502 What information must be provided when registering an IRB?

The following information must be provided to HHS when registering an IRB:

(a) The name, mailing address, and street address (if different from the mailing address) of the institution or organization operating the IRB(s); and the name, mailing address, phone number, facsimile number, and electronic mail address of the senior officer or head official of that institution or organization who is responsible for overseeing activities performed by the IRB.

(b) The name, mailing address, phone number, facsimile number, and electronic mail address of the contact person providing the registration information.

(c) The name, if any, assigned to the IRB by the institution or organization, and the IRB's mailing address, street address (if different from the mailing address), phone number, facsimile number, and electronic mail address.

(d) The name, phone number, and electronic mail address of the IRB chairperson.

(e)(1) The approximate numbers of:

(i) All active protocols; and

(ii) Active protocols conducted or supported by HHS.

(2) For purpose of this regulation, an ``active protocol'' is any protocol for which the IRB conducted an initial review or a continuing review at a convened meeting or under an expedited review procedure during the preceding twelve months.

(f) The approximate number of full-time equivalent positions devoted to the IRB's administrative activities.

§46.503 When must an IRB be registered?

An IRB must be registered before it can be designated under an assurance approved for federalwide use by OHRP under §46.103(a).

IRB registration becomes effective when reviewed and accepted by OHRP.

The registration will be effective for 3 years.

§46.504 How must an IRB be registered?

Each IRB must be registered electronically through http://ohrp.cit.nih.gov/efile unless an institution or organization lacks the ability to register its IRB(s) electronically. If an institution or organization lacks the ability to register an IRB electronically, it must send its IRB registration information in writing to OHRP.

§46.505 When must IRB registration information be renewed or updated?

(a) Each IRB must renew its registration every 3 years.

(b) The registration information for an IRB must be updated within 90 days after changes occur regarding the contact person who provided the IRB registration information or the IRB chairperson. The updated registration information must be submitted in accordance with §46.504.

(c) Any renewal or update that is submitted to, and accepted by, OHRP begins a new 3-year effective period.

(d) An institution's or organization's decision to disband a registered IRB which it is operating also must be reported to OHRP in writing within 30 days after permanent cessation of the IRB's review of HHS-conducted or -supported research.

APPENDIX F

Code of Federal Regulations

TITLE 21
FOOD AND DRUGS

CHAPTER I
FOOD AND DRUG ADMINISTRATION, DEPARTMENT OF HEALTH AND HUMAN SERVICES.

SUBCHAPTER A
GENERAL

PART 50
PROTECTION OF HUMAN SUBJECTS

***

Subpart A General Provisions

Sec.

50.1 Scope.

50.3 Definitions.

Subpart B Informed Consent of Human Subjects

50.20 General requirements for informed consent.

50.23 Exception from general requirements.

50.24 Exception from informed consent requirements for emergency research.

50.25 Elements of informed consent.

50.27 Documentation of informed consent.

Subpart C [Reserved]

Subpart D Additional Safeguards for Children in Clinical Investigations

50.50 IRB duties.

50.51 Clinical investigations not involving greater than minimal risk.

50.52 Clinical investigations involving greater than minimal risk but presenting the prospect of direct benefit to individual subjects.

50.53 Clinical investigations involving greater than minimal risk and no prospect of direct benefit to individual subjects, but likely to yield generalizable knowledge about the subjects' disorder or condition.

50.54 Clinical investigations not otherwise approvable that present an opportunity to understand, prevent, or al leviate a serious problem affecting the health or wel fare of children.

50.55 Requirements for permission by parents or guardians and for assent by children.

50.56 Wards.

Authority: 21 U.S.C 321, 343, 346, 346a, 348, 350a, 350b, 352, 353, 355, 360, 360c-360f, 360h-360j, 371, 379e, 381; 42 U.S.C. 216, 241, 262, 263b-263n.

Source: 45 FR 36390, May 30, 1980, unless otherwise noted.

Subpart A General Provisions

§ 50.1 Scope.

(a) This part applies to all clinical investigations regulated by the Food and Drug Administration under sections 505(i) and 520(g) of the Federal Food, Drug, and Cosmetic Act, as well as clinical investigations that support applications for research or marketing permits for products regulated by the Food and Drug Administration, including foods, including dietary supplements, that bear a nutrient content claim or a health claim, infant formulas, food and color additives, drugs for human use, medical devices for human use, biological products for human use, and electronic products. Additional specific obligations and commitments of, and standards of conduct for, persons who sponsor or monitor clinical investigations involving particular test articles may also be found in other parts (e.g., parts 312 and 812). Compliance with these parts is intended to protect the rights and safety of subjects involved in investigations filed with the Food and Drug Administration pursuant to sections 403, 406, 409, 412, 413, 502, 503, 505, 510, 513-516, 518-520, 721, and 801 of the Federal Food, Drug, and Cosmetic Act and sections 351 and 354-360F of the Public Health Service Act.

(b) References in this part to regulatory sections of the Code of Federal Regulations are to chapter I of title 21, unless otherwise noted.

[45 FR 36390, May 30, 1980; 46 FR 8979, Jan. 27, 1981, as amended at 63 FR 26697, May 13, 1998; 64 FR 399, Jan. 5, 1999; 66 FR 20597, Apr. 24, 2001]

§ 50.3 Definitions.

As used in this part:

(a) *Act* means the Federal Food, Drug, and Cosmetic Act, as amended (secs. 201-902, 52 Stat. 1040 et seq. as amended (21 U.S.C. 321-392)).

(b) *Application for research or marketing permit* includes:

(1) A color additive petition, described in part 71.

(2) A food additive petition, described in parts 171 and 571.

(3) Data and information about a substance submitted as part of the procedures for establishing that the substance is generally recognized as safe for use that results or may reasonably be expected to result, directly or indirectly, in its becoming a component or otherwise affecting the characteristics of any food, described in §§ 170.30 and 570.30.

(4) Data and information about a food additive submitted as part of the procedures for food additives permitted to be used on an interim basis pending additional study, described in § 180.1.

(5) Data and information about a substance submitted as part of the procedures for establishing a tolerance for unavoidable contaminants in food and food-packaging materials, described in section 406 of the act.

(6) An investigational new drug application, described in part 312 of this chapter.

(7) A new drug application, described in part 314.

(8) Data and information about the bioavailability or bioequivalence of drugs for human use submitted as part of the procedures for issuing, amending, or repealing a bioequivalence requirement, described in part 320.

(9) Data and information about an over-the-counter drug for human use submitted as part of the procedures for classifying these drugs as generally recognized as safe and effective and not misbranded, described in part 330.

(10) Data and information about a prescription drug for human use submitted as part of the procedures for classifying these drugs as generally recognized as safe and effective and not misbranded, described in this chapter.

(11) [Reserved]

(12) An application for a biologics license, described in part 601 of this chapter.

(13) Data and information about a biological product submitted as part of the procedures for determining that licensed biological products are safe and effective and not misbranded, described in part 601.

(14) Data and information about an in vitro diagnostic product submitted as part of the procedures for establishing, amending, or repealing a standard for these products, described in part 809.

(15) An *Application for an Investigational Device Exemption*, described in part 812.

(16) Data and information about a medical device submitted as part of the procedures for classifying these devices, described in section 513.

(17) Data and information about a medical device submitted as part of the procedures for establishing, amending, or repealing a standard for these devices, described in section 514.

(18) An application for premarket approval of a medical device, described in section 515.

(19) A product development protocol for a medical device, described in section 515.

(20) Data and information about an electronic product submitted as part of the procedures for establishing, amending, or repealing a standard for these products, described in section 358 of the Public Health Service Act.

(21) Data and information about an electronic product submitted as part of the procedures for obtaining a variance from any electronic product performance standard, as described in § 1010.4.

(22) Data and information about an electronic product submitted as part of the procedures for granting, amending, or extending an exemption from a radiation safety performance standard, as described in § 1010.5.

(23) Data and information about a clinical study of an infant formula when submitted as part of an infant formula notification under section 412(c) of the Federal Food, Drug, and Cosmetic Act.

(24) Data and information submitted in a petition for a nutrient content claim, described in § 101.69 of this chapter, or for a health claim, described in § 101.70 of this chapter.

(25) Data and information from investigations involving children submitted in a new dietary ingredient notification, described in § 190.6 of this chapter.

(c) *Clinical investigation* means any experiment that involves a test article and one or more human subjects and that either is subject to requirements for prior submission to the Food and Drug Administration under section 505(i) or 520(g) of the act, or is not subject to requirements for prior submission to the Food and Drug Administration under these sections of the act, but the results of which are intended to be submitted later to, or held for inspection by, the Food and Drug Administration as part of an application for a research or marketing permit. The term does not include experiments that are subject to the provisions of part 58 of this chapter, regarding nonclinical laboratory studies.

(d) *Investigator* means an individual who actually conducts a clinical investigation, i.e., under whose immediate direction the test article is administered or dispensed to, or used involving, a subject, or, in the event of an investigation conducted by a team of individuals, is the responsible leader of that team.

(e) *Sponsor* means a person who initiates a clinical investigation, but who does not actually conduct the investigation, i.e., the test article is administered or dispensed to or used involving, a subject under the immediate direction of another individual. A person other than an individual (e.g., corporation or agency) that uses one or more of its own employees to conduct a clinical investigation it has initiated is considered to be a sponsor (not a sponsor-investigator), and the employees are considered to be investigators.

(f) *Sponsor-investigator* means an individual who both initiates and actually conducts, alone or with others, a clinical investigation, i.e., under whose immediate direction the test article is administered or dispensed to, or used involving, a subject. The term does not include any person other than an individual, e.g., corporation or agency.

(g) *Human subject* means an individual who is or becomes a participant in research, either as a recipient of the test article or as a control. A subject may be either a healthy human or a patient.

(h) *Institution* means any public or private entity or agency (including Federal, State, and other agencies). The word facility as used in section 520(g) of the act is deemed to be synonymous with the term institution for purposes of this part.

(i) *Institutional review board* (IRB) means any board, committee, or other group formally designated by an institution to review biomedical research involving humans as subjects, to approve the initiation of and conduct periodic review of such research. The term has the same meaning as the phrase institutional review committee as used in section 520(g) of the act.

(j) *Test article* means any drug (including a biological product for human use), medical device for human use, human food additive, color additive, electronic product, or any other article subject to regulation under the act or under sections 351 and 354-360F of the Public Health Service Act (42 U.S.C. 262 and 263b-263n).

(k) *Minimal risk* means that the probability and magnitude of harm or discomfort anticipated in the research are not greater in and of themselves than those ordinarily encountered in daily life or during the performance of routine physical or psychological examinations or tests.

(l) *Legally authorized representative* means an individual or judicial or other body authorized under applicable law to consent on behalf of a prospective subject to the subject's particpation in the procedure(s) involved in the research.

(m) F*amily member* means any one of the following legally competent persons: Spouse; parents; children (including adopted children); brothers, sisters, and spouses of brothers and sisters; and any individual related by blood or affinity whose close association with the subject is the equivalent of a family relationship.

(n) *Assent* means a child's affirmative agreement to participate in a clinical investigation. Mere failure to object may not, absent affirmative agreement, be construed as assent.

(o) *Children* means persons who have not attained the legal age for consent to treatments or procedures involved in clinical investigations, under the applicable law of the jurisdiction in which the clinical investigation will be conducted.

(p) *Parent* means a child's biological or adoptive parent.

(q) *Ward* means a child who is placed in the legal custody of the State or other agency, institution, or entity, consistent with applicable Federal, State, or local law.

(r) *Permission* means the agreement of parent(s) or guardian to the participation of their child or ward in a clinical investigation. Permission must be obtained in compliance with subpart B of this part and must include the elements of informed consent described in § 50.25.

(s) *Guardian* means an individual who is authorized under applicable State or local law to consent on behalf of a child to general medical care when general medical care includes participation in research. For purposes of subpart D of this part, a guardian also means an individual who is authorized to consent on behalf of a child to participate in research.

[45 FR 36390, May 30, 1980, as amended at 46 FR 8950, Jan. 27, 1981; 54 FR 9038, Mar. 3, 1989; 56 FR 28028, June 18, 1991; 61 FR 51528, Oct. 2, 1996; 62 FR 39440, July 23, 1997; 64 FR 399, Jan. 5, 1999; 64 FR 56448, Oct. 20, 1999; 66 FR 20597, Apr. 24, 2001]

Subpart B Informed Consent of Human Subjects

Source: 46 FR 8951, Jan. 27, 1981, unless otherwise noted.

§ 50.20 General requirements for informed consent.

Except as provided in §§ 50.23 and 50.24, no investigator may involve a human being as a subject in research covered by these regulations unless the investigator has obtained the legally effective informed consent of the subject or the subject's legally authorized representative. An investigator shall seek such consent only under circumstances that provide the prospective subject or the representative sufficient opportunity to consider whether or not to participate and that minimize the possibility of coercion or undue influence. The information that is given to the subject or the representative shall be in language understandable to the subject or the representative. No informed consent, whether oral or written, may include any exculpatory language through which the subject or the representative is made to waive or appear to waive any of the subject's legal rights, or releases or appears to release the investigator, the sponsor, the institution, or its agents from liability for negligence.

[46 FR 8951, Jan. 27, 1981, as amended at 64 FR 10942, Mar. 8, 1999]

§ 50.23 Exception from general requirements.

(a) The obtaining of informed consent shall be deemed feasible unless, before use of the test article (except as provided in paragraph (b) of this section), both the investigator and a physician who is not otherwise participating in the clinical investigation certify in writing all of the following:

(1) The human subject is confronted by a life-threatening situation necessitating the use of the test article.

(2) Informed consent cannot be obtained from the subject because of an inability to communicate with, or obtain legally effective consent from, the subject.

(3) Time is not sufficient to obtain consent from the subject's legal representative.

(4) There is available no alternative method of approved or generally recognized therapy that provides an equal or greater likelihood of saving the life of the subject.

(b) If immediate use of the test article is, in the investigator's opinion, required to preserve the life of the subject, and time is not sufficient to obtain the independent determination required in paragraph (a) of this section in advance of using the test article, the determinations of the clinical investigator shall be made and, within 5 working days after the use of the article, be reviewed and evaluated in writing by a physician who is not participating in the clinical investigation.

(c) The documentation required in paragraph (a) or (b) of this section shall be submitted to the IRB within 5 working days after the use of the test article.

(d)(1) Under 10 U.S.C. 1107(f) the President may waive the prior consent requirement for the administration of an investigational new drug to a member of the armed forces in connection with the member's participation in a particular military operation. The statute specifies that only the President may waive informed consent in this connection and the President may grant such a waiver only if the President determines in writing that obtaining consent: Is not feasible; is contrary to the best interests of the military member; or is not in the interests of national security. The statute further provides that in making a determination to waive prior informed consent on the ground that it is not feasible or the ground that it is contrary to the best interests of the military members involved, the President shall apply the standards and criteria that are set forth in the relevant FDA regulations for a waiver of the prior informed consent requirements of section 505(i)(4) of the Federal Food, Drug, and Cosmetic Act (21 U.S.C. 355(i)(4)). Before such a determination may be made that obtaining informed consent from military personnel prior to the use of an investigational drug (including an antibiotic or biological product) in a specific protocol under an investigational new drug application (IND) sponsored by the Department of Defense (DOD) and limited to specific military personnel involved in a particular military operation is not feasible or is contrary to the best interests of the military members involved the Secretary of Defense must first request such a determination from the President, and certify and document to the President that the following standards and criteria contained in paragraphs (d)(1) through (d)(4) of this section have been met.

(i) The extent and strength of evidence of the safety and effectiveness of the investigational new drug in relation to the medical risk that could be encountered during the military operation supports the drug's administration under an IND.

(ii) The military operation presents a substantial risk that military personnel may be subject to a chemical, biological, nuclear, or other exposure likely to produce death or serious or life-threatening injury or illness.

(iii) There is no available satisfactory alternative therapeutic or preventive treatment in relation to the intended use of the investigational new drug.

(iv) Conditioning use of the investigational new drug on the voluntary participation of each member could significantly risk the safety and health of any individual member who would decline its use, the safety of other military personnel, and the accomplishment of the military mission.

(v) A duly constituted institutional review board (IRB) established and operated in accordance with the requirements of paragraphs (d)(2) and (d)(3) of this section, responsible for review of the study, has reviewed and approved the investigational new drug protocol and the administration of the investigational new drug without informed consent. DOD's request is to include the documentation required by § 56.115(a)(2) of this chapter.

(vi) DOD has explained:

(A) The context in which the investigational drug will be administered, e.g., the setting or whether it will be self-administered or it will be administered by a health professional;

(B) The nature of the disease or condition for which the preventive or therapeutic treatment is intended; and

(C) To the extent there are existing data or information available, information on conditions that could alter the effects of the investigational drug.

(vii) DOD's recordkeeping system is capable of tracking and will be used to track the proposed treatment from supplier to the individual recipient.

(viii) Each member involved in the military operation will be given, prior to the administration of the investigational new drug, a specific written information sheet (including information required by 10 U.S.C. 1107(d)) concerning the investigational new drug, the risks and benefits of its use, potential side effects, and other pertinent information about the appropriate use of the product.

(ix) Medical records of members involved in the military operation will accurately document the receipt by members of the notification required by paragraph (d)(1)(viii) of this section.

(x) Medical records of members involved in the military operation will accurately document the receipt by members of any investigational new drugs in accordance with FDA regulations including part 312 of this chapter.

(xi) DOD will provide adequate followup to assess whether there are beneficial or adverse health consequences that result from the use of the investigational product.

(xii) DOD is pursuing drug development, including a time line, and marketing approval with due diligence.

(xiii) FDA has concluded that the investigational new drug protocol may proceed subject to a decision by the President on the informed consent waiver request.

(xiv) DOD will provide training to the appropriate medical personnel and potential recipients on the specific investigational new drug to be administered prior to its use.

(xv) DOD has stated and justified the time period for which the waiver is needed, not to exceed one year, unless separately renewed under these standards and criteria.

(xvi) DOD shall have a continuing obligation to report to the FDA and to the President any changed circumstances relating to these standards and criteria (including the time period referred to in paragraph (d)(1)(xv) of this section) or that otherwise might affect the determination to use an investigational new drug without informed consent.

(xvii) DOD is to provide public notice as soon as practicable and consistent with classification requirements through notice in the *Federal Register* describing each waiver of informed consent determination, a summary of the most updated scientific information on the products used, and other pertinent information.

(xviii) Use of the investigational drug without informed consent otherwise conforms with applicable law.

(2) The duly constituted institutional review board, described in paragraph (d)(1)(v) of this section, must include at least 3 nonaffiliated members who shall not be employees or officers of the Federal Government (other than for purposes of membership on the IRB) and shall be required to obtain any necessary security clearances. This IRB shall review the proposed IND protocol at a convened meeting at which a majority of the members are present including at least one member whose primary concerns are in nonscientific areas and, if feasible, including a majority of the nonaffiliated members. The information required by § 56.115(a)(2) of this chapter is to be provided to the Secretary of Defense for further review.

(3) The duly constituted institutional review board, described in paragraph (d)(1)(v) of this section, must review and approve:

(i) The required information sheet;

(ii) The adequacy of the plan to disseminate information, including distribution of the information sheet to potential recipients, on the investigational product (e.g., in forms other than written);

(iii) The adequacy of the information and plans for its dissemination to health care providers, including potential side effects, contraindications, potential interactions, and other pertinent considerations; and

(iv) An informed consent form as required by part 50 of this chapter, in those circumstances in which DOD determines that informed consent may be obtained from some or all personnel involved.

(4) DOD is to submit to FDA summaries of institutional review board meetings at which the proposed protocol has been reviewed.

(5) Nothing in these criteria or standards is intended to preempt or limit FDA's and DOD's authority or obligations under applicable statutes and regulations.

(e)(1) Obtaining informed consent for investigational in vitro diagnostic devices used to identify chemical, biological, radiological, or nuclear agents will be deemed feasible unless, before use of the test article, both the investigator (e.g., clinical laboratory director or other responsible individual) and a physician who is not otherwise participating in the clinical investigation make the determinations and later certify in writing all of the following:

(i) The human subject is confronted by a life-threatening situation necessitating the use of the investigational in vitro diagnostic device to identify a chemical, biological, radiological, or nuclear agent that would suggest a terrorism event or other public health emergency.

(ii) Informed consent cannot be obtained from the subject because:

(A) There was no reasonable way for the person directing that the specimen be collected to know, at the time the specimen was collected, that there would be a need to use the investigational in vitro diagnostic device on that subject's specimen; and

(B) Time is not sufficient to obtain consent from the subject without risking the life of the subject.

(iii) Time is not sufficient to obtain consent from the subject's legally authorized representative.

(iv) There is no cleared or approved available alternative method of diagnosis, to identify the chemical, biological, radiological, or nuclear agent that provides an equal or greater likelihood of saving the life of the subject.

(2) If use of the investigational device is, in the opinion of the investigator (e.g., clinical laboratory director or other responsible person), required to preserve the life of the subject, and time is not sufficient to obtain the independent determination required in paragraph (e)(1) of this section in advance of using the investigational device, the determinations of the investigator shall be made and, within 5 working days after the use of the device, be reviewed and evaluated in writing by a physician who is not participating in the clinical investigation.

(3) The investigator must submit the written certification of the determinations made by the investigator and an independent physician required in paragraph (e)(1) or (e)(2) of this section to the IRB and FDA within 5 working days after the use of the device.

(4) An investigator must disclose the investigational status of the in vitro diagnostic device and what is known about the performance characteristics of the device in the report to the subject's health care provider and in any report to public health authorities. The investigator must provide the IRB with the information required in

§ 50.25 (except for the information described in § 50.25(a)(8)) and the procedures that will be used to provide this information to each subject or the subject's legally authorized representative at the time the test results are provided to the subject's health care provider and public health authorities.

(5) The IRB is responsible for ensuring the adequacy of the information required in section 50.25 (except for the information described in § 50.25(a)(8)) and for ensuring that procedures are in place to provide this information to each subject or the subject's legally authorized representative.

(6) No State or political subdivision of a State may establish or continue in effect any law, rule, regulation or other requirement that informed consent be obtained before an investigational in vitro diagnostic device may be used to identify chemical, biological, radiological, or nuclear agent in suspected terrorism events and other potential public health emergencies that is different from, or in addition to, the requirements of this regulation.

[46 FR 8951, Jan. 27, 1981, as amended at 55 FR 52817, Dec. 21, 1990; 64 FR 399, Jan. 5, 1999; 64 FR 54188, Oct. 5, 1999; 71 FR 32833, June 7, 2006; 76 FR 36993, June 24, 2011]

§ 50.24 Exception from informed consent requirements for emergency research.

(a) The IRB responsible for the review, approval, and continuing review of the clinical investigation described in this section may approve that investigation without requiring that informed consent of all research subjects be obtained if the IRB (with the concurrence of a licensed physician who is a member of or consultant to the IRB and who is not otherwise participating in the clinical investigation) finds and documents each of the following:

(1) The human subjects are in a life-threatening situation, available treatments are unproven or unsatisfactory, and the collection of valid scientific evidence, which may include evidence obtained through randomized placebo-controlled investigations, is necessary to determine the safety and effectiveness of particular interventions.

(2) Obtaining informed consent is not feasible because:

(i) The subjects will not be able to give their informed consent as a result of their medical condition;

(ii) The intervention under investigation must be administered before consent from the subjects' legally authorized representatives is feasible; and

(iii) There is no reasonable way to identify prospectively the individuals likely to become eligible for participation in the clinical investigation.

(3) Participation in the research holds out the prospect of direct benefit to the subjects because:

(i) Subjects are facing a life-threatening situation that necessitates intervention;

(ii) Appropriate animal and other preclinical studies have been conducted, and the information derived from those studies and related evidence support the potential for the intervention to provide a direct benefit to the individual subjects; and

(iii) Risks associated with the investigation are reasonable in relation to what is known about the medical condition of the potential class of subjects, the risks and benefits of standard therapy, if any, and what is known about the risks and benefits of the proposed intervention or activity.

(4) The clinical investigation could not practicably be carried out without the waiver.

(5) The proposed investigational plan defines the length of the potential therapeutic window based on scientific evidence, and the investigator has committed to attempting to contact a legally authorized representative for each subject within that window of time and, if feasible, to asking the legally authorized representative contacted for consent within that window rather than proceeding without consent. The investigator will summarize efforts made to contact legally authorized representatives and make this information available to the IRB at the time of continuing review.

(6) The IRB has reviewed and approved informed consent procedures and an informed consent document consistent with § 50.25. These procedures and the informed consent document are to be used with subjects or their legally authorized representatives in situations where use of such procedures and documents is feasible. The IRB has reviewed and approved procedures and information to be used when providing an opportunity for a family member to object to a subject's participation in the clinical investigation consistent with paragraph (a)(7)(v) of this section.

(7) Additional protections of the rights and welfare of the subjects will be provided, including, at least:

(i) Consultation (including, where appropriate, consultation carried out by the IRB) with representatives of the communities in which the clinical investigation will be conducted and from which the subjects will be drawn;

(ii) Public disclosure to the communities in which the clinical investigation will be conducted and from which the subjects will be drawn, prior to initiation of the clinical investigation, of plans for the investigation and its risks and expected benefits;

(iii) Public disclosure of sufficient information following completion of the clinical investigation to apprise the community and researchers of the study, including the demographic characteristics of the research population, and its results;

(iv) Establishment of an independent data monitoring committee to exercise oversight of the clinical investigation; and

(v) If obtaining informed consent is not feasible and a legally authorized representative is not reasonably available, the investigator has committed, if feasible, to attempting to contact within the therapeutic window the subject's family member who is not a legally authorized representative, and asking whether he or she objects to the subject's participation in the clinical investigation. The investigator will summarize efforts made to contact family members and make this information available to the IRB at the time of continuing review.

(b) The IRB is responsible for ensuring that procedures are in place to inform, at the earliest feasible opportunity, each subject, or if the subject remains incapacitated, a legally authorized representative of the subject, or if such a representative is not reasonably available, a family member, of the subject's inclusion in the clinical investigation, the details of the investigation and other information contained in the informed consent document. The IRB shall also ensure that there is a procedure to inform the subject, or if the subject remains incapacitated, a legally authorized representative of the subject, or if such a representative is not reasonably available, a family member, that he or she may discontinue the subject's participation at any time without penalty or loss of benefits to which the subject is otherwise entitled. If a legally authorized representative or family member is told about the clinical investigation and the subject's condition improves, the subject is also to be informed as soon as feasible. If a subject is entered into a clinical investigation with waived consent and the subject dies before a legally authorized representative or family member can be contacted, information about the clinical investigation is to be provided to the subject's legally authorized representative or family member, if feasible.

(c) The IRB determinations required by paragraph (a) of this section and the documentation required by paragraph (e) of this section are to be retained by the IRB for at least 3 years after completion of the clinical investigation, and the records shall be accessible for inspection and copying by FDA in accordance with § 56.115(b) of this chapter.

(d) Protocols involving an exception to the informed consent requirement under this section must be performed under a separate investigational new drug application (IND) or investigational device exemption (IDE) that clearly identifies such protocols as protocols that may include subjects who are unable to consent. The submission of those protocols in a separate IND/IDE is required even if an IND for the same drug product or an IDE for the same device already exists. Applications for investigations under this section may not be submitted as amendments under §§ 312.30 or 812.35 of this chapter.

(e) If an IRB determines that it cannot approve a clinical investigation because the investigation does not meet the criteria in the exception provided under paragraph (a) of this section or because of other relevant ethical concerns, the IRB must document its findings and provide these findings promptly in writing to the clinical investigator and to the sponsor of the clinical investigation. The sponsor of the clinical investigation must promptly disclose this information to FDA and to the sponsor's clinical investigators who are participating or are asked to participate in this or a substantially equivalent clinical investigation of the sponsor, and to other IRB's that have been, or are, asked to review this or a substantially equivalent investigation by that sponsor.

[61 FR 51528, Oct. 2, 1996]

§ 50.25 Elements of informed consent.

(a) *Basic elements of informed consent.* In seeking informed consent, the following information shall be provided to each subject:

(1) A statement that the study involves research, an explanation of the purposes of the research and the expected duration of the subject's participation, a description of the procedures to be followed, and identification of any procedures which are experimental.

(2) A description of any reasonably foreseeable risks or discomforts to the subject.

(3) A description of any benefits to the subject or to others which may reasonably be expected from the research.

(4) A disclosure of appropriate alternative procedures or courses of treatment, if any, that might be advantageous to the subject.

(5) A statement describing the extent, if any, to which confidentiality of records identifying the subject will be maintained and that notes the possibility that the Food and Drug Administration may inspect the records.

(6) For research involving more than minimal risk, an explanation as to whether any compensation and an explanation as to whether any medical treatments are available if injury occurs and, if so, what they consist of, or where further information may be obtained.

(7) An explanation of whom to contact for answers to pertinent questions about the research and research subjects' rights, and whom to contact in the event of a research-related injury to the subject.

(8) A statement that participation is voluntary, that refusal to participate will involve no penalty or loss of benefits to which the subject is otherwise entitled, and that the subject may discontinue partici-

pation at any time without penalty or loss of benefits to which the subject is otherwise entitled.

(b) *Additional elements of informed consent.* When appropriate, one or more of the following elements of information shall also be provided to each subject:

(1) A statement that the particular treatment or procedure may involve risks to the subject (or to the embryo or fetus, if the subject is or may become pregnant) which are currently unforeseeable.

(2) Anticipated circumstances under which the subject's participation may be terminated by the investigator without regard to the subject's consent.

(3) Any additional costs to the subject that may result from participation in the research.

(4) The consequences of a subject's decision to withdraw from the research and procedures for orderly termination of participation by the subject.

(5) A statement that significant new findings developed during the course of the research which may relate to the subject's willingness to continue participation will be provided to the subject.

(6) The approximate number of subjects involved in the study.

(c) When seeking informed consent for applicable clinical trials, as defined in 42 U.S.C. 282(j)(1)(A), the following statement shall be provided to each clinical trial subject in informed consent documents and processes. This will notify the clinical trial subject that clinical trial information has been or will be submitted for inclusion in the clinical trial registry databank under paragraph (j) of section 402 of the Public Health Service Act. The statement is: "A description of this clinical trial will be available on http://www.ClinicalTrials.gov, as required by U.S. Law. This Web site will not include information that can identify you. At most, the Web site will include a summary of the results. You can search this Web site at any time."

(d) The informed consent requirements in these regulations are not intended to preempt any applicable Federal, State, or local laws which require additional information to be disclosed for informed consent to be legally effective.

(e) Nothing in these regulations is intended to limit the authority of a physician to provide emergency medical care to the extent the physician is permitted to do so under applicable Federal, State, or local law.

[46 FR 8951, Jan. 27, 1981, as amended at 76 FR 270, Jan. 4, 2011]

§ 50.27 Documentation of informed consent.

(a) Except as provided in § 56.109(c), informed consent shall be documented by the use of a written consent form approved by the IRB and signed and dated by the subject or the subject's legally authorized representative at the time of consent. A copy shall be given to the person signing the form.

(b) Except as provided in § 56.109(c), the consent form may be either of the following:

(1) A written consent document that embodies the elements of informed consent required by § 50.25. This form may be read to the subject or the subject's legally authorized representative, but, in any event, the investigator shall give either the subject or the representative adequate opportunity to read it before it is signed.

(2) A *short form* written consent document stating that the elements of informed consent required by § 50.25 have been presented orally to the subject or the subject's legally authorized representative. When this method is used, there shall be a witness to the oral presentation. Also, the IRB shall approve a written summary of what is to be said to the subject or the representative. Only the short form itself is to be signed by the subject or the representative. However, the witness shall sign both the short form and a copy of the summary, and the person actually obtaining the consent shall sign a copy of the summary. A copy of the summary shall be given to the subject or the representative in addition to a copy of the short form.

[46 FR 8951, Jan. 27, 1981, as amended at 61 FR 57280, Nov. 5, 1996]

Subpart C [Reserved]

Subpart D Additional Safeguards for Children in Clinical Investigations

Source: 66 FR 20598, Apr. 24, 2001, unless otherwise noted.

§ 50.50 IRB duties.

In addition to other responsibilities assigned to IRBs under this part and part 56 of this chapter, each IRB must review clinical investigations involving children as subjects covered by this subpart D and approve only those clinical investigations that satisfy the criteria described in § 50.51, § 50.52, or § 50.53 and the conditions of all other applicable sections of this subpart D.

§ 50.51 Clinical investigations not involving greater than minimal risk.

Any clinical investigation within the scope described in §§ 50.1 and 56.101 of this chapter in which no greater than minimal risk to children is presented may involve children as subjects only if the IRB finds and documents that adequate provisions are made for soliciting the assent of the children and the permission of their parents or guardians as set forth in § 50.55.

§ 50.52 Clinical investigations involving greater than minimal risk but presenting the prospect of direct benefit to individual subjects.

Any clinical investigation within the scope described in §§ 50.1 and 56.101 of this chapter in which more than minimal risk to children is presented by an intervention or procedure that holds out the prospect of direct benefit for the individual subject, or by a monitoring procedure that is likely to contribute to the subject's well-being, may involve children as subjects only if the IRB finds and documents that:

(a) The risk is justified by the anticipated benefit to the subjects;

(b) The relation of the anticipated benefit to the risk is at least as favorable to the subjects as that presented by available alternative approaches; and

(c) Adequate provisions are made for soliciting the assent of the children and permission of their parents or guardians as set forth in § 50.55.

§ 50.53 Clinical investigations involving greater than minimal risk and no prospect of direct benefit to individual subjects, but likely to yield generalizable knowledge about the subjects' disorder or condition.

Any clinical investigation within the scope described in §§ 50.1 and 56.101 of this chapter in which more than minimal risk to children is presented by an intervention or procedure that does not hold out the prospect of direct benefit for the individual subject, or by a monitoring procedure that is not likely to contribute to the well-being of the subject, may involve children as subjects only if the IRB finds and documents that:

(a) The risk represents a minor increase over minimal risk;

(b) The intervention or procedure presents experiences to subjects that are reasonably commensurate with those inherent in their actual or expected medical, dental, psychological, social, or educational situations;

(c) The intervention or procedure is likely to yield generalizable knowledge about the subjects' disorder or condition that is of vital importance for the understanding or amelioration of the subjects' disorder or condition; and

(d) Adequate provisions are made for soliciting the assent of the children and permission of their parents or guardians as set forth in § 50.55.

§ 50.54 Clinical investigations not otherwise approvable that present an opportunity to understand, prevent, or alleviate a serious problem affecting the health or welfare of children.

If an IRB does not believe that a clinical investigation within the scope described in §§ 50.1 and 56.101 of this chapter and involving children as subjects meets the requirements of § 50.51, § 50.52, or § 50.53, the clinical investigation may proceed only if:

(a) The IRB finds and documents that the clinical investigation presents a reasonable opportunity to further the understanding, prevention, or alleviation of a serious problem affecting the health or welfare of children; and

(b) The Commissioner of Food and Drugs, after consultation with a panel of experts in pertinent disciplines (for example: science, medicine, education, ethics, law) and following opportunity for public review and comment, determines either:

(1) That the clinical investigation in fact satisfies the conditions of § 50.51, § 50.52, or § 50.53, as applicable, or

(2) That the following conditions are met:

(i) The clinical investigation presents a reasonable opportunity to further the understanding, prevention, or alleviation of a serious problem affecting the health or welfare of children;

(ii) The clinical investigation will be conducted in accordance with sound ethical principles; and

(iii) Adequate provisions are made for soliciting the assent of children and the permission of their parents or guardians as set forth in § 50.55.

§ 50.55 Requirements for permission by parents or guardians and for assent by children.

(a) In addition to the determinations required under other applicable sections of this subpart D, the IRB must determine that adequate provisions are made for soliciting the assent of the children when in the judgment of the IRB the children are capable of providing assent.

(b) In determining whether children are capable of providing assent, the IRB must take into account the ages, maturity, and psychological state of the children involved. This judgment may be made for all children to be involved in clinical investigations under a particular protocol, or for each child, as the IRB deems appropriate.

(c) The assent of the children is not a necessary condition for proceeding with the clinical investigation if the IRB determines:

(1) That the capability of some or all of the children is so limited that they cannot reasonably be consulted, or

(2) That the intervention or procedure involved in the clinical investigation holds out a prospect of direct benefit that is important to the health or well-being of the children and is available only in the context of the clinical investigation.

(d) Even where the IRB determines that the subjects are capable of assenting, the IRB may still waive the assent requirement if it finds and documents that:

(1) The clinical investigation involves no more than minimal risk to the subjects;

(2) The waiver will not adversely affect the rights and welfare of the subjects;

(3) The clinical investigation could not practicably be carried out without the waiver; and

(4) Whenever appropriate, the subjects will be provided with additional pertinent information after participation.

(e) In addition to the determinations required under other applicable sections of this subpart D, the IRB must determine that the permission of each child's parents or guardian is granted.

(1) Where parental permission is to be obtained, the IRB may find that the permission of one parent is sufficient, if consistent with State law, for clinical investigations to be conducted under § 50.51 or § 50.52.

(2) Where clinical investigations are covered by § 50.53 or § 50.54 and permission is to be obtained from parents, both parents must give their permission unless one parent is deceased, unknown, incompetent, or not reasonably available, or when only one parent has legal responsibility for the care and custody of the child if consistent with State law.

(f) Permission by parents or guardians must be documented in accordance with and to the extent required by § 50.27.

(g) When the IRB determines that assent is required, it must also determine whether and how assent must be documented.

§ 50.56 Wards.

(a) Children who are wards of the State or any other agency, institution, or entity can be included in clinical investigations approved under § 50.53 or § 50.54 only if such clinical investigations are:

(1) Related to their status as wards; or

(2) Conducted in schools, camps, hospitals, institutions, or similar settings in which the majority of children involved as subjects are not wards.

(b) If the clinical investigation is approved under paragraph (a) of this section, the IRB must require appointment of an advocate for each child who is a ward.

(1) The advocate will serve in addition to any other individual acting on behalf of the child as guardian or in loco parentis.

(2) One individual may serve as advocate for more than one child.

(3) The advocate must be an individual who has the background and experience to act in, and agrees to act in, the best interest of the child for the duration of the child's participation in the clinical investigation.

(4) The advocate must not be associated in any way (except in the role as advocate or member of the IRB) with the clinical investigation, the investigator(s), or the guardian organization.

Form 1572

DEPARTMENT OF HEALTH AND HUMAN SERVICES PUBLIC HEALTH SERVICE FOOD AND DRUG ADMINISTRATION **STATEMENT OF INVESTIGATOR** ***(TITLE 21, CODE OF FEDERAL REGULATIONS (CFR) PART 312)*** (See instructions on reverse side.)	Form Approved: OMB No. 0910-0014. Expiration Date: September 30, 2002. *See OMB Statement on Reverse.* NOTE: No investigator may participate in an investigation until he/she provides the sponsor with a completed, signed Statement of Investigator, Form FDA 1572 (21 CFR 312.53(c)).

1. NAME AND ADDRESS OF INVESTIGATOR

2. EDUCATION, TRAINING, AND EXPERIENCE THAT QUALIFIES THE INVESTIGATOR AS AN EXPERT IN THE CLINICAL INVESTIGATION OF THE DRUG FOR THE USE UNDER INVESTIGATION. ONE OF THE FOLLOWING IS ATTACHED.

☐ CURRICULUM VITAE ☐ OTHER STATEMENT OF QUALIFICATIONS

3. NAME AND ADDRESS OF ANY MEDICAL SCHOOL, HOSPITAL OR OTHER RESEARCH FACILITY WHERE THE CLINICAL INVESTIGATION(S) WILL BE CONDUCTED.

4. NAME AND ADDRESS OF ANY CLINICAL LABORATORY FACILITIES TO BE USED IN THE STUDY.

5. NAME AND ADDRESS OF THE INSTITUTIONAL REVIEW BOARD (IRB) THAT IS RESPONSIBLE FOR REVIEW AND APPROVAL OF THE STUDY(IES).

6. NAMES OF THE SUBINVESTIGATORS *(e.g., research fellows, residents, associates)* WHO WILL BE ASSISTING THE INVESTIGATOR IN THE CONDUCT OF THE INVESTIGATION(S).

7. NAME AND CODE NUMBER, IF ANY, OF THE PROTOCOL(S) IN THE IND FOR THE STUDY(IES) TO BE CONDUCTED BY THE INVESTIGATOR.

FORM FDA 1572 (8/01) PREVIOUS EDITION IS OBSOLETE. **PAGE 1 OF 2**

8. ATTACH THE FOLLOWING CLINICAL PROTOCOL INFORMATION:

☐ FOR PHASE 1 INVESTIGATIONS, A GENERAL OUTLINE OF THE PLANNED INVESTIGATION INCLUDING THE ESTIMATED DURATION OF THE STUDY AND THE MAXIMUM NUMBER OF SUBJECTS THAT WILL BE INVOLVED.

☐ FOR PHASE 2 OR 3 INVESTIGATIONS, AN OUTLINE OF THE STUDY PROTOCOL INCLUDING AN APPROXIMATION OF THE NUMBER OF SUBJECTS TO BE TREATED WITH THE DRUG AND THE NUMBER TO BE EMPLOYED AS CONTROLS, IF ANY; THE CLINICAL USES TO BE INVESTIGATED; CHARACTERISTICS OF SUBJECTS BY AGE, SEX, AND CONDITION; THE KIND OF CLINICAL OBSERVATIONS AND LABORATORY TESTS TO BE CONDUCTED; THE ESTIMATED DURATION OF THE STUDY; AND COPIES OR A DESCRIPTION OF CASE REPORT FORMS TO BE USED.

9. COMMITMENTS:

I agree to conduct the study(ies) in accordance with the relevant, current protocol(s) and will only make changes in a protocol after notifying the sponsor, except when necessary to protect the safety, rights, or welfare of subjects.

I agree to personally conduct or supervise the described investigation(s).

I agree to inform any patients, or any persons used as controls, that the drugs are being used for investigational purposes and I will ensure that the requirements relating to obtaining informed consent in 21 CFR Part 50 and institutional review board (IRB) review and approval in 21 CFR Part 56 are met.

I agree to report to the sponsor adverse experiences that occur in the course of the investigation(s) in accordance with 21 CFR 312.64.

I have read and understand the information in the investigator's brochure, including the potential risks and side effects of the drug.

I agree to ensure that all associates, colleagues, and employees assisting in the conduct of the study(ies) are informed about their obligations in meeting the above commitments.

I agree to maintain adequate and accurate records in accordance with 21 CFR 312.62 and to make those records available for inspection in accordance with 21 CFR 312.68.

I will ensure that an IRB that complies with the requirements of 21 CFR Part 56 will be responsible for the initial and continuing review and approval of the clinical investigation. I also agree to promptly report to the IRB all changes in the research activity and all unanticipated problems involving risks to human subjects or others. Additionally, I will not make any changes in the research without IRB approval, except where necessary to eliminate apparent immediate hazards to human subjects.

I agree to comply with all other requirements regarding the obligations of clinical investigators and all other pertinent requirements in 21 CFR Part 312.

INSTRUCTIONS FOR COMPLETING FORM FDA 1572
STATEMENT OF INVESTIGATOR:

1. Complete all sections. Attach a separate page if additional space is needed.
2. Attach curriculum vitae or other statement of qualifications as described in Section 2.
3. Attach protocol outline as described in Section 8.
4. Sign and date below.
5. FORWARD THE COMPLETED FORM AND ATTACHMENTS TO THE SPONSOR. The sponsor will incorporate this information along with other technical data into an Investigational New Drug Application (IND).

10. SIGNATURE OF INVESTIGATOR	11. DATE

(**WARNING:** A willfully false statement is a criminal offense. U.S.C. Title 18, Sec. 1001.)

Public reporting burden for this collection of information is estimated to average 100 hours per response, including the time for reviewing instructions, searching existing data sources, gathering and maintaining the data needed, and completing reviewing the collection of information. Send comments regarding this burden estimate or any other aspect of this collection of information, including suggestions for reducing this burden to:

Food and Drug Administration
CBER (HFM-99)
1401 Rockville Pike
Rockville, MD 20852-1448

Food and Drug Administration
CDER (HFD-94)
12229 Wilkins Avenue
Rockville, MD 20852

"An agency may not conduct or sponsor, and a person is not required to respond to, a collection of information unless it displays a currently valid OMB control number."

Please **DO NOT RETURN** this application to this address.

FORM FDA 1572 (8/01) **PAGE 2 OF 2**

APPENDIX H

Directory of Health Associations

General Resources

The Center for Information and Study on Clinical Research Participation
56 Commercial Wharf East
Boston, MA 02110
(617) 725-2750
(617) 725-2753 (fax)
www.ciscrp.org

World Health Organization
Avenue Appia 20
1211 Geneva 27
Switzerland
(+41 22) 791 2111
(+41 22) 791 3111 (fax)
www.who.org

American Heart Association National Center
7272 Greenville Avenue
Dallas, TX 75231
(800) 242 8731
(214) 706 1341 (fax)
www.heart.org

Cardiology/Vascular Diseases:

Vascular Disease Foundation
550 M Ritchie Highway
PMB-281
Severna Park, MD 21146
(443) 261-5564
robert.greenberg@vdf.org
vasculardisease.org

WomenHeart: The National
Coalition for Women with Heart Disease
818 18th Street, NW
Suite 1000
Washington D.C. 20006
(202) 728-7199
(202) 728-7238 (fax)
mail@womenheart.org
http://www.womenheart.org/

National Lipid Association
6816 Southpoint Parkway
Suite 1000
Jacksonville, FL 32216
(904) 998-0854
(904) 998-0855 (fax)
aapdinfo@aapd.org
www.lipid.org

Dental/Oral Health:

The American Academy of Dentistry
211 East Chicago Avenue
Suite 1700
Chicago, IL 60611
(312) 337-2169
(312) 337-6329 (fax)
aapdinfo@aapd.org
www.aapd.org

American Dental Association
211 East Chicago Ave.
Chicago, IL 60611
(312) 440-2500
online@ada.org
www.ada.org

Oral Health America
410 North Michigan Avenue
Suite 352
Chicago, IL 60611
(312) 836-9900
(312) 836-9986 (fax)
info@oralhealthamerica.org
oralhealthamerica.org

Dermatology/Plastic Surgery

The American Academy of Dermatology
PO Box 4014
Schaumburg, IL 60618
(866) 503-7546
(847) 240-1859 (fax)
www.aad.org

National Psoriasis Foundation
6600 SW 92nd Avenue
Suite 300
Portland, OR 97223
(800) 723-9166
www.psoriasis.org

Melanoma Research Foundation
1411 K Street, NW
Suite 800
Washington D.C. 20005
(202) 347-9675
(202) 347-9678 (fax)
info@melanoma.org
www.melanoma.org

National Eczema Association
4460 Redwood Highway
Suite 16D
San Rafael, CA 94903
(415) 499-3474
info@nationaleczema.org
www.nationaleczema.org

Endocrinology:

American Diabetes Association
ATTN: Center for Information
1701 North Beauregard Street
Alexandria, VA 22311
(800) 342-2383
www.diabetes.org
Joslin Diabetes Center
One Joslin Place
Boston, MA 02215
(617) 732-2400
www.joslin.org

The Endocrine Society
8401 Connecticut Avenue
Suite 900
Chevy Chase, MD 20815
(301) 941-0200
www.endocrine.org

Gastroenterology:

American Association for The Study of Liver Diseases
1001 North Fairfax Street
Suite 400
Alexandria, VA 22314
(703) 299-9766
(703) 299-9622 (fax)
aasld@aasld.org
www.aasld.org

American Board of Colon and Rectal Surgery
20600 Eureka Road
Suite 600
Taylor, MI 48180
(734) 282-9400
(734) 282-9402 (fax)
admin@abcrs.org
www.abcrs.org

The American Gastroenterological Association
4930 Del Ray Avenue
Bethesda, MD 20814
(301) 654-2055
(301) 654-5920 (fax)
member@gastro.org
www.gastro.org

American Liver Foundation
39 Broadway
Suite 2700
New York, NY 10006
(212) 668-1000
(212) 483-8179 (fax)
info@liverfoundation.org
www.liverfoundation.org

Crohn's and Colitis Foundation of America
(888) 694-8872
www.ccfa.org

Digestive Disease National Coalition
507 Capitol Court, NE
Suite 200
Washington, DC 20002
(202) 544-7497
(202) 546-7105 (fax)
www.ddnc.org

Gastro-Intestinal Reserach Foundation
70 East Lake Street
Suite 1015
Chicago, IL 60601
(312) 332-1350
(312) 332-4757 (fax)
www.girf.org

Cancer Patients Alliance
312 Fountain Avenue
Pacific Grove, CA 93950
(831) 658-0600
info@pancreatica.org
pancreatica.org

Gynecology:

Endometriosis Association
8585 N. 76th Place
Milwaukee, WI 53223
(414) 355-2200
(414) 355-6065 (fax)
www.endometriosisassn.org

Hematology:

National Heart, Lung, and Blood Institute
NHLBI Health Information Center
P.O. Box 30105
Bethesda, MD 20824-0105
(301) 592-8573
(301) 592-8563
nhlbiinfo@nhlbi.nih.gov
www.nhlbi.nih.gov

Sickle Cell Disease
Association of America
231 E. Baltimore Street
Suite 800
Baltimore, MD 21202
(800) 421.8453
(410) 528.1495 (fax)
www.sicklecelldisease.org

National Hemophilia
Foundation
116 West 32nd Street
11th Floor
New York, NY 10001
(212) 328-3700
(212) 328-3777 (fax)
handi@hemophilia.org
www.hemophilia.org

Immunology/Infectious Disease:

American Academy of Allergy, Asthma, &
Immunology
(414) 272-6071
www.aaaai.org

American Autoimmune
Related Diseases Association
22100 Gratiot Ave.
Eastpointe, MI 48021
(586) 776-3900
(586) 776-3903 (fax)
www.aarda.org

American Foundation for AIDS Research
120 Wall Street, 13th Floor
New York, NY 10005-3908
(212) 806-1600
(212) 806-1601 (fax)
www.amfar.org

American Sexual Health Association
PO Box 13827
Research Triangle Park, NC 27709
(919) 361-8400
(919) 361-8425 (fax)
info@ashastd.org
www.ashastd.org

Celiac Disease Foundation
20350 Ventura Boulevard
Suite 240
Woodland Hills, CA 91364
(818) 716-1513
(818) 267-5577
cdf@celia.org
www.celiac.org

Musculoskeletal:
National Osteoporosis Foundation
1150 17th Street NW
Suite 850
Washington D.C. 20036
(202) 223-2226
(202) 223-2237
www.nof.org

Arthritis Foundation
1330 W. Peachtree Street
Suite 100
Atlanta, GA 30309
(404) 872-7100
www.arthritis.org

The Restless Legs Syndrome Foundation
1610 14th St NW
Suite 300
Rochester, MN 55901
(507) 287-6465
(507) 287-6312 (fax)
rlsfoundation@rls.org
www.rls.org

Christopher & Dana Reeve Foundation
636 Morris Turnpike
Suite 3A
Short Hills, NJ 07078
(800) 225-0292
information@christopherreeve.org
www.ChristopherReeve.org

The MAGIC Foundation
6645 W. North Avenue
Oak Park, IL 60302
(708) 383-0808
(708) 383-0899 (fax)
ContactUs@magicfoundation.org
www.magicfoundation.org

Nephrology/Urology:

American Society of Nephrology
1510 H Street, NW
Suite 800
Washington D.C. 20005
(202) 640-4660
(202) 637-9793
email@asn-online.org
www.asn-online.org

Urology Care Foundation
1000 Corporate Boulevard
Linthicum, MD 21090
(410) 689-3700
(410) 689-3998 (fax)
info@urologycarefoundation.org
www.urologyhealth.org

Prostate Cancer Foundation
1250 Fourth Street
Santa Monica, CA 90401
(310) 570-4700
(310) 570-4701 (fax)
info@pcf.org
www.pcf.org

Neurology:

Alzheimer's Association
225 N. Michigan Ave., Floor 17
Chicago, IL 60601-7633
(800) 272-3900
(312) 335-8700
(312) 335-5886 (tdd)
(866) 699-1246 (fax)
www.alz.org

American Academy of Neurology
201 Chicago Avenue
Minneapolis, MN 55415
(800) 879-1960
(612) 454-2746 (fax)
memberservices@aan.com
www.aan.com

United Cerebral Palsy Association
1825 K Street NW
Suite 600
Washington D.C. 20006
(800) 872-5827
info@ucp.org
www.ucp.org

National Stroke Association
9707 E. Easter Lane, Suite B
Centennial, CO 80112
(800) STROKES
(800) 787-6537
(303) 649-1328 (Fax)
www.stroke.org

The Michael J. Fox Foundation for Parkinson's Research
Grand Central Station
P.O. Box 4777
New York, NY 10163
(800) 708-7644
(212) 509-2390 (fax)
info@michaeljfox.org
www.michaeljfox.org

Epilepsy Foundation
8301 Professional Place
Landover, MD 20785
(800) 332-1000
(301) 459-1569 (fax)
ContactUs@efa.org
www.epilepsyfoundation.org

The Foundation for Peripheral Neuropathy
485 Half Day Road
Suite 200
Buffalo Grove, IL 60089
(877) 883-9942
(847) 883-9960 (fax)
info@tffpn.org
www.foundationforpn.org

The National Fibromyalgia Association
2121 S. Towne Centre Place
Suite 300
Anaheim, CA 92806
(714) 921-0150
(714) 921-6920 (fax)
www.fmaware.org

Multiple Sclerosis Foundation
6520 North Andrews Avenue
Fort Lauderdale, FL 33309
(800) 225-6495
(954) 938-8708 (fax)
admin@msfocus.org
www.msfocus.org

Oncology:

National Cancer Institute
BG 9609 MSC 9760
9609 Medical Center Drive
Bethesda, MD 20892-9760
(800) 4-CANCER
(800) 422-6237
www.cancer.gov

American Cancer Society
250 Williams Street NW
Atlanta, GA 30303
(800) 227-2345
www.cancer.org

The Leukemia and Lymphoma Society
1311 Mamaroneck Avenue
Suite 310
White Plains, NY 10605
(914) 949-5213
(914) 949-6691 (fax)
http://www.lls.org

National Breast Cancer Foundation
2600 Network Blvd
Suite 300
Frisco ,TX 75034
(972) 248-9200
www.nbcf.org

Susan G. Komen for the Cure
5005 LBJ Freeway
Suite 250
Dallas, TX 75244
(877) 465-6636
ww5.komen.org

Opthalmology:

The Glaucoma Foundation
80 Maiden Lane
Suite 700
New York, NY 10038
(212) 285-0080
info@glaucomafoundation.org
www.glaucomafoundation.org

The Macular Degeneration Association (MDA)
P.O. Box 20256
Sarasota, FL 34276
(941) 870-4399
info@maculardegenerationassociation.org
www.maculardegenerationassociation.org

The Foundation of the American Academy of Ophthalmology
655 Beach Street
San Francisco, CA 94109
(877) 887-6327
(415) 561-8567 (fax)
faao@aao.org
www.faao.org

Otolaryngology:

American Tinnitus Association
P.O. Box 5
Portland, OR 97207-0005
(800) 634-8978
(503) 248-0024 (fax)
http://www.ata.org/

American Speech-Language-Hearing Association (ASHA)
2200 Research Boulevard
Rockville, MD 20850
(800) 638-8255
(301) 296-8580 (fax)
www.asha.org

Pediatrics/Neonatology:

March of Dimes
National Children's Cancer Society
One South Memorial Drive
Suite 800
St. Louis, MI 63102
(314) 241-1600
(314) 241-1996 (fax)
www.thenccs.org

Pediheart
www.pediheart.org.cy

Academic Pediatric Association
6728 Old McLean Village Drive
McLean, VA 22101
(703) 556-9222
(703) 556-8729 (fax)
info@academicpeds.org
www.ambpeds.org

Psychiatry/Psychology:

National Alliance on Mental Illness
3803 N. Fairfax Drive
Suite 100
Arlington, VA 22203
(703) 524-7600
(703) 524-9094 (fax)
www.nami.org

National Sleep Foundation
1010 N. Glebe Road
Suite 310
Arlington, VA 22201
(703) 243-1697
nsf@sleepfoundation.org
www.sleepfoundation.org

American Psychological Foundation
750 First Street NE
Washington, DC 20002
(202) 336-5843
(202) 336-5812 (fax)
foundation@apa.org
www.apa.org

Mental Health America
2000 N. Beauregard Street
6th Floor
Alexandria, VA 22311
(703) 684-7722
(703) 684-5968 (fax)
info@mentalhealthamerica.net
www.mentalhealthamerica.net

Anxiety and Depression Association of America
8701 Georgia Avenue
#412
Silver Spring, MD 20910
(240) 485.1001
(240) 485-1035 (fax)
information@adaa.org
www.adaa.org

Pulmonary/Respiratory Diseases:

American Lung Association
1301 Pennsylvania Avenue NW
Suite 800
Washington D.C 20004
(202) 785 3355
(202) 452 1805 (fax)
www.lung.org

National Heart, Lung, and Blood Institute
NHLBI Health Information Center
P.O. Box 30105
Bethesda, MD 20824-0105
(301) 592-8573
(301) 592-8563 (fax)
nhlbiinfo@nhlbi.nih.gov
www.nhlbi.nih.gov

Asthma and Allergy Foundation of America
8201 Corporate Drive
Suite 1000
Landover, MD 20785
(800) 727-8462
Info@aafa.org
www.aafa.org

American Academy of Allergy, Asthma, &
Immunology
(414) 272-6071
www.aaaai.org

COPD Foundation
20 F Street NW
Suite 200A
Washington D.C. 20001
(866) 731-2673
info@copdfoundation.org
www.copdfoundation.org

Coalition for Pulmonary Fibrosis
10866 W. Washington Boulevard
Suite 343
Culver City, CA 90232
(888) 222-8541
info@coalitionforpf.org
www.coalitionforpf.org

Arthritis Foundation
1330 W. Peachtree Street
Suite 100
Atlanta, GA 30309
(404) 872-7100
www.arthritis.org

S.L.E. Lupus Foundation
330 Seventh Avenue
Suite 1701
New York, NY 10001
(212) 685-4118
(212) 545-1843 (fax)
Lupus@LupusNY.org
www.lupusny.org

The CFIDS Association of America
PO Box 220398
Charlotte, NC 28222
(704) 365-2343
cfids@cfids.org
www.cfids.org

Rheumatology:

American College of Rheumatology
2200 Lake Boulevard NE
Atlanta, GA 30319
(404) 633-3777
(404) 633-1870 (fax)
ref@rheumatology.org
www.rheumatology.org

APPENDIX I

Directory of Pharmaceutical and Biotechnology Companies

3M Pharmaceuticals
3M Center
Building 275-6W-13
St. Paul, MN 55144
Phone: (888) 364-3577
www.mmm.com

Aastrom Biosciences
24 Frank Lloyd Wright Drive
PO Box 376
Ann Arbor, MI 48106
Phone: (734) 930-5555
www.aastrom.com

Abbott Laboratories
100 Abbott Park Road
Abbott Park, IL 60064
Phone: (847) 937-6100
www.abbott.com

Academic Pharmaceuticals
21 N. Skokie Valley Highway
Suite G3
Lake Bluff, IL 60044
Phone: (847) 735-1170

Access Pharmaceuticals
2600 Stemmons Freeway
Suite 176
Dallas, TX 75207
Phone (214) 905-5100
www.accesspharma.com

Acorda Therapeutics
420 Saw Mill River Road
Ardsley, NY 10502
Phone: (914) 347-4300
www.acorda.com

Actavis
Morris Corporate Center III
400 Interpace Parkway
Parsippany, NJ 07054
Phone: (862) 261-7000
www.actavis.com

Actelion Pharmaceuticals
Gewerbestrasse 16
CH-4123 Allschwil
Switzerland
Phone: +41 61 565 65 65
www.actelion.com

Acusphere
99 Hayden Avenue
Suite 385
Lexington, MA 2421
Phone: (617) 648-8800
www.acusphere.com

Adamis Pharmaceuticals Corp
11455 El Camino Real
San Diego, Ca 92130
www.adamispharmaceuticals.com

Alere Inc.
51 Sawyer Road
Suite 200
Waltham, MA 02453-3448
Phone: (781) 647-3900

AMAG Pharmaceuticals
100 Hayden Avenue
Lexington, MA 02421
Phone: (617) 498–3300
www.amagpharma.com

Advanced Tissue Sciences
7003 Valley Ranch Drive
Little Rock, AR 72223
Phone: (866) 217-9900
www.advtis.com

Aeterna Laboratories
1405 Par-Technologique Blvd.
Quebec, Canada G1P 4P5
Phone: (418) 652-8525
www.aezsinc.com

Affymax Research Institute
4001 Miranda Avenue
Palo Alto, CA 94304
Phone: (650) 812-8700
www.affymax.com

Ajinomoto U.S.A -
North American Headquarters
400 Kelby Street
Fort Lee, NJ 07024
Phone: (201) 292-3200
www.ajinomoto-usa.com

Akorn
1925 West Field Court
Lake Forest, IL 60045
Phone: (800) 932-5676
www.akorn.com

Alcon
6201 South Freeway
Ft. Worth, TX 76134
Phone: (817) 293-0450
www.alconlabs.com

Alexion Pharmaceuticals
352 Knotter Drive
Cheshire, CT 06410
Phone: (203) 272-2596
www.alxn.com

Alfacell
300 Atrium Drive
Somerset, NJ 08873
Phone: (732) 652-4525
www.alfacell.com

Alkermes
852 Winter Street
Waltham, MA 02451
Phone: (781) 609-6000
www.alkermes.com

Allergan
2525 DuPont Drive
PO Box 19534
Irvine, CA 92623-9534
Phone: (714) 246-4500
www.allergan.com

Alliance Pharmaceutical
17 Lee Boulevard
Malvern, PA 19355
Phone: (610) 296 3152
www.alliancepharmaco.com

Amarillo Biosciences
Clinical Trials Area
4134 Business Park Drive
Amarillo, TX 79100
Phone: (806) 376-1741
www.amarbio.com

Amgen, Inc.
One Amgen Center Drive
Thousand Oaks, CA 91320-1799
Phone: (805) 447-1000
www.amgen.com

Amylin Pharmaceuticals
9360 Towne Center Drive
San Diego, CA 92121
Phone: (858) 552-2200
www.amylin.com

Andrulis Pharmaceuticals
11800 Baltimore Avenue
Beltsville, MD 20705
Phone: (301) 419-2400

Angiotech Pharmaceuticals, Inc.
355 Burrard Street
Suite 1100
Vancouver, BC
Canada V6C 2G8
Phone: (604) 221-7676
www.angiotech.com

Angstrom Pharmaceuticals
990 Highland Drive
Suite 314
Solana Beach, CA 92075
Phone: (858) 314-2356
www.angstrominc.com

Anika Therapeutics
32 Wiggins Avenue
Bedford, MA 01730
Phone: (781) 457-9000
www.anikatherapeutics.com

Annovis
34 Mount Pleasant Drive
Aston, PA 19014
Phone: (610) 579-1200
www.annovis.com

Anthra Pharmaceuticals
103 Carnegie Center
Suite 102
Princeton, NJ 08540
Phone: (609) 514-1060

Agennix AG
101 College Road East
Princeton, NJ 08540
Phone: (609) 524-1000
www.agennix.com

Agenus Bio
3 Forbes Road
Lexington, MA 02421-7305
Phone: (781) 674 -4400
www.agenusbio.com

Akela Pharma (Formex)
11011 Torreyana Road
Suite 100
San Diego, CA 92121
Phone: (855) 436-7639
www.pharmaform.com

Ampliphi Biosciences Corporation
800 E. Leigh Street
Suite 54
Richmond, VA 23219
Phone: (800) 985-3730
www.apliphibio.com

Apricus Bio
11975 El Camino Real
Suite 300
San Diego, CA 92130
Phone: (858) 222-8041
www.apricusbio.com

Aptalis Pharma
22 Inverness Center Parkway
Birmingham, AL 35242
Phone: (800) 472-2634
www.aptalispharma.com

Aradigm Corporation
3929 Point Eden Way
Hayward, CA 94545
Phone: (510) 265-9000
www.aradigm.com

Ardea Biosciences Inc.
4939 Directors Place
San Diego, CA 92121
Phone: (858) 652-6500
www.ardeabio.com

Arena Pharmaceuticals
6166 Nancy Ridge Drive
San Diego, CA 92121
Phone: (858) 453-7200
www.arenapharm.com

Ariad Pharmaceuticals
26 Landsdowne Street
Cambridge, MA 02139
Phone: (617) 494-0400
www.ariad.com

Arkios BioDevelopment International
421 S. Lynnhaven Road
Suite 101
Virginia Beach, VA 23452
Phone: (757) 631-2114
www.arkios.com

Arqule
19 Presidential Way
Woburn, MA 01801-5140
Phone: (781) 994-0030
www.arqule.com

Aspen
Aspen Park
98 Armstrong Avenue
La Lucia Ridge
Durban, 4019
South Africa
Phone: +27 31 5808600
www.aspenpharma.com

Astellas
1 Astellas Way
Northbrook, IL 60062
Phone: (800) 888-7704
www.astellas.com

AstraZeneca Pharmaceuticals
P.O Box 15437
Wilmington, DE 19850-5437
Phone: (302) 886-3000
www.astrazeneca.com

AtheroGenics
8995 Westside Parkway
Alpharetto, GA 30004
Phone: (678) 336-2500
www.artherogenics.com

AuRX, Inc.
Elkridge, MD 21075
Phone: (410) 590-7610
www.aurx.com

AutoImmune Technologies
1010 Common Street
Suite 1705
New Orleans, LA 70112
Phone: (504) 529-9944
www.autoimmune.com

AVANIR Pharmaceuticals
20 Enterprise
Suite 200
Aliso Viejo, CA 92656
Phone: (949) 389-6700
www.avanir.com

AVAX Technologies
2000 Hamilton Street
Suite 204
Philadelphia, PA 19130
Phone: (215) 241-9760
www.avax-tech.com

Bausch & Lomb Pharmaceuticals
8500 Hidden River Parkway
Tampa, FL 33637
Phone: (813) 975-7770
www.bausch.com

Baxter Healthcare
One Baxter Parkway
Deerfield, IL 60015
Phone: (847) 948-2000
www.baxter.com

Bayer
100 Bayer Road
Pittsburgh, PA 15205
Phone: (412) 777-2000
www.bayerus.com

Berlex Laboratories
340 Changebridge Road
PO Box 1000
Montville, NJ 07045-1000
Phone: (973) 487-2000
www.berlex.com

Biocodex
7, Avenue Gallieni
Gentilly Cedex, France 94257
Phone: 33 (0)1 41 24 30 00
www.biocodex.com

BioCryst Pharmaceuticals
2190 Parkway Lake Drive
Birmingham, Al 35244
Phone: (205) 444-4600
www.biocryst.com

Biogen Idec
133 Boston Post Road
Weston, MA 02493
Phone: (781) 464-2000
www.biogenidec.com

Biomedical Frontiers
1000 Westgate Drive
Suite 100
St. Paul, MN 55114
Phone: (612) 375-1283
www.biomedicalfrontiers.com

BioNumerik Pharmaceuticals
8122 Datapoint Drive
Suite 1250
San Antonio, TX 78229
Phone: (210) 614-1701
www.bionumerik.com

Biosante Pharmaceuticals Inc.
111 Barclay Boulevard
Lincolnshire, IL 60069
Phone: (847) 478-0500
www.biosantepharma.com

Biospecifics Technologies
35 Wilbur Street
Lynbrook, NY 11563
Phone: (516) 593-7000
www.biospecifics.com

Biosyn
5939 Darwin Courts
Suite 114
Carlsbad, CA 92008
Phone: (760) 929-9352
www.biosyncorp.com

Biota Pharmaceuticals, Inc.
12270 Wilkins Avenue
Rockville, MD 20852
Phone: (800) 685-5579
www.biotapharma.com

Bio-Technology General
Be'er Tuvia Industrial Zone
P.O Box 571
Kirya Malachi 83104
Israel
Phone: (972) 8 861 2020
www.btgil.com

Biotherapies, Inc.
5692 Plymouth Road
Ann Arbor, MI 48105
Phone: (734) 996-9040

BioTime
1301 Harbor Bay Parkway
Alameda, CA 94502
Phone: (510) 521-3390

Boehringer Ingelheim Pharmaceuticals
900 Ridgebury Road
P.O. Box 368
Ridgefield, CT 06877
Phone: (203) 798-9988
www.boehringer-ingelheim.com

Boston Life Sciences
85 Main Street
Hopkinton, MA 01748
Phone: (508) 497-2360
www.bostonlifesciences.com

Bristol-Myers Squibb
345 Park Avenue
New York, NY 10154
Phone: (212) 546-4000
www.bms.com

Bryan Corporation
4 Plympton Street
Woburn, MA 01801
Phone: (800) 343-7711
www.bryancorporation.com

BSD Medical
2188 West 2200 South
Salt Lake City, UT 84119
Phone: (801) 972-5555
www.bsdmc.com

BTG International
Five Tower Bridge
Suite 800
300 Barr Harbor Drive
West Conshohocken, PA 19428
Phone: (610) 278-1660
www.btgplc.com

Cambridge Neuroscience
Phone: +44 (0) 1223 337733
www.neuroscience.cam.ac.uk

Capstone Therapeutics
1275 Washington Street
Suite 101
Tempe, AZ 85281
Phone: (800) 937-5520
www.capstonethx.com

Cardinal Health
7000 Cardinal Place
Dublin, OH 43017
Phone: (614) 757-5000
www.cardinal.com

Cardium Therapeutics
11750 Sorrento Valley Road
Suite 250
San Diego, CA 92121
Phone: (858) 436-1000
www.cardiumthx.com

Carrington Laboratories
2001 Walnut Hill Lane
Irving, TX 75038
Phone: (972) 518-1300
www.carringtonlabs.com

Cato Research
Westpark Corporate Center
4364 South Alston Avenue
Durham, NC 27713-2280
Phone: (919) 361-2286
www.cato.com

Celgene Corporation
86 Morris Avenue
Summit, NJ 07901
Phone: (908) 673-9000
www.celgene.com

Cell Therapeutics
3101 Western Avenue
Seattle, WA 98121
Phone: (206) 282-7100
www.celltherapeutics.com

Celldex Therapeutics, Inc.
119 Fourth Avenue
Needham, MA 02494-2725
Phone: (781) 433-0771
www.celldextherapeutics.com

CEL-SCI Corporation
8229 Boone Boulevard
Suite 802
Vienna, VA 22182
Phone: (703) 506-9460
www.cel-sci.com

Cephalon
41 Moores Road
Frazer, PA 19355
Phone: (610) 344-0200
www.cephalon.com

Cerus Corporation
2550 Stanwell Drive
Concord, CA 94520
Phone: (925) 288-6000
www.cerus.com

Ciba Vision
11460 Johns Creek Parkway
Duluth, GA 30097
Phone: (678) 415-3937
www.cibavision.com

Columbia Laboratories
354 Eisenhower Parkway
Second Floor – Plaza 1
Livingston, NJ 07039
Phone: (973) 994-3999
www.columbialabs.com

Cortex Pharmaceuticals
7700 Irvine Center Drive
Suite 750
Irvine, CA 92618
Phone: (949) 727-3157
www.cortexpharm.com

CSL
45 Poplar Road
Parkville, Victoria 3052
Australia
Phone: +61 3 9389 1911
www.csl.com.au

Cubist Pharmaceuticals
65 Hayden Avenue
Lexington, MA 02421
Phone: (781) 860-8660
www.cubist.com

Curis
4 Maguire Road
Lexington, MA 02421
Phone: (617) 503-6500
www.curis.com

Cyclacel Pharmaceuticals
200 Connell Drive #1500
Berkeley Heights, NJ 07922
Phone: (908) 517-7330
www.cyclacel.com

CytoDyn
5 Centerpointe Drive
Suite 400
Lake Oswego, OR 97035
Phone: (971) 204-0382
www.cytodyn.com

CytRx Corporation
11726 San Vicente Boulevard
Suite 650
Los Angeles, CA 90049
Phone: (310) 826-5648
www.cytrx.com

Daiichi Pharmaceutical
2 Hilton Court
Parsippany, NJ 07054
Phone: (973) 359-2600
www.daiichius.com

Dainippon Sumitomo
6-8, Doshomachi 2-chome,
Chuo-ku
Osaka, Japan
Phone: +81-6-6203-5321
www.ds-pharma.com

Demegen
100 Technology Drive
Suite 440B
Pittsburgh, PA 15219
Phone: (412) 621-9625
www.demegen.com

Dendreon Corporation
1301 Second Avenue
Suite 3200
Seattle, WA 98101
Phone: (877) 256-4545
www.dendreon.com

Discovery Laboratories
2600 Kelly Road
Suite 100
Warrington, PA 18976-3622
Phone: (215) 488-9300
www.discoverylabs.com

DJO, LLC
1430 Decision Street
Vista, CA 92081
Phone: (760) 727-1280
www.djoglobal.com

Draxis Health
16751 Trans-Canada Highway
Kirkland, Quebec
Canada H9H 4J4
Phone: (888) 633-5343
www.draximage.com

Eisai, Inc
100 Tice Boulevard
Woodcliff Lake, NJ 07677
www.eisai.com

Eli Lilly
Lilly Corporate Center
Indianapolis, IN 46285
Phone: (317) 276-2000
www.lilly.com

EMD Serono, Inc.
One Technology Place
Rockland, MA 02370
Phone: (800) 283-8088
www.emdserono.com

Emerald BioStructures
7869 NE Day Road West
Bainbridge Island, WA 98110
Phone: (206) 780-8900
www.emeraldbiostructures.com

Emergent Biosolutions
2273 Research Boulevard
Suite 400
Rockville, MD 20850
Phone: (301) 795-1800
www.emergentbiosolutions.com

Endo Pharmaceuticals
1400 Atwater Drive
Malvern, PA 19355
Phone: (484) 216-0000
www.endo.com

EntreMed
9620 Medical Center Drive
Suite 300
Rockville, MD 20850
Phone: (240) 864-2600
www.entremed.com

Enzo Biochem
527 Madison Avenue
New York, NY 10022
Phone: (212) 583-0100
www.enzo.com

Enzon
20 Kingsbridge Road
Piscataway, NJ 08854
Phone: (732) 980-4500
www.enzon.com

EpiCept Corporation
777 Old Saw Mill River Road
Tarrytown, NJ 10591
Phone: (914) 606-3500
www.epicept.com

Exocell
1880 JFK Boulevard
Suite 200
Philadelphia, PA 19103
Phone: (800) 234-3962
www.exocell.com

Exponential Biotherapies
248 East 44th Street
2nd Floor
New York, NY 10017
Phone: (347) 767-6945
www.expobio.com

Fibro Gen
409 Illinois Street
San Francisco, CA 94158
Phone: (415) 978-1200
www.fibrogen.com

Forest Laboratories, Inc.
909 Third Avenue
New York, NY 10022
Phone: (212) 421-7850
www.frx.com

Galderma Laboratories
14501 N. Freeway
Fort Worth, TX 76177
Phone: (866) 735-4137
www.galdermausa.com

Genelabs Technologies
505 Penobscot Drive
Redwood City, CA 94063-4738
Phone: (650) 369-9500
www.genelabs.com

Genentech
1 DNA Way
South San Francisco, CA 94080-4990
Phone: (650) 225-1000
www.gene.com

GenVec
65 West Watkins Mill Road
Gaithersburg, MD 20878
Phone: (240) 632-0740
www.genvec.com

Genzyme Corporation
500 Kendall Street
Cambridge, MA 02142
Phone: (617) 252-7500
www.genzyme.com

Gilead
333 Lakeside Drive
Foster City, CA 94404
Phone: (650) 574-3000
www.gilead.com

GlaxoSmithKline
One Franklin Plaza
P.O Box 7929
Philadelphia, PA 19101
Phone: (888) 825-5249
www.gsk.com

Grifols, Inc.
2410 Lillyvale Avenue
Los Angeles, CA 90032-3514
Phone: (800) 421-0008
www.grifolsusa.com

Gynetics
10300 West McNab Road
Tamarac, FL 33321
Phone: (239) 206-4285
www.gynetics.com

Hi-Tech Pharmacal
369 Bayview Avenue
Amityville, NY 11701
Phone: (631) 789-8228
www.hitechpharm.com

Hoffman La Roche
Roche Pharmaceuticals USA
Nutley, NJ
Phone: (973) 235-5000
www.rocheusa.com

Hospira
Lake Forest, IL
Phone: (877) 946-7747
www.hospira.com

Idera Pharmaceuticals
167 Sidney Street
Cambridge, MA 02139
Phone: (617) 679-5500
www.iderapharma.com

ImClone Systems
450 East 29th Street
New York, NY 10016
Phone: (212) 645-1405
www.imclone.com

ImmunoGen, Inc
830 Winter Street
Waltham, MA 02451-1477
Phone: (781) 895-0600
www.immunogen.com

Immunomedics
300 The American Road
Morris Plains, NJ 07950
Phone: (973) 605-8200
www.immunomedics.com

Incyte Pharmaceuticals
Route 141 & Henry Clay Road
Building E336
Wilmington, DE 19880
Phone: (302) 498-6700
www.incyte.com

Inovio Biomedical
11949 Sorrento Valley Road
San Diego, CA 92121-1318
Phone: (858) 597-6006
www.inovio.com

Insite Vision
965 Atlantic Avenue
Alameda, CA 94501
Phone: (510) 865-8800
www.insitevision.com

Insmed Pharmaceuticals
9 Deer Park Drive, Suite C
Monmouth Junction, NJ 08852
Phone: (732) 997-4600

Intellipharmaceutics International, Inc.
30 Worcester Road
Toronto, Ontario
Canada M9W 5X2
Phone: (416) 798-3001
www.intellipharmaceutics.com

Isis Pharmaceuticals
2855 Gazelle Court
Carlsbad, CA 92010
www.isispharm.com

iTherX
P.O. Box 262309
San Diego, CA 92196-2309
Phone: (858) 222-1568
www.itxpharma.com

Janssen Pharmaceuticals Inc.
1125 Trenton-Harbourton Road
P.O. Box 200
Titusville, NJ 08560
Phone: 1-800-526-7736
www.janssenpharmaceuticalsinc.com

Janssen Biotech, Inc.
800 Ridgeview Road
Horsham, PA 19044
Phone: (800) 526-7736
www.janssenbiotech.com

Jazz Pharmaceuticals
3180 Porter Drive
Palo Alto, CA 94304
Phone: (650) 496-3777
www.jazzpharma.com

Johnson & Johnson
One Johnson and Johnson Plaza
New Brunswick, NJ 08933
Phone: (800) 950-5089
www.jnj.com

Johnson Matthey Pharma Services
25 Patton Road
Devens, MA 01434
Phone: (978) 784-5000
www.jmpharmaservices.com

King Pharma
132 Windsor Road
Tenafly, NJ 07670
Phone: (888) 689-7917
www.king-pharma.com

Kyowa Hakko Kirin
212 Carnegie Center, Suite 101
Princeton, NJ 08540
Phone: (609) 919-1100
www.kyowa-kirin-pharma.com

La Jolla Pharmaceuticals
4370 La Jolla Village Drive
Suite 400
San Diego, CA 92122-1249
Phone: (858) 207-4264
info@ljpc.com

Ligand Pharmaceuticals
11119 North Torrey Pines Road
Suite 200
La Jolla, CA 92037
Phone: (858) 550-7500
BD@ligand.com

Lonza
8066 El Rio Street
Houston, TX 77054
Phone: (713) 568-6190
www.lonza.com

Lorus Theraputics Inc.
2 Meridian Road
Toronto, Ontario
Canada M9W 4Z7
Phone: (416) 798-1200
www.lorusthera.com

Lundbeck Research USA, Inc.
215 College Road
Paramus, NJ 07652-1431
Phone: (201) 261-1331
www.lundbeck.com

Mallinckrondt
675 McDonnell Boulevard
Hazelwood, MO 63042
Phone: (800) 325-8888
www.mallinckrodt.com

MedImmune
One Medimmune Way
Gaithersburg, MD 20878
Phone: (301) 398-0000
www.medimmune.com

Medinox
6120 Paseo Del Norte
Suite B-2
Carlsbad, CA 92009
Phone: (760) 603-8989
www.medinox.com

Menarini
Via Dei Sette Santi 1/3
50131
Florence, Italy
Phone: +39 (055) 56.80.1
www.menarini.com

Merck & Co.
One Merck Drive
P.O. Box 100
Whitehouse Station, NJ 08889-0100
Phone: (908) 423-1000
www.merck.com

Merrimack Pharmaceuticals
One Kendall Square
Suite B7201
Cambridge, MA 02139
Phone: (617) 441-1000
www.merrimackpharma.com

Merz
P.O. Box 18806
Greensboro, NC 27419
Phone: (888) 637-9872
www.merzusa.com

Metabolex
3876 Bay Center Place
Hayward, CA 94545
Phone: (510) 293-8800
www.metabolox.com

Mikart
1750 Chattahoochee Avenue
Atlanta, GA 30318
Phone: (404) 351-4510
www.mikart.com

Millenium Pharmaceuticals
40 Lansdowne Street
Cambridge, MA 02139
Phone: (617) 679-7000
www.mlnm.com

Mission Pharmacal
San Antonio, TX 78230-1355
Phone: (210) 696-7000
www.missionpharmacal.com

Mitsubishi Tanabe Pharma America Inc.
525 Washington Boulevard
Suite 400
Jersey City, NJ 07310
www.mt-pharma-america.com

Monsanto
800 N. Lindbergh Boulevard
St. Louis, MO 63167
Phone: (314) 694-6000
www.monsanto.com

Mylan Pharmaceuticals
1500 Corporate Drive
Suite 400
Canonsburgh, PA 15317
Phone: (724) 514-1800
www.mylan.com

Myriad Genetics
320 Wakara Way
Salt Lake City, UT 84108
Phone: (801) 584-3600
www.myriad.com

Marina Biotech
Phone: (425) 892-4322
www.marinabio.com

Nektar Therapeutics
455 Mission Bay Boulevard
San Francisco, CA
94158
Phone: (415) 482-5300
www.nektar.com

Neurogen
35 NE Industrial Road
Branford, CT 06405
Phone: (203) 488-8201
www.neurogen.com

Northwest Biotherapeutics
4800 Montgomery Lane
Suite 800
Bethesda, MD 20814
Phone: (240) 497-9024
www.nwbio.com

NovaDel Pharma Inc
1200 Route 22 East
Suite 2000
Bridgewater, NJ 08807
Phone: (908) 203-4640
www.novadel.com

Novartis Pharmaceutical Corporation
230 Park Avenue
21st Floor
New York, NY 10169
Phone: (888) 669-6682
www.novartis.com

Novartis Vaccines & Diagnostics
230 Park Avenue
21st Floor
New York, NY 10169
Phone: (888) 669-6682
www.us.novartis.com

Novavax
9920 Belward Campus Drive
Rockville, MD 20850
Phone: (240) 268-2000
www.novavax.com

Novelos Therapeutics
One Gateway Center
Suite 504
Newton, MA 02458
Phone: (617) 244-1616
www.novelos.com

Noven Pharmaceuticals
11960 SW 144th Street
Miami, FL 33186
Phone: (305) 253-5099
www.noven.com

Novo Nordisk Inc.
100 College Road
West Princeton, NJ 08540
Phone: (609) 987-5800
www.novonordisk-us.com

NPS Pharmaceuticals
550 Hills Drive
Bedminster, NJ 07921
Phone: (908) 450-5300
www.npsp.com

Nymox Pharmaceuticals
9900 Cavendish Boulevard
Suite 306
St. Laurent, Quebec
Canada H4M 2V2
Phone: (800) 936-9669
www.nymox.com

Onco Genx Pharmaceuticals
1522 217th Place SE
Bothell, WA 98021
Phone: (425) 686-1500
www.oncogenex.com

OPK Biotech
11 Hurley Street
Cambridge, MA 02141
Phone: (617) 234-6500
opkbiotech.com

Orexo AB
P.O. Box 303
Uppsala, Sweden SE-751 05
www.orexo.com

Organogenisis
85 Dan Road
Canton, MA 02021
Phone: (781) 575-0775
www.organogenesis.com

Osiris Therapeutics
7015 Albert Einstein Drive
Columbia, MD 21046
Phone: (443) 545-1800
www.osiris.com

Otsuka America Pharmaceuticals
2001 Aliceanna Street
Baltimore, MD 21231-3043
Phone: (410) 522-5005
www.otsuka-us.com

OxiGENE
701 Gateway Boulevard
Suite 210
South San Francisco, CA 94080
Phone: (650) 635-7000
www.oxigene.com

Oxygen Biotherapeutics
ONE Copley Parkway
Suite 490
Morrisville, NC 27560
Phone: (919) 855-2100
www.oxybiomed.com

OXIS International
468 N. Camden Drive
2nd Floor
Beverly Hills, CA 90210
Phone: (310) 860-5184
www.oxisresearch.com

Palatin Technologies
4-C Cedar Brook Drive
Cedar Brook Corporate Center
Cranbury, NJ 08512
Phone: (609) 495-2200
www.palatin.com

Par Pharmaceutical
300 Tice Boulevard
Woodcliff Lake, NJ 07677
Phone: (800) 828-9393
www.parpharm.com

Parnell Pharmaceuticals
3070 Kerner Boulevard
Suite A
San Rafael, CA 94901
Phone: (800) 457-4276
www.parnellpharm.com

PDL BioPharma Inc.
932 Southwood Boulevard
Incline Village, NV 89451
Phone: (775) 832-8500
www.pdl.com

Pediatric Pharmaceuticals
120 Wood Avenue South
Suite 300
Iselin, NJ 08830
Phone: (732) 603-7708
www.pediatricpharm.com

Perdue
One Stamford Forum
201 Tresser Boulevard
Stamford, CT 06901-3431
Phone: (203) 588-8000
www.purduepharma.com

Peregrine Pharmaceuticals Inc.
14272 Franklin Avenue
Trustin, CA 92780
Phone: (714) 508-6000
www.peregrineinc.com

Perrigo
515 Eastern Avenue
Allegan, MI 49010
Phone: (269) 673-8451
www.perrigo.com

Pfizer
235 East 42nd Street
NY, NY 10017
Phone: (212) 573-2323
www.pfizer.com

Pharmaceutical Product Development (PPD)
929 North Front Street
Wilmington, NC 28401-3331
Phone: (910) 251-0081
www.ppdi.com

Pharmacyclics
995 East Arques Avenue
Sunnyvale, CA 94085
Phone: (408) 774-0330
www.pcyc.com

Pharmascience
6111 Avenue Royalmount
Suite 100
Montreal, Quebec
Canada H4P 2T4
Phone: (514) 340-9800
www.pharmascience.com

Pherin Pharmaceuticals
4962 El Camino Real
Los Altos, CA 94022
Phone: (650) 961-2703
www.pherin.com

Polydex Pharmaceuticals Limited
421 Comstock Road
Toronto, ON
Canada M1L 2H5
Phone: (242) 322-8571
www.polydex.com

Praecis Pharmaceuticals
830 Winter Street
Waltham, MA 02451-1420
Phone: (984) 798-1122
www.praecis.com

Protein Sciences
1000 Research Parkway
Meriden, CT 06450
Phone: (800) 488 -7099
www.proteinsciences.com

Purdue Pharma L.P.
One Stamford Forum
201 Tresser Boulevard
Stamford, CT 06901
Phone: (203) 588-8000
www.purduepharma.com

QLT Inc.
2579 Midpoint Drive
Fort Collins, CO 80525
Phone: (604) 707-7000
www.qltinc.com

Questcor
26118 Research Road
Hayward, CA 94545
Phone: (510) 400-0700
www.questcor.com

Regeneron Pharmaceuticals
777 Old Saw Mill River Road
Tarrytown, NY 10591
Phone: (914) 847-7000
www.regeneron.com

Repligen Corporation
41 Seyon Street
Building 1, Suite 100
Waltham, MA 02453
Phone: (781) 250-0111
www.repligen.com

Repros Therapeutics
2408 Timberloch Place B-7
The Woodlands, TX 77380
Phone: (281) 719-3400
www.reprosrx.com

Research Corporations Technologies
5210 East Williams Circle
Suite 240
Tucscon, AZ 85711-4410
Phone: (520) 748-4400
www.rctech.com

Roche Bioscience – Genentech (of Roche Group)
1 DNA Way
South San Francisco, CA 94080
Phone: (800) 626-3553
www.gene.com

Romark Laboratories
3000 Bayport Drive
Suite 200
Tampa, FL 33607
Phone: (813) 282-8544
www.romark.com

Roxane Laboratories
P.O Box 16532
Columbus, OH 43216
Phone: (800) 962-8364
www.roxane.com

Salix Pharmaceuticals, Inc
8510 Colonnade Center Drive
Raleigh, NC 27615
Phone: (919) 862-1000
www.salix.com

Sanofi-Aventis
55 Corporate Drive
Bridgewater, NJ 08807
Phone: (800) 981-2491
www.sanofi.us.com

Santarus, Inc.
3611 Valley Centre Drive
Suite 400
San Diego, CA 92130
Phone: (858) 314-5700
www.santarus.com

Sarepta Therapeutics
245 First Street
Suite 1800
Cambridge, MA 02142
Phone: (617) 444-8424
www.sareptatherapeutics.com

SciClone Pharmaceuticals, Inc.
950 Tower Lane
Suite 900
Foster City, CA 94404-2125
Phone: (650) 358-3456
www.sciclone.com

Seattle Genetics
21823 30th Drive S.E.
Bothell, WA 98021
Phone: (425) 527-4000
www.seattlegenetics.com

Selective Genetics
11545 Sorrento Valley Road
Suite 310
San Diego, CA 92121
Phone: (858) 793-6641
www.selectivegenetics.com

Sepracor
84 Waterford Drive
Marlborough, MA 01752
Phone: (508) 481-6700
www.sepracor.com

Servier
Neuilly-sur-Seine
France
www.servier.com

Shionogi
300 Campus Drive
Florham Park, NJ 07932
Phone: (973) 966-6900
www.shionogi.com

Shire
725 Chesterbrook Boulevard
Chesterbrook, PA 19087
Phone: (484) 595-8903
www.shire.com

SIGA Technologies
35 East 62nd Street
New York, NY 10065
Phone: (212) 672-9100
www.siga.com

Sigma-Tau Pharmaceuticals
9841 Washingtonian Boulevard
Suite 500
Gaithersburg, MD 20878
Phone: (301) 948-1041
www.sigmatau.com

Soligenix
29 Emmons Drive
Suite C-10
Princeton, NJ 08540
Phone: (609) 538-8200
www.soligenix.com

Spectrum Pharmaceuticals
11500 S. Eastern Avenue #240
Henderson, NV 89052
Phone: (702) 835-6300
www.sppirx.com

Stiefel Laboratories
20 T.W. Alexander Drive
Research Triangle Park, NC 27709
Phone: (305) 443-3800
www.stiefel.com

Stryker Corporation
2825 Airview Boulevard
Kalamazoo, MI 49002
Phone: (269) 385-2600
www.strykercorp.com

Synageva
128 Spring Street
Suite 520
Lexington, MA 02421
Phone: (781) 357-9900
www.synageva.com

Synsorb Biotech
1167 Kensington Crescent NW
Suite 410
Calgary, Alberta
Canada T2N 1X7
Phone: (403) 283-5900
www.synsorb.com

Takeda Pharmaceuticals North America
One Takeda Parkway
Deerfield, IL 60015
Phone: (224) 554-6500
www.tpna.com

Tekmira Pharmaceuticals Co.
100 - 8900 Glenlyon Parkway
Burnaby, British Columbia
Canada V5J 5J8
Phone: (604) 419-3200
www.tekmirapharm.com

Telik
700 Hansen Way
Palo Alto, CA 94304
www.telik.com

Teva Pharmaceutical Industries
5 Basel Street
Petach Tikva 49131
Israel
Phone: +972-3-9267267
www.tevapharm.com

Theratechnologies Inc.
2310 Alfred-Nobel Boulevard
Montreal, Quebec
Canada H4S 2B4
Phone: (514) 336-7800
www.theratech.com

Titan Pharmaceuticals, Inc.
400 Oyster Point Boulevard
Suite 505
S. San Francisco, CA
94080-1921
Phone: (650) 244-4990
www.titanpharm.com

Transgenomic
12325 Emmet Street
Omaha, NE 68164
Phone: (402) 452-5400
www.transgenomic.com

UCB
1950 Lake Park Drive
Smyrna, GA 30080
Phone: 800-477-7877
www.ucb-usa.com

United Therapeutics
1040 Spring Street
Silver Spring, MD 20910
Phone: (301) 608-9292
www.unither.com

Upsher-Smith Laboratories
6701 Evenstad Drive
Maple Grove, MN 55369
Phone: (763) 315-2000
www.upsher-smith.com

Valeant Pharmaceuticals
700 Route 202/206 North
Bridgewater, NJ 08807
Phone: (866) 246-8245
www.valeant.com

Valentis
Molėtų pl. 11, LT-08409
Vilnius, Lithuania
Phone: 370-5-270-1222
valentis@valentis.lt

Vaxgen
1000 Marina Boulevard
Suite 200
Brisbane, CA 94005
Phone: (650) 624-1000
www.vaxgen.com

Vertex Pharmaceuticals
130 Waverly Street
Cambridge, MA 02139
Phone: (617) 341-6100
www.vrtx.com

Vical
10390 Pacific Center Court
San Diego, CA 92121-4340
Phone: (858) 646-1100
www.vical.com

Viropharma
730 Stockton Drive
Exton, PA 19341
Phone: (610) 458-7300
www.viropharma.com

Vivus
351 E. Evelyn Avenue
Mountain View, CA 94041
Phone: (650) 934-5200
www.vivus.com

Warner Chillcott
1 Grand Canal Square
Docklands, Dublin 2, Ireland
Phone: 353 1 897 2000
www.wcrx.com

XOMA Corporation
2910 Seventh Street
Berkeley, CA 94710
Phone: (510) 204-7200
www.xoma.com

ABOUT CISCRP

Founded in 2003, the Center for Information and Study on Clinical Research Participation (CISCRP) is an independent, Boston-based, nonprofit organization dedicated to providing outreach and education about clinical research to the public and patients around the world. CISCRP's portfolio of educational initiatives include:

- AWARE for All events—Clinical Research Education programs—designed to introduce individuals to their local research community through sessions, workshops, and free health screenings. Between 2003 and 2013, these live and online programs have reached 429,000 households in cities across the United States.

- Medical Heroes—a public service campaign—portrays medical heroes in everyday situations to illustrate the point that the brave individuals who give the gift of participation are all around us. CISCRP's Medical Heroes communications generate over 120 million impressions quarterly.

- Educational books, DVDs, and brochures cover a wide range of topics for research participants, in culturally sensitive 6th- to 8th-grade reading-level language, and are translated into two dozen languages. Since 2004, investigative sites and pharmaceutical companies have distributed nearly one million copies.

- SearchClinicalTrials.org is a service designed to manually search for relevant clinical trials on behalf of patients, family, and friends overwhelmed by the online search process. CISCRP performs searches for nearly 2,000 unique requests annually.

- Research on public and patient attitudes, behaviors, and experiences. CISCRP regularly conducts studies that provide valuable insights into actionable ways that clinical research professionals can better understand, and more effectively engage with, the public and study volunteers.

- CISCRP's communicating clinical trials results program involves the translation of technical clinical trial results into lay-language non-technical summaries for study volunteers who participated in those trials. CISCRP is now collaborating with dozens of major pharmaceutical companies to provide these clinical trial results summaries.

- New in 2015—CISCRP will be launching an educational exhibit appropriate for science museums and children's museums. The purpose of this traveling exhibit is to demystify clinical research, to show what research participation is all about through the eyes of study volunteers, and to celebrate and appreciate the profound gift that volunteers make to advance public health.

For more information, contact CISCRP at 617-725-2750 or visit our web site at www.ciscrp.org

ABOUT THE AUTHOR

Kenneth Getz is the founder and chairman of CISCRP and the director of sponsored research programs, associate professor at the Center for the Study of Drug Development at Tufts University's School of Medicine.

A well-known speaker at conferences, symposia, universities, and corporations, Ken has published hundreds of articles in peer-review and trade journals, as well as ten book chapters including one entitled *The Science of Medicine and Clinical Trials* published in the Merck Manual. Ken is also the author of two nationally recognized books for patients and their families: *Informed Consent* and *The Gift of Participation: A Guide to Making Informed Decisions about Volunteering for a Clinical Trial.*

Ken received the 2006 "Innovator in Clinical Research" award from the Association of Clinical Research Professionals and was named one of the 100 most inspiring individuals in the life sciences in 2007. Ken has served on a variety of boards and committees including the Institute of Medicine's Clinical Research Roundtable, the Consortium to Examine Clinical Research Ethics at Johns Hopkins University, and the Clinical Trials Transformation Initiative. He is on the editorial boards of *Pharmaceutical Medicine* and *Therapeutic Innovation and Regulatory Science* and writes a bi-monthly column for *Applied Clinical Trials* that was nominated for a Neal Award in 2010.

Ken holds an MBA from the J. L. Kellogg Graduate School of Management at Northwestern University and an undergraduate degree from Brandeis University. He lives with his wife Debra, their three children, and a curly-coated retriever named Ketcher in Southern Massachusetts and Northern Maine.

Notes

Notes

Notes